Role Theory

Role Theory
PERSPECTIVES FOR
HEALTH PROFESSIONALS

MARGARET E. HARDY, PH.D., F.A.A.N.
Associate Professor, School of Nursing
Boston University
Boston, Massachusetts

MARY E. CONWAY, PH.D., F.A.A.N.
Dean and Professor, School of Nursing
The University of Wisconsin-Milwaukee
Milwaukee, Wisconsin

APPLETON-CENTURY-CROFTS/NEW YORK

To Bill, Paul, and William

Copyright © 1978 by **APPLETON-CENTURY-CROFTS**
A Publishing Division of Prentice-Hall, Inc.

*All rights reserved. This book, or any parts thereof, may
not be used or reproduced in any manner without written
permission. For information, address Appleton-Century-Crofts,
292 Madison Avenue, New York, NY 10017*

79   80   81   82/   10   9   8   7   6   5   4   3   2

Prentice-Hall International, Inc., London
Prentice-Hall of Australia, Pty. Ltd., Sydney
Prentice-Hall of India Private Limited, New Delhi
Prentice-Hall of Japan, Inc., Tokyo
Prentice-Hall of Southeast Asia (Pte.) Ltd., Singapore
Whitehall Books Ltd., Wellington, New Zealand

Library of Congress Cataloging in Publication Data
Hardy, Margaret E., 1938 —
    Role Theory.
    Bibliography: p.
    Includes index.
    1. Medical personnel. 2. Social role. 3. Pro-
fessional socialization. I. Conway, Mary E., 1923-
joint author. II. Title.
R690. H37   301.5   78-13269
ISBN 0-8385-8471-3

Text Design: Carolyn Giacalone
Cover Design: Karin Batten

PRINTED IN THE UNITED STATES OF AMERICA

Contributors

BONNIE BULLOUGH, R.N., Ph.D. (Sociology), F.A.A.N.
Professor, Department of Nursing
California State University
Long Beach, California

MARY E. CONWAY, Ph.D. (Sociology), F.A.A.N.
Dean and Professor, School of Nursing
The University of Wisconsin-Milwaukee
Milwaukee, Wisconsin

SUZANNE HALSEY, R.N., M.S.N.
Head Nurse
New England Deaconess Hospital
Boston, Massachusetts

MARGARET E. HARDY, Ph.D. (Sociology), F.A.A.N.
Associate Professor, School of Nursing
Boston University
Boston, Massachusetts

ADA SUE HINSHAW, R.N., Ph.D. (Sociology), F.A.A.N.
Director of Research, College of Nursing
University Hospital
University of Arizona
Tucson, Arizona

BARBARA ANN HURLEY, R.N., Ph.D. (Sociology)
Assistant Professor, School of Nursing
University of North Carolina
Chapel Hill, North Carolina

MADELEINE LEININGER, Ph.D. (Anthropology), F.A.A.N.
Dean and Professor of Nursing
University of Utah College of Nursing
Salt Lake City, Utah

JEAN L. J. LUM, Ph.D. (Sociology), F.A.A.N.
Professor, School of Nursing
University of Hawaii at Manoa
Honolulu, Hawaii

SANDRA MACKAY, R.N., M.S.N. (Anthropology)
Doctoral student in Anthropology
Boston University;
Assistant Professor
Department of Community Medicine
Dartmouth College
Hanover, New Hampshire

MARY-'VESTA MARSTON, Ph.D. (Psychology), F.A.A.N.
Professor, School of Nursing
Boston University
Boston, Massachusetts

Contents

Introduction

Thought-provoking, stimulating questions of former students and the anticipated queries of future students played a significant part in our decision to
produce *Role Theory: Perspectives for Health Professionals.* In developing
and organizing this book we considered several approaches. One approach
would have been to organize the material around a prevailing paradigm
untilized by health professionals—if there were such a paradigm. We feel,
however, that there is no common agreement about such a metaparadigm;
the holistic model, the medical model, the psychoanalytic model, the public
health model, and the family interaction model are all among the common
paradigms health professionals presently employ, but not one of them has
total acceptance by health professionals. We then considered organizing the
book around the conceptualizations held by health professionals vis-à-vis the
person to be helped. Here, too, we found a number of orientations. These
included: patient, client, victim, occupant of the sick role, recipient, consumer, and informed decision maker. We finally turned to a consideration
of the commonalities that exist among health professionals, whether they be
nurses, physicians, medicial sociologists, social workers, occupational
therapists, or medical anthropologists. Persons in all of the health disciplines
use the clinical model, the public health model, the educational model, or
the scientific model. We believe these prevail across the entire health care
field. Furthermore, health professionals may occupy roles based on several
of these models simultaneously or move from one role to another during their
careers. We therefore decided to organize knowledge about roles—role
theory—into major areas which have gained the attention of scientists, which
have the strongest empirical support, which are most useful in health care
disciplines, and which are at a useful level of abstraction for health care
professionals. Accordingly, we have addressed the issue of theory develop-

ment, discussed the two prevailing perspectives in the field of role (functional and symbolic interaction), addressed key role areas, and have made reference to clinical situations to illustrate some theoretical perspectives. In addition, we have provided three chapters which analyze the hospital setting, the medical educational setting, and the interdisciplinary education setting from a role theory perspective. Because we believe that health professionals should contribute to the development of knowledge useful in their field, in addition to utilizing up-to-date knowledge, we begin with a chapter which focuses on knowledge development and end with a chapter on a newer methodology for measuring role attitudes. A brief overview of the chapters is provided as follows.

Chapter One provides a text-in-miniature of theory in science and the development of theory. Scientific knowledge is presented as advancing through slow and steady increments. (For a different—less rationalistic—approach based on T. Kuhn's theory of scientific revolutions see M. Hardy, "Perspectives on Nursing Theory," *Advances in Nursing Science* 1 (1978). This paper explores the development of metaparadigms and exemplar paradigms and their potential influence on the development of scientific knowledge in nursing. This chapter, by focusing on the traditional view of knowledge development, serves as a useful background for the study of those concepts and theories which are presented in subsequent chapters. The reader is provided with a précis of the characteristics of theories in general and a rationale and perspective for approaching the study of roles in health systems from a theoretical perspective. This introductory chapter sets a relatively high level of abstraction, one which is characteristic of most of the material in the text. Hardy defines science as a social system, thus: "Science as a social system refers to interrelated structures, processes, and activities which are common to groups of persons engaged in developing a substantive body of knowledge through the scientific method." An important contribution of this chapter is a set of criteria against which the student can assess the conceptual frameworks and hypotheses presented in the remaining chapters of the text. Thus, chapter one sets the stage for the study of roles and such related constructs as socialization, role strain, role-making, social exchange, and reference groups.

Chapter Two continues development of the theoretical background introduced in the first chapter. Conway gives an overview of the two major perspectives within which roles historically have been treated. These are the *functional* and the *symbolic interaction* perspectives. Consistent with the view of science as a social organization, roles are described not as being fixed, precisely defined entities but, rather, as systems' phenomena. An interaction between two individuals is viewed as a type of system; the initial act of one individual (his "output") becomes the "input" stimulating the response of an other. Attention is given to explication of symbolic interaction in the belief that this perspective allows more freedom for actors who wish to evolve selected roles. A distinction is made between role-making and role-taking—two concepts which have empirical implications for the professional practitioner who seeks to "make" a role rather than accept a role-as-given.

Chapter Three continues in logical sequence by providing an extensive treatment of the more recent literature on socialization. Here, as in chapter two, the symbolic interaction perspective is highlighted. Continuities and discontinuities between childhood and adult socialization processes are explicated by Hurley, who provides numerous references to encourage the student to explore primary sources in learning more about this important and rapidly evolving aspect of role theory.

The student will find that Chapter Four, which reviews and analyzes theory and research surrounding the concept of role strain, makes direct reference to role problems associated with the socialization process. Role strain is considered a pervasive aspect of many roles in complex societies. The lack of congruity between self perception and many professional and organizational norms is explored here Also highlighted are the conflicting norms held by professionals and those held by the organization in which the professional works. Of particular interest in this chapter are the strategies by which individuals can alter some of the role expectations held by others to reduce their role strain. Strategies of role bargaining and strategies based on social exchange are explored. Hardy explicates the theory of social exchange, providing both a theoretical treatment of the concept and examples of its application in health care settings.

In Chapter Five the focus shifts from the individual to the organization. The salient features of bureaucratic organizations are identified as are both the structural and social aspects of organizations which are of consequence for the actualization of professional roles. Findings from some of the more recent research on professionals within bureaucratic organizations are reviewed. Conway examines how organizations—their officials, that is—attempt to manage order, and she makes explicit the fact that organizations depend upon their professional employees to achieve the organization's goals. Contrary to a popular notion that the need of the organization to maintain its routine is a barrier to the work autonomy of professionals, Conway notes that the burden of evidence from recent research suggests that the organization may actually enhance the work autonomy of professionals.

The concept of socialization is developed further in Chapter Six. Reference groups and their contribution to socialization are the major topics. The role occupant looks beyond his immediate others for an evaluation of his behavior . . . he chooses as his evaluative reference point selected other persons or groups which provide him with cues for his behavioral responses. Reference groups are powerful constrainers of behavior; a so-called *normative* reference group may reward or punish an individual depending on whether the individual's behavior is consistent with the group's norms, or is deviant. The "rehearsing" of a role—anticipatory socialization—is one of the commonly employed methods by which individuals prepare themselves for new roles; for the professional, such rehearsal is a necessity if one is to take on the attitudes essential to successful actualization of a new role. While emphasizing that professional socialization is a life-long process, Lum brings out the complexity of the task facing the neophyte professional. This person must not only internalize the role of professional in a given discipline but, in a majority of instances, must simultaneously make a status transition from adolescent to adulthood. That some do not achieve both of these transitions with an equal degree of success is not surprising. Following Lum's review of selected research in which students preparing for medicine and nursing careers were subjects, one is prompted to ask: Does a learning environment which accepts the student as a junior "colleague" offer a superior socialization experience to the one which treats the student as a "novice"?

Chapter Seven introduces the concept of stratification. Bullough claims that "stratification systems within the health care delivery system are major determinants of the roles and behaviors of occupants of the system." The importance of an understanding of this concept for the would-be professional lies in large measure upon the fact that it is not one's competence alone that determines one's location within a hierarchy of professionals, but that other variables such as social class or sex may be more important determinants. Bullough suggests that there may be a dilemma in attempts to improve the health care system to the extent that such non-rational elements as historical dominance and professional elitism are not amenable to rational control.

Chapters Eight, Nine, and Ten present the research of three scholars: MacKay, Marston, and Halsey. MacKay and Halsey report on their own research. Each author examines how selected role occupants create, or recreate, their individual roles within complex health care settings. While Halsey deals with one role type—the *Queen Bee Syndrome*—MacKay provides descriptive evidence on the ways in which professionals *negotiate* their role functions and statuses within an innovative setting. A thoughtful reading of this chapter prompts the reader to ask: How powerful must incentives for change be in order to bring about both substantive and enduring alterations in a dysfunctional system of health care delivery? What kinds of negative and/or positive sanctions will be required for the profession of medicine, in particular, to alter its order of "doing business"?

Marston reviews the research which has been done surrounding the conditions under which individuals take, or fail to take, action to maintain health. For the health professional this chapter offers a wealth of information about the health belief system. The literature cited suggests that large-scale health education programs are minimally effective in bringing about recommended health behaviors. Becker's *Health Belief Model* is presented as the most comprehensive model existant from which testable theories for understanding health-behavior motivation may be derived.

Halsey in her chapter examines one pattern of role conflict resolution by females in administrative positions. She presents strong evidence that female professionals, as they move up the administrative ladder, resolve role conflict by developing a cluster of role-related antifeminist attitudes. Halsey suggests that this cluster of attitudes, the Queen Bee Syndrome—may prevent professional development and career mobility of younger female members of the nursing profession. This intriguing chapter raises questions as to how this syndrome affects the function of the work organization, the health care system, and female-dominated professions.

In Chapter Eleven Leininger draws on her years of experience in helping to bring about interdisciplinary learning among the health professions. Ethnocentrism—the propensity of professionals to adhere to the traditional norms of their individual professions—is identified as the chief obstacle to effective inter-disciplinary collaboration. Leininger's experiential observations on ethnocentrism receive some empirical support from MacKay's chapter, Chapter Eight. MacKay's evidence suggests the present strength of ethnocentric norms which constrain role behavior in spite of a structure that is intended to support both altered behavior and an innovative mode for the delivery of health care. Leininger identifies those economic and social incentives which appear to be moving—albeit slowly—the individual health sciences toward an eventual model of interdisciplinary student learning within institutions of higher education.

In the final chapter Hinshaw describes the application of a technique used in psychophysics for the measurement of role attitudes. This is the technique of *magnitude estimation*. This topic has special relevance for nurses, physicians, and other health care givers since role perceptions of the recipient vis-à-vis those of the provider are important determinants of both compliance and satisfaction with the care provided. Up until the present time there has been no reliable method for testing the *strength* of attitudes and, consequently, there have been only uncertain efforts at reducing role incongruency. Magnitude estimation is asserted by some, Hinshaw included, to produce a ratio scale of attitudes. Whether or not this assertion can be considered valid, it is apparent that magnitude estimation offers a new and potentially fruitful approach to assessing the strength of certain attitudes which are basic to understanding roles. For example, it should be possible to apply this technique to a variety of situations in which both practitioners and clients interact, and, based on the data generated, realign some role behaviors. Moving attitude research from the subjective domain to the objective domain is one of the most promising and exciting prospects in the field of role.

In ordering the chapters within the text we have chosen a sequence which we find useful but it should not be considered absolute. Each chapter may be considered individually; selected chapters such as Chapters 4 and 6 or 8, 9, 10 may be used in examining a particular aspect of role theory or several aspects. The entire text may be utilized in an altered sequence to complement course material. We urge that the readers consider their own unique learning needs in identifying which strategy would best serve their goals.

We believe that for the health practitioner the practical value of greater knowledge about self- and other roles cannot be overestimated. We have not intended that this role theory text be considered exhaustive, rather that it be a meaningful stimulus for the reader. We believe that serious students will discover for themselves the exciting possibilities of drawing from the theoretical constructs and practical examples in this text, knowledge which they can test and apply in the development of their own professional role.

1

Perspectives on Knowledge and Role Theory

MARGARET E. HARDY

The promotion and maintenance of health and the prevention of illness are goals for all health professionals. In attempting to meet these goals, health professionals may draw upon the steadily evolving knowledge base of the social sciences as one basis for understanding. This base, although relatively new, is a resource that may be used to improve the management and delivery of the unique services offered by each of the health professions. However, to skillfully extract and subsequently use the relevant knowledge, a practitioner must have a general understanding of the norms and goals of science. In addition, one must have a comprehension of the methods of scientific inquiry, of theory development, and of the pertinent criteria for evaluating theory. An understanding of these areas is essential to any practitioner who wishes to implement well-grounded knowledge or to contribute to the expansion of the knowledge base.

Although most health professionals are well aware that science is a continuous, self-correcting enterprise involving theory development, empirical testing, and subsequent refinement of theory, they are usually less aware that norms governing these activities are not necessarily congruent with the norms guiding their clinical practice. Therefore, this chapter is devoted to an exploration of the norms governing science. In addition, an overview of theory development and the criteria for assessing theory will

1

be discussed in order to provide the reader with a basis for critical reading and appreciation of the subsequent sections of this book.

SCIENCE AS A SOCIAL ORGANIZATION

There are several accepted meanings of the term *science*. Science may refer to a body of well-grounded knowledge, a method of inquiry, or a social system that generates knowledge. Science as a body of knowledge refers to a circumscribed set of theory and research findings which have accumulated over time, whereas science as a method of inquiry refers to an objective, empirical means for seeking "truth." Alternatively, science as a social system refers to the interrelated structures, processes, and activities that are common to groups of persons engaged in developing a substantive body of knowledge through the scientific method. In examining science as a social system, one focuses on the social norms and goals that guide the activities of scientists rather than on a set of substantive propositions or axioms, or on systematic methods of inquiry.

NORMS GOVERNING SCIENTIFIC ACTIVITY

Health professionals are influenced by a set of standards or norms that guide their behavior or professional conduct. The scientist likewise is guided by a general set of norms as he or she participates in activities such as theory construction, development of data-measuring devices, data collection and analysis, scientific reporting, and policy making. Individuals in the social system of science are committed to the common goals of expanding the boundaries of existing knowledge and improving its soundness; they are obligated to follow a common set of rules or norms.

Since the norms guiding scientific activity are different from those guiding clinical conduct, and since the norms of the system of science prescribe the meticulous and sometimes tedious reporting of scientific writing, an understanding of science norms can assist health professionals to critically read, assess, and implement existing knowledge. Furthermore, discussion of science norms may increase the health professional's awareness of the incongruity between some science and some professional norms. This awareness may aid the professional in determining when scientific knowledge can and cannot provide a reasonable basis for action.

A *norm*, a concept originating in role theory, refers to a set of rules or standards guiding behavior. The science norms that will be identified here are broad guidelines which make a significant impact on the work activities of the scientists. Such norms may not be totally independent of each other. The norms will be presented individually in this section for the sake of clarity. Identifying important norms, even if they overlap, makes it possible to develop a sounder understanding of the social system of science.

As in any area of behavior, some science norms are more mandatory than others. For example, severe sanctions are likely to follow discovery of the "fixing" of one's data, whereas the reporting of scientific knowledge in nonscientific journals is likely to receive minimal sanctions from the community of scientists.

The norm that is a major determinant of the behavior of social scientists is the rule stating that the *study of human behavior will be objective and empirical*. Although the idea of objectivity and of empirical validation is familiar, one should note the fact that theories and research that are made public must be testable and must be open to replication. Since the final test of a theory is objective, as opposed to subjective, both theoretical reasoning and research methods are made available for critical assessment by other scientists. Scientific work can then be examined for its plausibility and the degree of its empirical support. Not surprisingly, a pluralism of proposed theories and methods encourage the advancement of knowledge. Competing and complementary theories provide for objective, empirical testing and can be substantiated or withdrawn. For example, in the mental health literature, differing but plausible conceptions of schizophrenia have been examined. Whether schizophrenia is primarily genetically determined, has a primarily biochemical cause, or is socially induced is not clear because the empirical evidence is not yet sufficient. Although the different theoretical stances are plausible, they can not all simultaneously be true. At present, no one stance has emerged with acceptably strong empirical support; thus, the search and debate goes on.

Another norm holds that theory and research must be *critically scrutinized* and openly evaluated by members of the scientific community. The honest evaluation not only of one's own work but also the work of others upon which one's work is based is a highly valued means of generating valid knowledge. The critical assessment of the validity of accumulated knowledge is clearly seen in scientific review articles where areas of congruence and divergence in cumulative knowledge are identified and where those theoretical and methodologic problems that preclude the testability of a theory and the interpretation of empirical findings are explored. This norm serves to increase the likelihood that research will be replicated in order to examine the accuracy of empirical support claimed for theoretical predictions and that cumulative knowledge will be valid.

A related norm directs scientist to *share their work* with *colleagues*. This type of collegiality encourages not only sharing of research findings but the sharing of techniques and new ideas. Sharing knowledge of unsuccessful endeavors, dead-ends, and other theoretical and methodologic problems reduces wasted effort. This type of collegiality is intended to accelerate the growth of scientific knowledge. Communications relative to this norm occur both in publications and in professional meetings. An informal network often develops among persons working on similar problems or with similar theoretical orientations.

Another important norm is that the truth and value of scientific work depends only on *the merit of the work*. It is independent of the scientist's prestige, nationality, political views, and professional allegiance. It is also unrestricted by time and geographical location. Recognition is based on the credibility and significance of the work, not on the person, time, or place associated with the contribution.

A closely related norm encourages scientists to be *open to new developments and approaches* whenever research suggests this to be appropriate. Ideally, the scientist is not biased or committed to a specific theory or methodoloy to the extent that contradictory ideas, differing views, and conflicting empirical evidence are overlooked. He is committed to seeking the truth wherever the search leads. This norm suggests that the scientist be flexible, that he fairly evaluate the state of knowledge, and that he be informed of the most recent developments in his field.

These general norms guide the activities of scientists in all fields and their effects are seen in conceptual and methodologic debates commonly found at scientific meetings, in publications, and in the day-to-day activities of working scientists. Science is a continuous, self-correcting social activity; it is the only reliable method for advancing knowledge.

The cycle of developing ideas, recreating and reformulating them, and then testing hypotheses and refining theories and concepts in light of empirical evidence is a slow but dependable method. However, this slow self-correcting process may make scientifically based knowledge appear irrelevant to individuals in applied fields. The debate over the meaning of a specific concept, the various methodologic problems, and the conflicting empirical findings may seem unimportant when compared to the everyday problems facing the practitioner. If the health practitioner is frustrated by a lack of specific knowledge to solve an immediate problem, his frustration may be somewhat ameliorated by the knowledge that the social system of science has different norms and goals than does the social systems of the health professions.

THEORY DEVELOPMENT

Any substantive body of scientific knowledge from another discipline, such as role theory, needs to be analyzed and synthesized before it can be assessed for its relative value in clinical application. To do this, it may be useful for the reader to view theory as having stages of development. The early stages of substantive theory development are quite different from the later stages. Although the general goals of social science are to understand and explain social behavior, early contributions to role theory may not appear to directly contribute to these goals. In a similar manner, the scientist's general concern for conceptualizing social processes, labeling regularly occuring phenomena, and identifying regularities and diversities in social behavior may not be apparent in the early writings of the role theorists.

These activities of conceptualization, concept formation, and determination of lawful relationships need not occur simultaneously. In fact, it is likely that the early stages of a theory are concerned with conceptualization and concept formation, while later stages emphasize the identification of lawful relationships between concepts. The developmental stage of a particular theory is reflected in the type of work that the majority of that field's theoreticians and researchers are engaged in at that particular time.

STAGES OF THEORY DEVELOPMENT

Theories of social behavior first appeared as informal theories, presented in narrative form using everyday terms to describe behavior. For example, early writings on role theory employed terms such as role, conduct, habits, interaction, and self. Terms were often not defined at all, since they represented the common everyday meaning. *Role*, for example, was initially used as it was defined in the dictionary. The concept *role* used today has a more precise and restricted meaning. The development of concepts is discussed more fully in the next section. Here it is only important to note that the informal theories do not make use of specially defined concepts.

Typically in the early stage of theory development, interest groups form, associated with schools of thought or specific theoretical orientations, and informal communication networks are set up for discussing the "theory." Attempts are made to delineate the boundaries of the theory and to identify unique and fundamental concepts. Often, eager new supporters of emerging theories focus on the producer of the major ideas rather than the ideas themselves. In this early stage there may be considerable repetition in presenting ideas, looseness in formulating concepts, and a use of anecdotal observations to support fundamental conceptualizations. Concepts drawn from the everyday language are used without being clearly defined. This stage of establishing and clarifying a theoretical orientation involves individuals identifying with the "orientation" and attempting to convince others of its "rightness." The informal tradition of establishing and clarifying a theoretical orientation may almost be necessary as an initiation rite in the process of generating enough enthusiasm and motivation within the discipline to engage in the logical step-by-step rigor of scientific inquiry. In role theory the publication of Mead's work in 1934 ended the informal tradition (Kuhn, 1972, p.58) associated with symbolic interaction. In subsequent years, much creative conceptualization and research was undertaken.

The next stage of development of theory in a field may be one of grand conceptualization. In the role theory literature, it is not clear whether this stage developed after the conceptualization in everyday terminology or if there was an overlap in the stages. This second stage of "grand theory" or "general theory" is characterized by writings which attempt to describe the totality of behavior. These theories, including the work on social systems by Parsons and perhaps some of the stress formulations, are loosely constructed and contain vague and ill-defined concepts with questionable linkage between concepts. Such formulations could not be made sufficiently concrete to permit empirical testing, nor are these "theories" subject to falsification. In retrospect, it appears that early attempts at theory building have been overly ambitious attempts to develop all-inclusive conceptualizations. The task of empirically testing such grand conceptualizations is virtually impossible.

The stage of circumscribed or partial theories follows the stage of grand conceptualizations. It appears that scientists, recognizing the difficulty of empirically grounding and testing grand schemes, have turned to developing empirically testable theories which focus on limited aspects of social behavior. This stage of circumscribed theories may be seen as an attempt to make the discipline more scientific and conceptualizations of the discipline more amenable to research. Examples of circumscribed theories that may be relevant to the health professions include role theory, communication theory, behavioral modification theory, cognitive dissonance theory, and the health belief model. By developing conceptualizations which focus on only a segment of social behavior, it is expected that useful concepts can be identified and defined, hypotheses generated, and empirically tested. The development and testing of circumscribed theories leads to more carefully designed studies and usually results in accumulation of knowledge through experimental studies. By this method, empirically sound knowledge is expected to be developed more quickly than is possible with grand theories. However, in time some of these circumscribed theories may be combined to form more general theories that explain a larger domain of behavior.

THE STRUCTURE OF THEORY

In the scientific field we find two sets of vocabulary. One is substantive in nature, dealing with conceptualization and the theoretical concepts which circumscribe the field of study. The other pertains to the method of work—scientific inquiry. In the next section the terminology basic to scientific inquiry will be discussed. Subsequent chapters will focus on terminology or concepts in role theory.

Concepts

The most fundamental element in any theory is the concept. Since most social scientists are concerned with uncovering commonly occurring phenomena and general patterns, they identify and name or label such phenomena, rather than unique events or conditions. Concepts identify similarities in otherwise diverse empirical situations, entities, and properties. Role, status, socialization, and norms are all examples of concepts in role theory. Since concepts are central to the growth of knowledge, they must change as theories develop and empirical evidence accumulates. In time, a body of concepts becomes accepted as the rudiments of a particular theoretical orientation. Some concepts may take on a more specific and precise meaning than they originally had, while other concepts may be created when commonalities among initially disparate entities are identified. This advances the congruence of the concept with empirical findings.

The concept *role*, for example, has been made more specific through the creation of more definitive concepts such as role behavior, role expectations, role playing, and status. The general concept *role* still maintains its usefulness in linking individuals and society, but the additional modifying concepts add to the precision of the meaning and thereby facilitate understanding. On the other hand, the concept *role strain* was created to account for responses of military personnel, chaplains, nurses, patients, chiropractors, and other persons in the work force. This one concept identifies a process which occurs in diverse settings.

Concepts, once identified, may or may not be used identically by all writers in a given field. Some writers do not define their concepts in their writing; they assume that their meaning is well known and agreed upon. Unfortunately, such consensus is hard to reach. In attempting to achieve precision in their work, others carefully define their terms. Such careful defining may initially result in one concept having diverse meanings. The particular meaning of the concept will depend upon the scientist using it, his theoretical orientation, and the context in which the term is used. As concepts develop meaningfulness and usefulness within a body of knowledge their definitions usually become more precise and explicit while at the same time becoming less meaningful to "the man on the street." As concepts are defined more carefully, they gradually become part of a larger body of scientific knowledge. For example, the concept *role* has developed more restricted meaning for theorists today than for lay persons using the term.

The evolution of a concept may be illustrated by the historical development of the concept *role*. Although the systematic study of roles did not occur until the 1930s, the term *role* was part of the common language. An examination of early writings related to *role* reveals that concepts *similar* to the current concept of role were used. For example, early writers—such as James, Baldwin, Dewey, Thomas, Faris, Simmel, Cooley, Mead, Moreno, and Linton—wrote about self, habits, conduct, mores, social interaction, social forces, and personality. These early writers addressed phenomena that later became part of role theory. Their conceptualization came from everyday language; even though the concept *role*, when used, was not presented as a technical or scientific term, these writers have contributed significantly to the understanding and development of role and role-related concepts.

The writings of three of the early theoreticians in this period—Moreno, Mead, and Linton—illustrate the process of theory development and concept differentiation and refinement. A brief discussion of their works will give the reader a deeper appreciation of the process of developing meaningful concepts. A much fuller discussion of the development of role theory and the works of these theoreticians is presented by Thomas and Biddle (1968).

Moreno, who came to the United States from Germany in 1930, was a psychiatrist interested in changing individual behavior. He introduced sociometry and the concepts of psychosomatic roles, psychodramatic roles, social roles, role playing, and role-taking. His conceptualizations were articulated in numerous publications between 1934 and 1960 and are part of the modern role theory literature.

George Herbert Mead, who taught at the University of Chicago during the years 1893 through 1931, was concerned with maintaining social order; he was especially interested in the socially reflexive nature of behavior and in social interaction. He introduced such concepts as self, socialization, role-taking, and role-playing. (The latter two terms are defined differently than Moreno's concepts). The significance of the posthumous publication of his conceptualizations is that it ended a long era of an "oral tradition," an era when most of the germinating ideas were transmitted by word of mouth. The impact of his work is evident in the writings of the present-day *interactionists* such as Blumer, Becker, Cottrel, Goffman, Lindesmith, Rose, Strauss, and Turner.

Ralph Linton, an anthropologist, made a significant contribution to our understanding of social behavior through his publications during the 1930s and 1940s. A conceptualization developed by him which has carried over to modern role theory is the differentiation between the concepts *status* (position) and *role*. Role is the carrying out of the rights and obligations associated with a status.

In the strictest sense, it would be more accurate to talk about a role framework rather than a role theory, although most scientists and practitioners concerned with role-related issues utilize the latter. In this context, the term *theory* is used loosely to refer to a specific orientation toward social structure and social behavior, and to a selected body of concepts and research. In this book, the term *role theory* will be used in this fashion.

Theoretical Statements

It has been pointed out that concepts are the basic units in any theory. These units may be used singly or combined with others to form theoretical statements. Such statements may either by descriptive or predictive. A statement containing one concept—for example, role strain—may be descriptive; the statement may report on the extent of the role strain experienced by health practitioners. Two concepts, such as rank and role strain, may be combined to produce a theoretical statement that is analytical rather than descriptive; such statement may predict. For example, one might predict that the higher one's rank in the health care system, the less role strain he/she will experience. This type of statement is a theoretically based prediction which is amenable to testing; that is, the concepts of both rank and role strain may be operationalized or measured. The proposed link between the concepts makes it possible to test empirically whether the predicted relationship actually does exist. Such theoretical statements, when supported by empirical testing, form the substance of theories.

Besides empirically testing a theory, one should assess its internal consistency or *logical adequacy*. A theory consists of a set of interrelated concepts and theoretical statements; these units of the theory can be diagrammed to examine the structure of the theory rather than its substantive meaning. Diagramming permits a relatively objective assessment of the linkage between concepts. The process of determining logical adequacy is discussed more fully elsewhere (Hardy, 1974). Here it is sufficient to note diagramming as a vehicle for identifying gaps, overlaps, and contradictions within the theory. Furthermore, since hypotheses derived from the theory serve as an indirect test of the theory, the links between the theoretical concepts and constructs and the empirically testable hypotheses must be clear and consistent. Abstract symbols are used to represent the theory's terms and ± signs to depict the type of relationships between the terms; a ? signifies an unspecified linkage. For example, if an increase in *role overload* is associated with an increase in *role strain* and an increase in *role strain* is associated with a decrease in *cooperation* this could be diagrammed as:

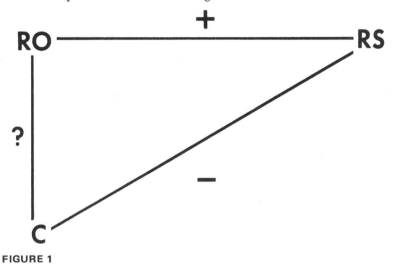

FIGURE 1

where RO = role overload, RS = role strain, and C = cooperation. The + sign indicates a positive relationship between role overload and role strain, the − sign indicates a negative relationship between role strain and cooperation, and the ? indicates the relationship between role overload and cooperation is unspecified. This type of diagramming facilitates an objective evaluation of the structure of a theory and the relationship of derived hypotheses to the theory itself. If these explicit steps are not taken, the practitioner or researcher may overlook internal weaknesses in the structure. This is especially likely to occur if the substantive focus or conclusions of the theory are in accord with the philosophy and experience of the practitioner.

The literature on theories contains a hierarchy of theoretical statements. The more common forms of statements are laws, axioms, postulates, propositions, hypotheses, theorems, and empirical generalizations. These various forms of statements all specify the type of link between concepts; for example, a linear, curvilinear, or power relationship between two or more concepts. The term *theoretical statements* is used in this chapter as a general term encompassing all of the hierarchical forms of statements linking theoretical concepts.

Theoretical statements have differing degrees of *generality* or numbers of phenomena they apply to, irrespective of time and place and the extent of empirical support. Propositions, for example, are relatively general and have strong empirical support, whereas hypotheses are less general and lack empirical support. Empirical generalizations are statements summarizing scientific data from numerous studies and as such are well substantiated; they are empirically grounded and thus do not have the degree of generality that propositions have.

In a substantive field such as role theory, it is important to progress from the stage of theoretical orientation in which one recognizes a cluster of concepts as important to the field, to a stage in which one develops theoretical statements linking the field's important concepts. The development of theoretical statements gives the theoretical approach plausibility and at the same time makes it possible to test the theory. It is vital that theories be tested. It is only with the testing of theoretical statements that have been developed from more general, theoretical statements that a field develops a body of empirically substantiated knowledge.

A proliferation and refinement of role-related terms occurred in the social science literature after World War II. For example, role may be defined to mean a *position* in a social structure, a set of *expectations* associated with a position in a social structure, or a set of *behaviors* associated with a position. The concept role has been used in a variety of ways. The growing interest in role theory is illustrated by the fact that while there were only 5 publications on the concept of role in the period from 1931 to 1935, during 1956 through 1960 there were over 35. In recent years there have been several significant publications addressing the major conceptual changes and conceptual problems in role theory (Biddle and Thomas, 1968; Kuhn, 1972; Neiman and Hughes, 1952; Sarbin, 1968). The influx of theoretical and research articles, as well as reviews and critiques, has added significantly to the understanding of the concept of role.

A theory is a selective symbolic representation of reality; it is not an exact replication of reality in all its complexity but presents a close approximation. A theory is a set of interrelated concepts and theoretical statements which are amenable to testing. A whole theory is not tested per se but is subjected to indirect testing. This occurs when hypotheses logically derived from the theory are empirically tested. A theory that is internally consistent and plausible and has strong empirical support is one which can be used with confidence by the health professional.

EVALUATION OF THEORY

When the problem of evaluating a theory is broached, the problem is metatheoretical rather than theoretical. The evaluation of a theory requires judgments to be made about how sound or "good" a theory is. It may also involve a judgment regarding which of two theories is "better." Evaluation implies the comparison of concepts and theoretical statements against some standard. Criteria are related to the structure of theory (discussed in preceding section), the nature of the theory's concepts and theoretical statements, and the goals of theory.

In assessing the "goodness" of a theory, one can examine the concepts used in the theory to determine the soundness of both their theoretical and operational definitions and the congruence of these two sets of definitions with each other and to the real world. The concepts may also be examined to determine the completeness with which they describe and classify the phenomena under study. In addition, the theoretical statements themselves may be examined for their plausibility and their predictive power. Of particular interest is the type of linkage specified between concepts; statements which clearly specify the direction and form of the relationship between concepts and have adequate empirical referents for the concepts as well, may serve as an indirect test of theory. These derived statements, with operational definitions of concepts, form the links between the theoretical world and the empirical world.

Although there are a variety of criteria utilized by theorists for assessing theory—such as scope, parsimony, abstractness, and testability—selected criteria for evaluating theory—such as the logical adequacy and empirical support for a theory, the plausibility of a theory, and exactness of prediction by the theory—are of importance to practitioners.

The scientist is interested in the expansion of knowledge while the practitioner's primary focus is usually on the applicability of the available knowledge. The use of theory to alter the health and lives of patients demands close analysis to see how empirically adequate the statements or theory are. The practitioner needs to ask whether there is sufficient empirical evidence to feel confident that the theory at hand is "sound." The empirical adequacy of a theory is of primary significance to anyone wishing to alter social events in accord with theoretical orientation; the strength of the empirical support indicates the validity of that particular theory.

Also of significance to the practitioner is the *plausibility* of a theory. The theory's statements, when taken as a whole, need to provide a reasonable and believable explanation concerning the phenomena of concern. The theory should present a credible and likely explanation. If role conflict is of concern, then the practitioner can ask if role theory provides a reasonable explanation for the occurrence of role conflict and of the consequences of role conflict. The theory in hand can likewise be assessed for the degree of understanding it communicates; a plausible explanation associated with a sense of *understanding* is of prime importance to practitioners. Only a theory that is plausible and conveys a sense of understanding should be considered for clinical use by practitioners.

Another important criterion for assessing a theory is the exactness of the *predictions* it provides. Theoretical statements that precisely identify the link between two or more concepts make exact predictions possible. In the earlier stages of theory development, theoretical relationships may be loosely stated; they may provide indefinite or imprecise links between concepts. For example, in role theory, there are statements such as "the more overload a person is exposed to, the more role strain he will experience." This type of statement links two concepts and indicates the linkage may be proportional. However, statements such as this one do not give a precise prediction of how may units of role overload will result in how many units of role strain. This is exactly the precision of prediction that is sought for from theory. This preciseness of prediction can be found in some aspects of the health sciences. Reasonably precise drug dosages are given to produce a precise range of biochemical or physiologic changes. Theories that could provide exact predictions of health-related social behavior do not exist at this time in the social sciences but are being actively sought. In the meantime, less precise statements that indicate the direction and form of a relationship can be tested. A statement that indicates that an increase in role overload is associated with an increase in role strain can be empirically tested and is of more value than a statement that only indicates that role overload and role strain are associated or that the two conditions coexist.

In determining the "goodness" of a theory, the health professional utilizes criteria used to evaluate theory and then makes some judgment as to how well the theory meets these criteria. This assessment is not an either/or activity; the judgment is neither that the theory is "good" nor that the theory is "bad" but rather an assessment using a number of criteria and judgment to determine the degree to which the theory adequately meets the criteria. Any final decision regarding the "relative goodness" of that theory should be derived from such an assessment.

The determination of which theory is the "best" to use requires an additional judgment on the part of the health professional. Any theory being considered for application must satisfactorily meet the standards for theory, but a question may be raised concerning which of two or more theoretical orientations should be selected and used. For example, a health practitioner working with a family may identify that the problem of concern is that a member of a family is not following a specified medical regimen. Role theory, social exchange theory, and the health belief model may be identified as the theories that are relatively "good" ones for analyzing the problem at hand. Choosing the "best" theory may involve decisions regarding the following: (1) which theory deals most adequately with the variables of concern to the health professional, (2) which variables central to the theory are the ones that the health professional can alter or modify to bring about the desired change; and (3) would such changes be strong enough or significant enough to make it worth implementing a plan of action based on the theory.

Although evaluation of theory is briefly presented in this chapter so that the reader may have an operational perspective for a reading and assessment of the adequacy of role theory, it should be recognized that the health professional plays a vital role in making judgments about the soundness of theories, their appropriateness for modifying behavior, and the appropriateness of modifying the behavior in the predicted direction. Evaluating existing theory is a serious and significant activity for health professionals. They may also wish to contribute to the development of the body of knowledge relevant to health care. Most importantly, the health professional must have sufficient expertise to evaluate knowledge for its soundness and for its appropriateness in improving the quality of health care and, ultimately, of the quality of life.

CONCLUSION

It is important to make a distinction between science as a human social activity and science as a body of knowledge or as a method of inquiry. In looking at science as a social activity, certain important goals and norms can be seen to operate. These goals and norms are not identical to those of health professionals. Scientists work primarily to accumulate a body of knowledge that can help us to understand and explain the world around us. The health professional is primarily engaged in the delivery of care to clients and in the improvement of this care. The scientist's work is guided by the norms of scientific inquiry, while the health professional's work is guided by professional codes of ethics. Although scientists and the health professionals may have similar perspectives on theory, the relative importance of criteria utilized by them to assess theory may differ according to whether the goal is to develop a body of knowledge or to solve a specific health-related problem. Theory development is an activity that both scientists and health professionals engage in as they attempt to explain phenomena. An understanding of science, theory development, the structure of theory, and selected criteria for evaluating theory is necessary for both the health professional who is to contribute to the body of scientific knowledge and to the health professional who is utilizing existing scientific knowledge. This understanding facilitates the generation of a body of scientific knowledge relevant to health care and the utilization of appropriate knowledge.

This chapter has presented science as a social organization with its own goals, norms and phases of theory development. The basic structure of theory and selected criteria for evaluating theory are also presented. The reader is encouraged to utilize material from this chapter to analyze and evaluate the subsequent chapters on role theory.

2

Theoretical Approaches to the Study of Roles

MARY E. CONWAY

We have used the words *role theory* in the title of this book. However, to the serious student who has learned that a theory is a set of logically interrelated concepts from which can be deduced testable hypotheses, the term *role theory* may seem a misnomer. Role theory represents a collection of concepts and a variety of hypothetical formulations that predict how actors will perform in a given role, or under what circumstances certain types of behaviors can be expected. The word *role* has its roots in theatrical usage, and refers to a part one plays or is assigned in a drama. It began to appear in behavioral science literature as early as the 1920s (Thomas and Biddle, 1966; p. 6), and from that time on its usage has increased rapidly with an associated body of terminology growing up around it.

The word *theory*, as it is used in this text and as it is construed by a number of authorities (Merton, 1968; Rose, 1962; Secord and Backman, 1964; Thomas and Biddle, 1966), refers to a large body of literature—much of it hypothetical discussion and somewhat less of it reporting empirical research—related to social behavior and both the overt and covert mechanisms which shape it. While the question of a single, unitary theory is debatable, it is unlikely that a coherent body of knowledge will emerge that is all-encompassing, or a "unique and total system of theory" (Merton, 1967, p. 64). As noted by Thomas and Biddle (1966, p. 18):

The field of role consists of many hypotheses and theories concerning particular aspects of its domain, but these propositions like the knowledge to which they relate, have yet to be reviewed and integrated. And even if the propositions were brought together in some organized form, they would undoubtedly not constitute a single, monolithic theory of the sort that the appellation role theory implies, nor would they always be distinguishable from other theoretical statements in such disciplines as psychology, sociology and anthropology.

In this chapter the two major perspectives from which roles and role performance have been studied in the behavioral sciences, and their relevance for health professionals in particular, will be considered. These two perspectives are the *functionalist* and the *interactionist* approaches (See Table 1, p. 21). The former derives its title from the underlying assumption that roles are more or less fixed positions within society to which are attached certain expectations and demands, and further, that these are enforced by sanctions—either negative or positive. (The interactionist perspective is also addressed in Hurley, "Socialization For Roles," Chapter 3, this volume.)

The interactionist perspective is the one which will be more fully developed here. It derives its name from the interpretation of human behavior as a response to the symbolic acts of others—notably gestures and speech—the response being in effect an "interpretation" of those acts. Symbolic interaction acknowledges society and its institutions as a framework within which actors make their roles explicit. This framework, however, is acknowledged only as a skeleton, so to speak, a skeleton within which the actor constructs or *organizes* social action (Bolton, 1967, p. 104). A major difference between the two perspectives is that the former conceives of social action as "learned responses" that are communicated during the process of socialization and reinforced in the individual by the approval or disapproval of significant others such as parents, teachers, or employers (Goslin, 1969, p. 6; LeVine, 1969, p. 508), while the latter posits that the individual engages in interactions with others and selects certain cues for action which, for him, have more relevance than others. Bolton (1967) perceives the "elements" of organic behavior in the social context as learned; but he holds, in addition, that human beings *conduct* their actions. Thus, social action is construed not simply as learned responses but as an organizing and interpreting of cues in one's environment.

Mead (1934, pp. 154-155) expressed an almost identical viewpoint

in his belief that the individual takes the attitudes of others toward himself as well as their general attitudes toward social institutions in constructing his own actions. Mead was the first social psychologist to introduce the idea of the self as *reflexive*; that is, the individual in the course of normal growth and development comes to take himself as both *subject* and *object* (Mead, 1934, pp. 136-137).

FUNCTIONAL PERSPECTIVE

The functional perspective holds that institutions arise in society because they fill a need for the society in question. An additional assumption of the functional perspective is that the division of labor within a given society is considered an expression of its state of development. That is, the more developed a society, the more complex are its structure and, accordingly, the more differentiated is its labor force (Parsons, 1951; Durkheim, 1964; Caplow, 1954) Durkheim, considered by some to be the earliest proponent of functionalism, made an analogy between the cohesiveness engendered by the division of labor and that which is characteristic of the biologic system. "Organic solidarity" is that patterning of roles and statuses that is characteristic of the division of labor (Durkheim, 1964, pp. 147-173). Inherent in the concept of a division of labor that is *organic* is the realization that as social forms evolve and change over time, so will the division of labor adjust or reconstruct itself to reflect these changes. An example in recent history of a profoundly reordered division of labor is the large body of professionals, technologists, and skilled laborers that "grew up" around the United States space exploration efforts.

In the functionalist view of society, roles as well as institutions, culture, and norms are treated as *social facts*—facts that are transmitted to each succeeding generation in the process of socialization as objective, real entities (Berger and Luckman, 1966). The individual's place in this scheme of things has been described as an egoism-altruism dichotomy, with egoism held to be less functional for society and altruism more functional (Simmel, 1950). Altruism involves subordination of the individual to society; he is a "mere part" of the all-important organic whole (Simmel, 1950, p. 59) and, further, the individual is expected to subordinate his personal orientation to the collectivity (Parsons, 1964, p. 97). If roles are to be construed as social facts—as the functional view casts them—then the behaviors of actors can be considered to be structurally determined by the social forces dominant in a given society at any point in time (Bandura and Walters, 1963; Brim, 1966).

While sanctions can be imposed for behaviors that violate norms, a consensual acceptance of these norms is the strongest force for maintaining adherence to them. This consensual acceptance has been called the "collective conscience" (Durkheim, 1964, pp. 287-297).

Roles, in the functionalist schema, are viewed as *primary mechanisms* serving essential functional prerequisites of the social system (Parsons, 1964, p. 115), and a relationship is held to exist between roles and the social structure that is similar to that which exists between organs and functions in the biologic system. While the conceptualization of roles as social facts suggests a kind of fixed or stable character, roles can be seen to change as the institutions of society evolve. Buckley holds that institutions undergo a developmental process over time in which they recreate themselves (Buckley, 1967, p. 137).

The particular social structure of a given society is one important determinant of the process of socialization—perhaps the most important determinant. Those norms and values that characterize the society's culture are the "social facts," as Durkheim puts it, that the younger members of that society will be expected to adopt as they take on adult roles. Consistent with the conceptualization of roles as social facts is the view that those roles which are considered appropriate for the individual as he progresses from infancy to childhood are *sequentially* made relevant for him as he matures (Bandura and Walters, 1963; Brim, 1966; Goslin, 1969; LeVine, 1969). That is, such roles as student, son, daughter, breadwinner, and the like are more or less age related. In addition to age-related roles, there are other broad aspects of the social structure that are relevant for an individual at any stage of the socialization process (Inkeles, 1969, pp. 615-632). These broad aspects have been identified as ecologic, economic, and political, and their relationship to a system of values (Inkeles, 1969, p. 618). The ecologic dimension has to do with the size and distribution of population; the economic refers to how goods and services are distributed; the political encompasses power relationships; and the value system deals with those values which predominate in the institutions of the society.

THE SYMBOLIC INTERACTION PERSPECTIVE

In contrast to the functional perspective, the symbolic interactionist interpretation of roles and role behavior focuses on the *meaning* which the acts and symbols of actors in the process of interaction have for each other. The theoretical formulations of this perspective derive from the writings and

TABLE 1

TWO PERSPECTIVES ON SOCIAL INTERACTION

Functionalist View*	Symbolic Interactionist View
1 Objects and persons are stimuli which act on an individual.	An individual constructs objects on the basis of his ongoing activity. He gives meaning to objects and makes decisions on the basis of his judgments.
2 Action is a release or response to what the situational norms demand.	The individual decides what he wishes to do and how he will do it. He takes account of external and internal cues, interpreting their significance for his action.
3 Environmental forces act to "produce" behavior.	By a process of self-indication, an individual accepts, rejects, or transforms the meaning (impact) of such forces.
4 Prescriptions for action, or norms, dictate appropriate behaviors. They are social facts.	Others' attitudes are the basis for individual lines of action.
5 An act is a unitary, bounded phenomenon; i.e., it starts and stops.	An act is disclosed over time and what the end of the act will be cannot be foretold at the start.
6 The act (of an actor) will be followed by the response of another with or without any interpretation taking place on the part of the other.	An act is validated by the response of an other.
7 Persons act on the basis of a generally objective reality; i.e., learned responses.	Reality is defined by each actor; one defines a situation as he "sees it" and acts on this perception.
8 Group action is the expression of societal demands and shared social values.	Group action is the expression of individuals confronting their life situations.

*For a more detailed explanation of numbers, 1, 2, and 8 see H. Blumer: "Society as Symbolic Interaction." In Rose, A. (ed.): Human Behavior and Social Processes. New York, Houghton Mifflin, 1962, pp. 179-192.

research of such social psychologists as Cooley (1964), Mead (1934), Thomas (1918), Goffman (1952), Turner (1962), Blumer (1962), and Webster and Sobieszek (1974), to name but a few. Symbolic interaction emphasizes the meanings significant symbols have for actors, rather than the normative constraints presumed to be exerted by the social structure (Blumer, 1962, p. 180; Turner, 1962, p. 23). Symbolic interactionism does not discard the belief that structure influences behavior within the context of the social system; rather, it holds that structure alone does not account for, nor can it predict, how persons will act in a set of specified circumstances (Cottrell, 1969, p. 548).

The symbolic interactionist approach to the study of behavior clearly has taken precedence over functional theory in the continuing attempts to "explain" human behavior (Blumer, 1962; Goffman, 1952; Rose, 1962; Webster and Sobieszek, 1974). One obvious reason for this is that functional theory—as it is generally understood—simply does not account well enough for the wide variations in behavior which take place within complex social structures. Presumably, if the social structure alone were the underlying determinant of behavior, all social action should be explainable and predictable on the basis of the norms governing the society in question. Developments in psychology, particularly those associated with the psychoanalytic tradition, have led to a recognition of the influence of individual personality and early socialization experiences as important determinants of the subsequent adaptive (or nonadaptive) behavior of individuals (Gewirtz, 1969, pp. 57-212; Piaget, 1968; Sullivan, 1953).

In seeking a more adequate explanation for social behavior, social scientists have joined other researchers in a trend toward conceptualizing problems in cybernetic terms—a trend which has permeated both sociology and psychology. While many find this a useful model, others (Bolton, 1967, for example) view it as sociologic reductionism. The cybernetic conception of behavior essentially views behaviors as a form of energy exchange which includes inputs, thruputs, outputs, feedback, and goal directedness (Buckley, 1967; Homans, 1974; Kuhn, 1974). For example, two persons can be perceived as representing a *system* of interaction in which the initial act is an input for the other; his (other's) response to the actor could be considered an example of feedback; and the subsequent act of the initial actor, a correction in the system based on its feedback. (For definitions of systems terminology the reader is referred to Chapter 8.)

Definition of Terms

Interaction: A situation in which at least two persons are involved in verbal or nonverbal communication (Kuhn, 1974, p. 139; Turner, 1962, p. 6).

Symbol: A stimulus that has a meaning for individuals and calls forth a response based on meaning rather than on some physical object (Turner, 1962; Mead, 1934).

Interpretation: The meaning an individual gives to the symbols used by an other during the course of interaction (Biddle and Thomas, 1966; Blumer, 1962; Turner, 1962).

Role-taking: The reflection of an understanding of the generalized attitudes of others in one's actions (Turner, 1962).

What may already be apparent from the above but which merits additional emphasis here is the fact that the interpretation actors in a given interaction assign to each other's responses may frequently differ from the interpretation which would be made by bystanders. For example, the bystander who sees two men gesticulating wildly and shouting at each other may be startled to observe the men suddenly halt their verbal exchange and embrace each other. And, in another hypothetical instance, two men might be observed talking quietly and earnestly to each other when one of them is seen to pull a gun from under his coat and shoot the other. Admittedly, this latter example is a somewhat dramatic one, but it is by no means beyond the range of possibility. The outcomes in each instance may puzzle the bystander and, further, the explanation given each situation by the observer may or may not correspond to the meanings the interaction had for the actors involved.

ROLE MODIFICATION
AS RESPONSE TO KNOWLEDGE EXPANSION

The body of scientific knowledge has grown markedly in recent years, and concomitantly the field of health care has experienced a proliferation of roles. In addition, the health care system is one of the most rapidly expanding and complex systems within society. In part, because of both the exponential increase in technology that has occurred within an extremely short time span and the expansion of the health care system itself, attempts to cope with related role changes have been identified as a major stressor. In coping with the demands associated with expansion of knowledge and the demands made by consumers seeking ready access to care, health professionals are faced with the continuing need to redefine and realign their roles. Role redefintion involves consideration of normative patterns of interaction in the relationships of professional to consumer and professional to professional. It is within the context of this impetus toward role redefinition and realignment that the theoretical framework of symbolic interaction offers a "map" for understanding the process of role change. This framework can be used to explain how roles evolve over time and, in addition, it suggests means by which present role patterns can intentionally be altered.

The term *role-making* best describes the process that takes place when role modification is consciously entered into. There are at least five distinct phases that can be isolated in the sequential process of role making. These five phases are: (1) initiator behavior, (2) other-response, (3) interpretation by actor and other, (4) altered response pattern, and (5) role validation (Table 2).

Both role-taking and role-making involve taking the attitudes of others who are involved in an interaction; that is, both actor and other endeavor to understand the meaning of each other's symbolic gestures. What is unique to role making, however, is the structuring of the interaction in such a way as to *modify* it and, in doing so, to make explicit certain aspects of the role (Turner, 1962, p. 22). As we have already observed, consistency is a feature of roles, and role participants can anticipate with a fair degree of predictability what the responses of their role partners will be. It is when the response of a role partner departs from the one anticipated in some phase of the interaction, and the other in the interaction accepts that departure (i.e., reciprocates in such a way as to *sustain the interaction*), that role making can be said to take place. That is, some *part* of the role was modified. The word "phase" is used deliberately (Turner uses the term "segment" in a similar though not identical sense) to convey the idea that an interaction consists of a sequential pattern of successive action/response episodes and to emphasize that any single episode of action/reponse must be considered incomplete within the context of the entire interaction.

The notion of phase is an appropriate and meaningful term for the empirical study of interactions for the reason that neither observers nor participants in a given interaction can predict on the basis of one, or even several, act/response sequences what the eventual meaning of the completed interaction will be. Let us take an example from a multiprofessional health team. The physician (who perceives himself to be the leader of the team) gives a directive to the physical therapist who has been providing passive exercise to a patient who has suffered a cerebral accident. The physical therapist (who perceives himself to be more knowledgeable than the physician about the extent of muscle atrophy that the patient has sustained) responds not by agreeing to follow the physician's directive, as might be expected, but instead suggests an alternative therapy. The physician (who momentarily may

TABLE 2

ROLE MAKING AS A SEQUENTIAL FIVE-PHASE PROCESS

1st Phase: **Initiator Behavior**	2nd Phase: **Other-Response**	3rd Phase: **Actor/Other** **Interpretation**	4th Phase: **Altered Response** **Pattern**	5th Phase: **Validation**
1. Actor initiates behavior. 2. Intent of actor may not be explicit. 3. Completion of interaction unpredictable.	1. Other responds on basis of established normative expectations. 2. Other may or may not be aware of actor's intent.	1. Act unfolds in successive symbolic expressions. 2. Successive act/responses are based on interpretation of each prior act/response unit.	1. Actor/other role relationship different from that which existed at onset of interaction.	1. Altered relationship acknowledged by behaviors of relevant others. 2. Revised normative expectations emerge for this altered relationship.

be surprised that his directive is not accepted) acquiesces to the therapist's suggested alternative. In this instance role-making can be said to have occurred. Let us examine what took place: (1) the initiator of the interaction exhibited a behavior generally consistent with that of physician; (2) the "other," i.e., physical therapist, responded with a behavior generally inconsistent with that of physical therapist—that is, his act "challenged" the authority of the physician; (3) the physician can be said to have interpreted the attitude conveyed by the therapist and on the basis of his response apparently accepted it as within the norms of his perception of physician-other role; (4) the therapist made explicit an aspect of his self-perceived role as an autonomous professional by defining the treatment he determined appropriate to the patient's need. If, over time, both physician and therapist were to continue in this altered pattern of response to the other's role and relevant others were to accept the realigned role relationship, it could be concluded that the therapist's *evolved* role was validated.

One example of an evolving health professional role is that of the nurse practitioner—a role also referred to as the *expanded* role of the nurse (Andrews and Yankauer, 1971; U.S. Department of Health, Education and Welfare, 1971). The nurse practitioner is trained to provide health supervision and health assessment of individuals through performing history taking and physical examination of clients—role functions that have previously been restricted to the physician. In one study of nurse practitioners, it was reported that clients were better satisfied with the health supervision provided by the nurse than that provided by the physician (Linn, 1976). Similarly, the role of occupational therapist is a role that is in the process of evolving from one of a dependent (vis-a-vis physician) provider of services to the disabled or mentally ill to a role in which the focus is on health promotion and prevention of disability within the community at large (Cermak, 1976). In addition, the role of the pharmacist shows a similar evolutionary trend. Pharmacists, emphasizing their in-depth knowledge of drugs and their chemistry, are moving beyond their traditionally defined role of compounders and dispensers of prescriptions to one of educators of the consumer (Salisbury, 1977). It is conceivable that at some not too distant time the pharmacist, rather than the physician, will be the legitimate prescriber of drugs. Given what seems to be a momentum toward still further role realignments within the total system of health delivery, we can assume that, in addition to the roles alluded to above, other health provider roles are undergoing, or will soon undergo, similar altered role functions and relationships.

SUMMARY

Two competing theoretical formulations for the study of roles and role behavior have been defined and briefly explicated. The point has been emphasized that, although many hypotheses have been advanced to explain social (role) behavior, empirical research is still far from complete and caution must be exercised in drawing generalizations. It is obvious that neither the functionalist nor the interactionist perspective alone is sufficiently comprehensive to account for the wide variety of responses possible in those infinitely numerous situations where human actors confront each other.

3

Socialization for Roles

BARBARA ANN HURLEY

THE NATURE OF SOCIALIZATION

Traditions in Socialization

The systematic study of the area which is today known as socialization emerged simultaneously from three different traditions, i.e., anthropology, psychology, and sociology. Although the focus, theories, and methodologies used by each of these fields differ substantially, each has endeavored from its perspective to delineate some aspect of how the human person develops within his social and cultural milieu. Anthropology, for example, has distinguished itself by focusing upon the broader culture, viewing socialization as an enculturation process in which the learner passively absorbs and internalizes the cultural norms and contents transmitted by the society of which he is a member. In contrast, psychology focuses upon the processes of learning and development. Studies of the processes of identification, motivation, and cognitive, psychosexual, language, and conscience development have reflected psychologists' varied theoretical positions on the inherent nature of man as a passive learner requiring control of intrinsic negative tendencies. In contrast to the psychologist's position, sociologists have in large part focused on the agencies of socialization (family, peers, school, institutions) and the processes involved in the acquisition of social skills, including modes of social control, development of the social self, the influences of social structure and value orientation on child-rearing practices, and social roles and role training (Clausen, 1968a, pp. 22-48; Goslin, 1969, p. 1; Levine, 1969, pp. 505-510; Zigler and Child, 1969, pp. 451-473; 1973, pp. 5-35).

Anthropology, psychology, and sociology have distinguished themselves by their divergent perspectives and approaches to a central phenomenon of interest, i.e., how is it that a human person acquires the prerequisite knowledge, skills, and motivation to become a functioning member of society? Anthropologists, psychologists, and sociologists differentiate themselves from one another in several respects on this matter. These include the theoretical and methodologic perspectives they adopt, the levels of analysis with which they treat the subject, the aspects of the socialization process upon which they focus, and, in particular, the positions they assume on major theoretical issues stemming from their adopted theoretical and methodologic approaches (Clausen, 1968a, pp. 47-52; Goslin, 1969, pp. 1-2). Such issues (as summarized by Goslin, 1969, pp. 1-2) include the relative importance of early as opposed to later experiences on socialization outcomes; the relative emphasis attached to individual needs, motives, and drives as opposed to environmental determinants of behavior; the relative importance attached to process as opposed to content in predicting the outcomes of social behavior; the emphasis placed upon the unique aspects of the socialization experience as opposed to its common properties; and, finally, the focus upon the processes promoting conformity to societal norms as opposed to the causes of deviations from these behavioral norms. Of particular relevance here are two further issues that distinguish psychologists from sociologists in studying the phenomenon of socialization; namely, differences in views regarding the characteristics of the learner and the learning process and differences in the conceptualization of socialization as an active or passive process (Dreitzel, 1973b, pp. 5-24; Goslin, 1969, pp. 3-5; Zigler and Child, 1969, pp. 468-470; 1973, pp. 28-31). Reference to several of these issues will recur throughout the chapter.

The Concept of Socialization

USAGE OF THE TERM

The term *socialization* has a history of varied use in the disciplines from which theory and research relevant to it emerged (Clausen, 1968a, pp. 18-46). First used in sociology in the mid-1890s by Simmel, the term *socialization* originally referred to "the process of group formation or development of the forms of association" (Clausen, 1968a, p. 22). From that time until the end of the 1920s, the term was used with markedly varied meanings, but eventually it was used to refer primarily to "the 'shaping' of the person and to the mechanisms whereby individuals were transformed into persons" (Clausen, 1968a, p. 24). Prior to the mid-1930s, much of the research focusing on the development of the person and of the personality that we currently refer to as socialization research was classified under the rubric "culture and personality" (Clausen, 1968a, p. 24). Although the term *socialization* retained vestiges of earlier usages, as evidenced in the writings of Park (1939) and Dollard (1939), it was not until approximately 1939 that it came to be used widely in its present sense (Clausen, 1968a, pp. 24-25).

Because the field of socialization has emerged from various traditions, it has been defined in numerous ways. Elkin and Handel (1972, p. 4) have defined socialization as "the process by which someone learns the ways of a given society or social group so that he can function within it." For Zigler and Child (1973, p. 36), "socialization is a broad term for the whole process by which an individual develops, through transactions with other people, his specific pattern of socially relevant behavior and experience." For Inkeles (1969, pp. 615-616), who takes a sociologic and societal point of view, "socialization refers to the process whereby individuals acquire the personal system properties—the knowledge, skills, attitudes, values, needs and motivations, cognitive, affective and conative patterns which shape their adaptation to the physical and sociocultural setting in which they live."

Various theoretical perspectives give the concept of socialization differing connotations. Despite this variety, all definitions seem to encompass basic elements of this process. Common to the definitions is an attempt to delineate what is learned, how it is learned, why it is learned, and what are its expected outcomes. Ultimately, all theories attempt to account for individual variation (differences) in characteristics or performance.

VIEWS ON SOCIALIZATION

Perhaps one of the issues that most clearly distinguishes positions on socialization is the question of whether the socializee is viewed as an active or passive agent in his own socialization. Those investigators who advocate the position that the socializee is a passive recipient of cultural norms and contents assume that the effect of socializers is unidirectional. However, as Dreitzel (1973b, pp. 5-24), Goslin (1969, pp. 5-10), and Zigler and Child (1973, pp. 28-31) point out, there has been a shift in emphasis from a passive to an active view of the socializee as a result of empirical evidence gathered during the mid-1960s. Increasingly, socialization has come to be viewed as an interactional and reciprocal process in which the socializee and socializer are mutually influenced. Such an emphasis on the socializee as an active participant in his own socialization is an issue which most clearly differentiates positions on socialization. Sociologists and psychologists who hold this position employ different theoretical and methodologic approaches in order to systematically study socialization as an interactive process.

Socialization can also be viewed both from the perspective of the individual being socialized and from that of the society. From the individual perspective, the process of socialization encompasses the learning of motor and language skills, the acquisition of self-other systems, and the learning of social roles and moral norms and values, as well as affective and cognitive modes of functioning (Clausen, 1968b, p. 4; Inkeles, 1968, p. 83). From the societal perspective, the goals of socialization focus primarily upon the attainment of some form of competence that the society accepts as appropriate for adult performance, as well as an internalized commitment to continuing responsible participation in society (Elkin and Handel, 1972, pp. 29-32).

In order to attain these ultimate goals, society uses its socializing agents (family, peers, institutions) as means of transmitting to the socializee the kinds of social learning that ultimately have relevance for adult role performance, i.e., the development of motor and language skills, the teaching of social roles, the development of the social self, and the teaching of moral norms and values, as well as affective and cognitive modes of functioning. The word *transmitting* is used broadly here, since socialization has come to be viewed more and more as an interactional process in which the socializer and socializee are mutually influenced.

Viewed in this context, that is, socialization as an interactional process, individual and societal perspectives are interrelated, with both the socializers and the socializees influencing the acquisition of those types of social learning requisite for adequate and socially acceptable adult role performance (Clausen, 1968c, pp. 139-146; Inkeles, 1968, pp. 78-83).

Broadly conceived, socialization has been viewed as including a variety of processes that prepare the socializee for adult performance. Such an encompassing view takes the socialization process to be not only efforts of socialization agents to transmit existing norms, motives, and values to the socializee through child-rearing practices but also as efforts to transmit the learning that is required for marriage, parenthood, and occupational roles, as well as the kinds of social learning leading the individual to acquire the knowledge, skills, and dispositions appropriate to an individual of a particular age, sex, and social status (Clausen, 1968b, p. 7).

Because socialization is viewed as the societal means of attaining and maintaining social and cultural continuity, the adequacy of the socialization process is assessed in terms of the criterion of adequate adult performance. Adequate adult performance is seen to include the attainment of socially accepted competencies, as well as a motivated commitment to continued participation in the society. From a societal perspective, the socialization process is seen as a method utilized to establish the standards by which the socializee is expected to pattern achievements and developments in skills, emotional expression, intellectual activity, and relations with significant others (Clausen, 1968b, p. 5; Elkin and Handel, 1972, pp. 29-32; Inkeles, 1968, p. 75).

Frequently, the socialization process is viewed as implying that the socializee is induced in some measure to conform willingly to the norms and values transmitted to him by society's designated socialization agents. Inherent in this view is the assumption that norms and values transmitted to the socializee are internalized, becoming standards for behavior in the absence of internal or external sanctions (Clausen, 1968b, pp. 5-10).

QUESTIONS SOCIALIZATION ADDRESSES

There is no single theory of socialization. As previously indicated, the theories and research of the various traditions treat different aspects of the process at different levels of analysis, focusing upon various issues pertinent to their theoretical perspective and methodology. Thus, the various theoretical perspectives may be viewed as addressing different questions, which taken together comprise the whole area of socialization. These questions include some of the following: (1) What is learned, i.e., what is the content learned through the process of socialization? (2) How is the content learned, i.e., what is the learning process associated with the process of socialization? (3) Why is the content learned and subsequently enacted, i.e., what motivates the learner to both learn the content and subsequently utilize it in role performance? (4) What is the outcome of socialization desired by society? (5) What accounts for individual differences as opposed to conformity to social norms as a result of the socialization process? (6) What methods are used by society to ensure learning of social norms? (7) What are the preconditions for socialization? (8) What are the prerequisites for the learning of social roles? (9) What is the overall process through which socialization occurs?

THE NATURE OF SOCIALIZATION
FROM A ROLE PERSPECTIVE

Socialization for Roles

Among sociologists, one of the traditions that has focused upon the phenomenon of socialization has been role theory. From the role theorist's perspective, the nature of socialization has largely been defined in terms of the learning of social roles that prepare the socializee for adult role performance. In large part, role theorists studying the phenomenon of socialization have focused primarily upon adult socialization for occupational, marital, and parental roles. However, as Brim (1960, p. 127; 1966, p. 7), Clausen (1968c, pp. 133-138), and Goslin (1969, p. 6) point out, the conceptualization of socialization from a role perspective provides a mechanism for viewing socialization as a continuous and cumulative process. Viewed as a continuous and cumulative process, how social roles are learned by children and adults permits the joining of these seemingly disparate areas of interest within the socialization literature (Brim, 1966, pp. 5-7; Maccoby, 1959, pp. 239-252; 1961, pp. 493-503; Sewell, 1970, pp. 568-572).

Brim (1960, 1966) has given us two definitions of socialization from a role perspective. In the first, he defined socialization "as a process of learning through which an individual is prepared with varying degrees of success, to meet the requirements laid down by other members of society for his behavior in a variety of situations" (1960, p. 128). In Brim's second definition (1966, p. 3), which is the most frequently quoted, "socialization refers to the process by which persons acquire the knowledge, skills, and dispositions that make them more or less able members of their society."

In each of these definitions, socialization refers to the learning of those social roles that facilitate the socializee's participation and adequate adult performance in the ongoing society of which he is a member. In his first definition, Brim identified the content of socialization, i.e., what is learned, as the "requirements laid down by other members of society," namely, role prescriptions and role behaviors. In his second definition, he more specifically identified the content of socialization or what is learned as the "knowledge, skills, and dispositions," i.e., role demands attached to positions or statuses within the social structure of the society. Thus, the content learned includes not only the role prescriptions and role behaviors with their associated feeling modes but additionally the positions or statuses to which these role demands are attached. In each definition, Brim specified that the content of socialization, "knowledge, skills, and dispositions," is acquired through a process of learning that occurs within an interactional context. Further, each definition specifies that the socializees will learn the content of socialization with "varying degrees of success," and will fulfill the function and outcome of the socialization process by becoming "more or less able members of their society."

Brim's definitions of socialization and his discussions of the nature of socialization from a role perspective (Brim, 1960, pp. 127-159; 1962, pp. 176-180; 1966, pp. 1-50; 1968a, pp. 555-562; 1968b, pp. 182-226) address and elaborate upon many of the questions on which theorists and investigators from various disciplines in the area of socialization focus. Each of these aspects of socialization developed from the role perspective,

—including content, processes, motivation, outcomes, and individual differences—will be addressed in the discussion that follows. Brim's and other role theorists' conceptualizations of the nature of socialization will be used as the organizing framework for the discussion of each of these aspects. Contributions of theorists and investigators from various other disciplines will be included only as these deal with the process of socialization at different levels of analysis or focus upon aspects of the socialization process minimally addressed by the role perspective.

WHAT CONTENT IS LEARNED?

From a role perspective, the content or what is learned in the process of socialization includes both knowledge and understanding of the status structure of the society, as well as the role prescriptions and role behaviors attached to the various statuses or positions within the social structure (Brim, 1957, p. 345; 1960, p. 128; 1966, pp. 4-5).

Members of a society develop both prescriptive and performance aspects of roles in order to regulate the behavior of members so that the functions of the society will be successfully discharged. These normative prescriptions specify the feelings which the socializee occupying a particular status within the society should have, the behavior he should perform, and the effects he should produce (Brim, 1957, p. 345).

Since role prescriptions are based on implicit or explicit theories about human behavior, changes in role prescriptions will occur either when the underlying theory of human nature changes or when there are changes in the functions of society. Discrepancies or conflicts in what constitutes the content of role prescriptions result either from differences in underlying theories of human behavior or from differences in conceptions of what constitutes adequate, competent adult role performance (Brim, 1957, p. 345).

Role prescriptions for the occupant of a particular status not only explicitly specify how that individual is to behave, but implicitly specify as well the behaviors of persons in related positions toward the occupant of that particular status. It is generally the case that occupants of particular positions or statuses within the society know both the explicitly stated role prescriptions attached to their respective positions and the implicit reciprocal prescriptions guiding the role behaviors of others toward them (Brim, 1957, pp. 345-347).

Because the ultimate purpose of prescribed behavior is fulfillment of the functions of the society, societal role prescriptions are based on theories which incorporate into the role prescriptions the motives of the status incumbent, his overt behavior, and the effects of his behavior. Viewed in a causal sequence, motives are considered to result in behavior, which produces certain effects (Brim, 1957, pp. 348-349).

Whether role analysis involves motives, overt behavior, or effects of such behavior as the units of analysis, one or more descriptive properties of the role are required. Thus one may analyze the amount of dependence or aggression shown or the degree to which some other characteristic is demonstrated. It is equally important to analyze roles in terms of such variables as sex, ordinal position within the family, size of family, absence of statuses within the family system, and so forth (Brim, 1957, pp. 350-354; 1960, p. 148).

The preceding discussion of role prescriptions may lead the reader to believe that roles are always clearly prescribed and perceived by occupants of different positions as congruent. However, the role prescriptions perceived by occupants of similar or different statuses will differ considerably depending upon the source from which information about the role has been derived, i.e., formal laws, opinions, special interest groups, individuals, and so forth (Brim, 1957, pp. 351-354). Thus, it may be concluded that while some positions or statuses within society have highly specified role prescriptions regulating motives, behaviors, and the behavioral effects of the occupant of the status and of the expected behavior of related status holders, there are many positions for which role prescriptions are extremely vague and open to wide variation in interpretation and in enactment.

HOW IS THE CONTENT LEARNED?

The content of socialization, i.e., knowledge of the status structure of the society and of the role prescriptions and role behaviors attached to the various statuses, is acquired through two simultaneously occurring processes: interactional processes and learning processes that involve different agents or agencies of socialization (family, peers, school, other institutions).

Interactional Processes Through Which Socialization Occurs. Heiss (1976, p. 4) makes an initial distinction between two distinct role theory traditions: the structural tradition emerging from the work of Linton (1936, 1945) and the sociopsychologic branch emerging from the work of George Herbert Mead (1934). In essence, this distinction is made on the basis of whether or not socialization is viewed as a unidirectional or a two-way process. Linton, cited in Hollander and Hunt (1972, p. 112), used the term "role to designate the sum total of the culture patterns associated with a particular status . . . [which] includes the attitudes, values and behavior ascribed by the society to any and all persons occupying this status." From this perspective, role performance consists of the enactment of a prescribed role, a socially agreed upon specific script in which the actor plays out a series of role behaviors that he has learned through the process of socialization.

As analyzed by Turner (1962, p. 32), this model of "role as conformity," based on Linton's definitions of status and role, specifies that the individual enacts the prescribed set of expectations appropriate to individuals in relevant other statuses, conforms to others' expectations, and receives in return some indications of approval (Turner, 1962, pp. 32-33). Viewed from this perspective, socialization is a unidirectional process in which the socializee is a passive recipient and enactor of cultural norms and contents.

In contrast to the "enacting of a prescribed role" inherent in Linton's perspective, a Meadian view of *role* similarly defined as "prescriptions for interpersonal behavior associated with . . . statuses" (Heiss, 1976, p. 3) emphasizes the principle of role reciprocity, in which the individual devises his role performance on the basis of the role that he imputes to the other, i.e., the individual improvises a performance based on immediate cues (Heiss, 1976, p. 13). From this symbolic interactionist or Meadian perspective, interaction proceeds as roles are identified and given content, that is, self and other roles are created and modified as the process of interaction unfolds (Turner, 1962, pp. 21-23). From this viewpoint the learning of roles or role making is a two-way process in which the socializee and the socializer are active participants in an interactional process in which they are mutually influenced (Goslin, 1969, pp. 5-10; Rheingold, 1969, pp. 779-790; Turner, 1962, pp. 21-23).

Mead's concept of role learning through the process of interaction is described in more detail by Brim (1958, pp. 1-16; 1966, pp. 7-17), Elkin and Handel (1972, pp. 27-63), Goslin (1969, pp. 5-10), Heiss (1976, pp. 16-25), Hewitt (1976), Kerckhoff (1972, pp. 17-38), and Turner (1968b, pp. 95-97). Role theorists following Mead make two assumptions: (1) that roles are learned in the process of social interaction and (2) that in the interactional process the individual sees himself and the other as occupants of particular statuses and responds accordingly with appropriate role behaviors. But what is the mechanism by which roles are learned through interaction?

Through the process of interaction with members of the *primary group* (Cooley, 1962, pp. 23-31), the individual learns those role behaviors appropriate to his position within the group. The members of the primary group, holding normative beliefs about what constitutes the role, use reward and punishment to assist the individual to learn both the correct and incorrect actions appropriate to his role. The socializee becomes involved in a series of complex interpersonal relationships with a number of people who, because of their frequency of contact, their primacy, and their control over rewards and punishment, orient the child toward those role prescriptions and role behaviors that are expected outcomes of the socialization process (Brim, 1958, p. 1; 1966, pp. 8-9). Because of their intense contact and influence upon the socializee, the family members and particularly the mother are called *significant others*. When the child matures, the potential set of significant others enlarges, with teachers and peers becoming of more importance to the socializee (Kerckhoff, 1972, pp. 18-20).

In essence, from a Meadian point of view, socialization for roles begins with the personal attachment established between mother and child. For the child the relationship with the mother is his first encounter with what it means to be human; it is through her that he is presented with his first expectations of the social world and with her that he first begins to experience his sense of himself. Through being cared for and through evoking responses and being responded to by the mother, the child learns both the sense of himself and that of another person (Elkin and Handel, 1972, pp. 37-41). Although the mother is the first emotionally significant person with whom the child may establish a relationship in the course of his life, other significant others including the father, siblings, and peers will make different contributions to his socialization because of their different statuses and roles within the social structure (Elkin and Handel, 1972, pp. 40-41).

Goslin's (1969, p. 6) conceptualization of socialization in role-developmental terms adds further to our understanding of socialization as a two-way process. Goslin proposes that the process of interaction through which socialization occurs is one of role negotiation in which each participant influences the behavior of each other participant in significant ways, with the result that the behavior of each is altered to some degree.

Even though socialization is viewed as a process of role negotiations, numerous factors affect the extent to which the behavior of individuals may be subject to negotiation (Goslin, 1969, p. 7). As an occupant of a particular social position, the individual is involved in responding both to the expectations of others and in exercising his right to expect certain behaviors from related status holders. In the interactional situation, this involves an agreement or *contract* between participants as to what one may expect of the other. Deviations from prescribed expectations may vary considerably depending upon the institutionalized nature of the situation in which the participants interact. In the highly institutionalized situation, both participants have little opportunity for role negotiation since the rights and duties of each are specified in advance, allowing little room for negotiation of a new contract. Socialization under this highly institutionalized situation consists primarily in learning the existing role prescriptions for reciprocal roles (Goslin, 1969, p. 7).

When there are very general institutional prescriptions, such as in cases of friendships or casual social situations, societal norms or prescriptions are relatively unspecified and large variations in role enactment may be anticipated. For interaction to proceed in such situations, the pair of participants must create reciprocal roles through the process of role negotiation in which both must establish and maintain situational identities (roles) and recognize the identities (roles) of the other (Goslin, 1969, pp. 7-8).

With respect to role negotiation, Goslin (1969, pp. 8-10) makes several significant points that follow from his position that socialization is a two-way process. First, in the establishment of every interactional relationship, regardless of how highly institutionalized its roles may be, some negotiation is possible and necessary. This role negotiation goes on whether one or all the parties to the interaction are aware or unaware of the process and whether they perceive the possibility that aspects of their roles are subject to negotiation (Rheingold, 1969, pp. 779-790). Those participants able to accurately assess the negotiability of a situation are at a distinct advantage.

Acquisition of awareness that roles can be negotiated is fostered by nonauthoritarian child-rearing practices in which children are encouraged to express their own feelings and in which their rights as children are given explicit recognition (Goslin, 1969, p. 8). In nonauthoritarian child-rearing situations not only does the child develop an awareness of the possibility of role negotiation, but he also develops specific techniques for handling himself in role-bargaining situations. There are distinct advantages and disadvantages for the child who acquires both the awareness that roles can be negotiated and the specific techniques of role-bargaining, as well as for the child who learns neither of these skills. For those children who have experienced the freedom to utilize bargaining techniques in various situations with frequent success, situations in which role negotiation is not possible may be viewed as frustrating and intolerable. This is particularly true when these children have not learned to distinguish between situations in which role negotiation is and is not possible (Goslin, 1969, p. 9).

Those children who have had little experience in role negotiation, that is, who have neither learned of the possibility nor developed negotiation techniques, are at a distinct disadvantage when they become involved in situations where negotiation is necessary or desirable (Goslin, 1969, p. 9).

As Goslin further points out, the distribution of power in an interactional system is of extreme importance in role negotiation. With respect to power, control of resources is a particularly critical factor, as the member possessing the greater resources has considerably greater bargaining power, regardless of the formality or informality of the power structure (Goslin, 1969, p. 9).

Finally, Goslin makes the point that the absolute freedom to negotiate one's role may be significantly restricted by the individual's internalization of values and standards of conduct that inhibit his exercise of personal power in situations that are negotiable (Goslin, 1969, p. 10).

Through the process of interaction, the child learns not only the social structure of statuses and their accompanying role prescriptions and role behaviors but also the prerequisites necessary for learning of role demands. The outcomes of the interactional process which are also prerequisites for the learning of roles include (1) the learning of verbal or language skills, (2) the learning of role-taking skills, (3) the genesis or development of the self, and (4) the learning of the presentation of self or interpersonal competence. Because of the importance of each of these prerequisite outcomes or elements to the learning of roles, each will be discussed with respect to its importance in relation to role-learning and its interrelationships with the others (Brim, 1966, pp. 7-15; Elkin and Handel, 1972, pp. 9-63; Goslin, 1969, pp. 10-12 Heiss, 1976, pp. 6-16; Hewitt, 1976, pp. 21-104; Kerckhoff, 1972, pp. 17-38).

Verbal or Language Skills. The acquisition of language, i.e., verbal skills, is a prerequisite for learning of most roles (Goslin, 1969, p. 10) and plays an important part in socialization because it facilitates learning other skills required for role acquisition (Jenkins, 1969, p. 663).

Within the last 40 years, four models representing a range of views of psychologists regarding the acquisition of language have been popular: language as words, language as strings of words or classes, language as utterances, and language as a structural system (Jenkins, 1969, p. 663). Although it seems obvious that language is made up of words, word-based systems, with some notable exceptions (e.g., Chinese), have been replaced by more efficient alphabetic systems. If language is thought of as words, its acquisition is seen to consist of two processes: development of the motor skills involved in saying words and the cognitive skill of getting the words attached to meanings (Jenkins, 1969, p. 663). Viewed from this perspective, language involves a combination of instrumental learning and classical conditioning that permits the learning of both semantic and emotional meanings (Jenkins, 1969, pp. 663-669).

When language is viewed as a string of words, the sequences and the exact pattern of sequences in which words are ordered or combined are of critical importance (Jenkins, 1969, p. 667). Two general approaches have been proposed to account not only for the words but for their ordering in sentences, both as they are spoken and as they are understood. In the first approach, it is assumed that humans engage in probabilistic learning in which words subsequently become probabilistically linked in productive arrangements. The second approach proposes that words are learned as members of classes, with certain sequences of classes forming permissible sequences. It has been suggested that these two approaches can be fused into a joint model in which there is the probabilistic linking of classes or words with varying probabilities of words having memberships in classes (Jenkins, 1969, pp. 666-672).

Language viewed as utterances stems from B. F. Skinner's prospect that language is behavior reinforced by others. Language, like any other behavior, is seen as developing through operant conditioning. Skinner divides verbal behaviors into two functional classes, *mands* and *tacts*. Mands refer to verbal behaviors controlled by the organism's state of deprivation; their purpose is to command some specific reinforcement for the organism. Mands, which are "shaped" and maintained by reinforcement, will be extinguished when no longer reinforced. Tacts, on the other hand, refer to verbal behaviors that report something about the state of the world and are maintained by generalized reinforcement (Jenkins, 1969, pp. 672-675).

The fourth model of language acquisition focuses on language as a rule system. This position, championed by modern linguistics, and Chomsky in particular, argues that since language is infinitely variable, productive rules are learned rather than words of particular sentence orders. The learning of these productive rules permits the individual to produce a variety of sentences and to understand a variety of sentences as well (Jenkins, 1969, p. 675). However, little is known about how the child actually acquires the rules of language. It is suggested that the child starts with "pivot grammars" that subsequently become more complex (Jenkins, 1969, pp. 675-682).

From a sociologic role perspective, language develops through interactional processes between mother and infant. Initially, social interaction between mother and infant is preverbal. Nonetheless, the infant and mother do communicate at a rudimentary level, with the mother interpreting the infant's cries and responding with activities that she hopes will restore him to a state of comfort. Not only does the mother interpret the infant's cries, but subsequent to her intervention she evaluates from the infant's response whether her interpretation was correct. Although the mother possesses the capacity to interpret the infant's communication and to represent to herself what the infant may be trying to communicate, the newborn must develop this capacity through interaction with the mother. Gradually the infant becomes able to anticipate his mother's appearance, learning in his relationship with the mother how to emit meaningful sounds. Basically, this occurs through a process of operant learning in which the child learns to associate his vocal sounds and his mother's reinforcing responses. With his increasing capacity to emit vocal sounds, which are reinforced by the mother, the infant learns to make sounds in the mother's absence. Gradually, through vocal interaction between mother and child, the child develops the ability to associate a specific sound with a specific desired circumstance, and this subsequently leads to a building up of vocabulary and to the use of an increasingly complex set of shared symbols (Elkin and Handel, 1972, pp. 41-44; Kerckhoff, 1972, pp. 23-24).

The acquisition of language accelerates socialization and is of enormous importance as one of the component processes of role learning. With the gradual acquisition of language and the use of common gestures, the infant acquires the ability to symbolize, i.e., to specifically identify things, persons, and feelings to himself. Once he has acquired the ability to present to himself the same symbol for an object that is presented to others, the child makes great strides toward the regulation of his own behavior and simultaneously toward responsive participation with others. Having entered into the social world of shared symbols, the child has gained the capacity to move beyond the mother-infant relationship into the larger social world of family, peers, school, and so forth (Elkin and Handel, 1972, pp. 41-44).

Role-taking. Another prerequisite to the learning of roles is the development of the capacity to take the role of the other. Turner (1956, p. 316) has defined role-taking in its most general form as "a process of looking at or anticipating another's behavior by viewing it in the context of a role imputed to that other." Role-taking has been defined by others as "the process by which the actor imagines what the other person's response would be to any one of a number of things he might do" (Kerckhoff, 1972, p. 32); "the ability to imagine oneself in the place of the other and to see things as he sees them" (Heiss, 1976, p. 6); "the imaginative construction of the other's role" (Turner, 1956, p. 317, after Coutu, 1951). Common to these and many other definitions of role-taking is the fact that the individual anticipates the response of the other to his own behavior, i.e., self-consciously views himself from the standpoint of the other in terms of relative social location (position, status), reflects upon his own performance or appraises his own behavior in view of the other's response, and enacts or performs his own role accordingly (Brim, 1966; Coutu, 1951; Heiss, 1976; Hewitt, 1976; Kerckhoff, 1972; Lauer and Boardman, 1971). The role of the other may be inferred through observation of the behavior of the other, supplying in imagination the role of which the behavior is indicative. The role may also be inferred by knowledge of the situation through projection, i.e., imputing the role to the other, or through prior knowledge of the other obtained from previous experiences with the individual or those like him, with the other's behavior in similar situations, or with behavior of individuals in comparable situations (Turner, 1956, p. 318).

The manner in which the inferred other-role shapes the enactment of the self-role depends on what standpoint the individual adopts in taking the role of the other and on whether the role-taking is reflexive or non-reflexive (Turner, 1956, p. 319). Taking the role of the other need not include taking the standpoint of the other. When the standpoint of the other is adopted, however, one acts from the standpoint of the other in taking the role of the other. When the standpoint of the other is not adopted in role-taking, other factors would then determine what influence taking the role of the other will have on the individual's behavior (Turner, 1956, p. 319).

Taking the role of the other is not the same as taking the standpoint of the other. Taking the standpoint of the other refers to the individual's ability to imaginatively take the role of the other while at the same time maintaining his own personal identity (Turner, 1956, p. 319). This distinction between taking the role of the other and taking the standpoint of the other is not made by children in early role-taking activity. As the child gradually engages in more complex behavior, role-taking becomes divested of identification, i.e., taking the standpoint of the other. Such situations arise when the individual becomes simultaneously concerned with multiple others and is unable to simultaneously take the standpoint of each; when there are conflicting standpoints in the varied roles with which the individual becomes involved; or when needs or purposes gradually lead the individual to adopt role-taking in an adaptive context (Turner, 1956, p. 319). Thus, in taking the role of the other, the individual may adopt the other's standpoint as his own, with an automatically resulting indentification with the other-role, which serves as a guide to self-behavior; the individual may adopt a third-party standpoint, in which the role of the other is viewed from the standpoint of some personalized third party or depersonalized norm; or the individual may take, in an adaptive context, a standpoint consisting of a purpose or objective (Turner, 1956, p. 321).

The manner in which the inferred other-role shapes the enactment of the self-role is also determined by whether role taking is reflexive or nonreflexive. In reflexive role-taking, the role of the other serves as a mirror reflecting the expectations and/or evaluations of the self as seen by the other, i.e., Cooley's "looking-glass-self." From this perspective, the role-taker is focused upon the way he appears to the other and shapes the behavior of the self accordingly. More attention will be given to this aspect of role-taking when we consider the genesis of the self. In nonreflexive role-taking, other-attitudes, expectations or evaluations are not directed toward the self and thus are not relevent to the determination of the individual's behavior (Turner, 1956, p. 321).

By using the concepts of reflexive and nonreflexive role-taking in combination with the three general standpoints which may be adopted in role-taking, we can more sharply delineate the different ways in which self-other relationships can determine behavior (Turner, 1956, p. 322). First, when role-taking is nonreflexive and involves taking the standpoint of the other, the individual's behavior is determined by identification with the standpoint of the other. When role-taking is reflexive and the standpoint of the other is adopted, the individual desires to conform to the other's expectations and shapes his self-behavior into conformity with the other. When role-taking is reflexive and a third-party standpoint is adopted, the individual is able to act discriminatively toward the other in determining which aspirations and attitudes he will use for himself. When role-taking is reflexive and the actor adopts the standpoint of the third party, the actor is enabled to react selectively to his audience, accepting some of their evaluations as legitimate while rejecting those expectations which lack legitimacy. When role-taking occurs in an adaptive context and is reflexive, the other manipulates his own self-image as a means of achieving his ends. In contrast, when role-taking is nonreflexive, the other may endeavor to establish a false image of himself in order to modify the behavior of the self in the anticipated direction (Turner, 1956, pp. 322-323).

These types of role-taking are important because in each the individual finds himself in a somewhat different relationship with the other whose role he is attempting to take, and in combination, the effect on self-role behavior is different (Turner, 1956, p. 323).

Taking the role of the other occurs through the process of social interaction and is clearly related to cognitive development (Kerckhoff, 1972, p. 57). Through interaction the individual learns both his own responses to others and the responses of those others with whom he interacts (Brim, 1966, p. 10). In learning self-other roles, the individual gets needed information by direct instruction, by observing interaction as a participant, or by observing interaction as a bystander (Heiss, 1976, pp. 6-7).

Several factors affect the individual's role-taking ability. The actor's ability to take a particular role is largely determined by (1) the extent of his social experience; (2) the extent of his experiences with a particular role as actor, other, or observer; (3) the adequacy of his memory of his experiences; (4) the recency of relevant experiences; and (5) the extent to which the individual "paid attention" during the interaction (Heiss, 1976, p. 7). When the individual finds himself in a situation that he has not previously experienced, he must not only draw upon prior experience but apply information that he has previously obtained. Skill in perceiving the essential differences in situations previously experienced depends upon the ability of the individual to develop, through a process of trial and error, implicit hypotheses concerning the differences between past and present circumstances, and to take the role of the other on this basis; usually, the role taken is that of the *generalized other*. The individual's ability to take the role of the *generalized other* is based upon his ability to take into account the statuses of the others involved in the interaction, take all of their roles in turn, and then develop a conception of the probable group reactions or responses (Heiss, 1976, pp. 7-8).

Development of the Self.   The development or genesis of the self is both a product of social interaction and prerequisite for social interaction and the learning of social roles. The self, which is not initially present at birth, arises through the process of interaction with *significant others*, particularly the mother. Preverbal social interaction that precedes the acquisition of language takes place through a process that Mead termed a *conversation of gestures* (Mead, 1934, pp. 135-141). Differential responses on the part of parents, siblings, and others communicate to the infant whether or not his behavior is appropriate, and in so doing they lay the groundwork for the child's self-evaluation. Since language is essential for the development of the self, the child's increasing ability to use language enables the socialization process and the development of the self to proceed with greater rapidity and depth (Brim, 1966, p. 11).

From a Meadian viewpoint, the self is a process in which the individual first becomes an object to himself by taking the attitudes of others toward himself. This ability to take the attitude of others toward the self is made possible through the development of language. The self, which is essentially a social process, arises in social experience, allowing the self to be an object to himself (Mead, 1934, pp. 138-140).

The *conversation of gestures* that the individual comes to carry on within himself is the beginning of communication. With the increasing ability of the child to use language, the symbol that the child uses arouses in the self the same response that it arouses in other individuals. As the child develops, he begins to use larger segments of behavior, even whole roles, and engages in what Mead has referred to as *play*. Through play the child may actively and dramatically play the role of parent, teacher, or policeman; as he plays each role he builds up a repertoire of roles that assist him to participate in a variety of situations.

With encouragement from the culture to play roles that may subsequently be required for adult role performance, the child learns the statuses or positions within the social structure of the society, as well as the role prescriptions and role behaviors required of occupants of specific positions. The child also learns those role behaviors and prescriptions that should be avoided. Since play occurs under conditions that are viewed as practice sessions for future role performances, the atmosphere is a nonpunitive one where there is little censure. This early-role play, which occurs in learning situations that are essentially unrelated, is essentially transient and unorganized.

As the child grows older, he finds himself involved in more complex situations that require him to take the roles of several individuals simultaneously in order to enact his role. Mead referred to this advanced state of development as the *game*. In contrast to the play situation, in the game the self must take into account the attitude of everyone else involved in the game, taking into account as well the relationships of each of the varying roles to the other. Essentially, this period of time or activity that Mead calls *the game* is the situation through which the self incorporates the *generalized other*, i.e., the attitude of the whole community of which he is a part.

It is under the conditions of play and the game that the self arises as an object to itself. To develop the self to its fullest extent the individual must not only take on the attitudes of the other individuals toward himself and toward one another within the process of social interaction and bring the whole social process into his individual experience, but he must also take on the attitude of the generalized other, which is the attitude of the whole community of which he is a part. It is through the process of incorporating the generalized other that the individual's behavior is influenced and the community exercises control over the conduct of its members.

Thus, the development of the self involves two general stages. The first, designated by Mead as *play*, involves the self being constituted through incorporating the attitudes of particular individuals toward himself and one another in specific social acts in which the individual participates with those individuals. In the second stage, which Mead termed the *game*, the self is organized not only by the particular attitudes of individuals but also by the organization of the social attitudes of the generalized other, the social group, or community to which the individual belongs (Mead, 1934, p. 158). The game is simply an illustration of the process through which the self is developed by continually taking the attitudes of those about him, by taking the roles of those who in some sense are the controllers of his behavior and upon whom he depends (Mead, 1934, p. 160.).

Both the acquisition of language and the taking on of the role of the other are prerequisites for play, in which the individual takes the role of the individual other, and for the game, in which the individual incorporates the attitudes of the generalized other. Taking on the role of the other occurs essentially through the use of language, and it is through language that the individual is able to arouse in himself the same attitudes that he arouses in the other (Mead, 1934, pp. 160-161).

What constitutes the self as viewed by Mead is the organization of the attitudes that are common to the group of which the individual is a part. By putting himself in the place of the generalized other, the individual is guided and controlled by principles. It is only through the relationship of the self to other selves that the self can exist (Mead, 1934, p. 164). The individual becomes a self only in so far as he is able to take the attitude of the other and act toward himself as others act toward him (Mead, 1934, p. 171). This implies the preexistence of a group with whom the individual can interact. The self is a reflexive and cognitive phenomenon rather than an emotional one. Its essence lies in its capacity to carry on an internalized conversation of gestures which constitutes thinking (Mead, 1934, p. 173). The *I* consists of the response of the individual to the attitudes of the other, while the *Me* is the organized set of attitudes, the "generalized other," which the individual assumes (Mead, 1934, p. 175). The *I* and the *Me* constitute phases of the self. Essential to the self in its full expression are the *I* and the *Me* (Mead, 1934, p. 199). Although all selves are constituted by means of social interaction with significant others, the individual self has its own peculiar individuality and uniqueness.[1]

Presentation of Self and Interpersonal Competence.   Equally important for the acquisition of roles is the learning of interpersonal competence (Weinstein, 1969, pp. 753-775) and presentation of self (Goffman, 1959) through the process of social interaction. Interpersonal competence is the ability of the actor to control the response of the other through the use of interpersonal tactics, an ability which ultimately depends upon the development of language.

Intelligence and cue sensitivity underly the individual's capacities for developing interpersonal competence. Cue sensitivity, meanings of common gestures, facial expressions, and voice inflections are learned through a social conditioning process as part of language acquisition. Heightened cue sensitivity is necessary to the individual in order to recognize and discriminate differences in meaning between individuals and for the same individuals in differing situations.

The genesis for developing interpersonal competence is found in the capacity that the individual develops to distinguish self from non-self. Projective and positional role-taking, personality sterotyping, individuation, and autistic projection are types of role-taking that have their beginnings during the early school years and continue developing subsequently.

Several conditions promote the development of interpersonal competence, including exposing the child to a breadth and variety of social relationships, role-playing, and parental practices that orient the child toward projective role-taking. Highly authoritarian child-rearing practices tend to inhibit role-taking accuracy.

Interpersonal competence, the "ability to control the responses of others" (Weinstein, 1969, p. 764), depends both upon the development of more self-conscious of interpersonal tactics and upon the development of language. The learning of role prescriptions and role behaviors and how these are enacted in varying situations is fundamental to the learning of interpersonal tactics. The individual must learn the tactics of interpersonal bargaining as well as techniques for both establishing and maintaining his situational identity, and *altercasting* or assigning situational identity to others (Weinstein, 1969, p. 757).

Effective participation in social exchange requires awareness of exchange as an approach to the pursuit of personal goals, the learning of exchange tactics, and the development of the ability to differentiate situations in which tactics may not be equally effective for interpersonal control.

The development of reciprocity in exchange is believed to have its foundations early in socialization, peer influence probably having a major importance. Through interaction with peers, the individual learns that advantageous exchange means maximizing one's outcomes in terms of the balance of rewards and costs for the individual actor.

For the adult, much interaction focuses upon establishing and maintaining situational identities, which may change from encounter to encounter. Situational identities or the ways in which one presents oneself to others are the basis for lines of action and interpersonal tasks. In establishing which self is to be presented, the individual learns the cues that need to be given in establishing his identity through direct claim, by adoption of the particular sets and demeanor associated with the desired identity, shading and coloration, and by directing others to assume or play roles through the use of sanctions or through altercasting.

Several personal tendencies may enhance or inhibit the individual's ability and freedom to be interpersonally competent. Role rigidity, particularly as it relates to being rule bound, and rigidity in certain aspects of one's self-concept interfere with interpersonal competence. Personal motivations also affect the individual's motivation for interpersonal competence, with feelings of alienation resulting in low motivation, internal locus of control resulting in high motivation, and external locus of control resulting in reduced motivation. Failure also affects motivation for interpersonal competence. When an individual assumes a failure-avoidance orientation, the result is reduced flexibility in the bargaining process. The underlying basis for the failure-avoidance orientation is probably low self-esteem enhanced by parental rejection (Weinstein, 1969, pp. 753-775).

From the point of view of Meadian role theory, a socialization process is necessary to teach the individual what self he should present in specific situations and how he is to go about presenting an image of himself that is consistent with his actual self-image. The processes by which the individual learns to present the correct self-image, sometimes termed management of impressions, are basically the same processes as those utilized in socialization for roles. The difference is essentially in the content learned rather than in the process by which the learning occurs.

According to Elkin (1976, pp. 356-358), the child goes through several stages in learning impression management or presentation of self. Using the work of Goffman (1959), Elkin proposes that through the process of socialization, i.e., interaction with significant others, the child learns the parts or roles which he should present before certain audiences and in certain settings as well as those behaviors permitted in "back regions" which are not open to the audience. Elkin maintains that the learning required for presentation of self, i.e., role performance behavior, begins very early in the child's life, even before the development of the self. Ultimately, the ability to learn to manage impressions requires both the development of the self and the ability to take the role of the other, i.e., to take the attitude of the other person with respect to one's own behavior. Once the child has developed a self and is capable of taking the role of the other, others take greater care in the presentation of the self that they enact before the child.

The Learning Processes
Through Which Socialization Occurs

The main emphasis of Meadian role theorists has been upon the interactional processes through which socialization occurs rather than upon the learning processes through which socialization is achieved. Although these theories conceptualize the learner as an active participant in his own socialization, they acknowledge that socialization involves both conscious and unconscious learning processes in which the socializee may be viewed under varying circumstances as either an active or passive participant in the process of role learning and role enactment (Goslin, 1969, p. 12). In the earlier discussion of the interactional processes through which socialization occurs, several learning processes were identified as necessary for the learning of verbal or language skills, the learning of role-taking skills, the genesis or development of the self, the learning of the presentation of the self or interpersonal competence, and the learning of social roles. These learning mechanisms included: (1) operant learning; (2) direct instruction; (3) observational learning; (4) imitation; (5) role-taking; (6) role-playing; (7) modeling; (8) trial and error; (9) identification; and (10) role negotiation.[2] Although a theory of social learning is thus necessarily inherent in the role theorists' position that socialization occurs through interactional processes, this learning theory has not as yet been specifically delineated.

As indicated earlier, psychologists have focused upon processes of learning and development, taking varied theoretical perspectives with respect to the processes of identification, motivation, and cognitive, language, psychosexual, and moral development. Learning theorists have also taken theoretical positions regarding the acquisition of sex role identities and sex role standards (D'Andrade, 1966, pp. 173-203; Kagan, 1964, pp. 137-167; Kohlberg, 1966, pp. 82-172; Mischel, 1966, pp. 56-81; Mussen, 1969, pp. 707-731; Spencer, 1967, pp. 193-205), which are pertinent to the sociologist's interest in the mechanisms through which role prescriptions and role behaviors are learned.

With respect to learning theories and learning mechanisms in general, Gewirtz (1969, pp. 57-212) emphasizes the operant conditioning paradigm and uses imitation-identification and dependence-attachment as the two key social-learning processes (Gewirtz, 1969, pp. 136-182). In contrast, Bandura (1969, pp. 213-262) proposes a social-learning theory of identificatory processes that is much in keeping with the Meadian role theorists' position on learning processes. In Bandura's theory, the terms " 'identification,' 'imitation,' and 'observational learning' are employed interchangeably to refer to behavioral modification resulting from exposure to modeling stimuli" (Bandura, 1969, p. 219). Bandura proposes that the basic learning process underlying identification is observational learning, which involves imagery formation and verbal coding of observed events. The proposed modeling phenomenon consists of four components: attentional, retentional, motoric reproduction, and incentive or motivational processes. In order to reproduce modeling stimuli, Bandura proposes that the individual must (1) attend to, recognize, and differentiate the distinctive features of the model's responses; (2) retain the coded modeling events over time through covert role-practice of modeled responses that produce rewarding outcomes; (3) utilize symbolic representations of modeled responses in the form of imagery and verbal coding to guide overt role performances; and (4) respond to favorable or reinforcing incentive conditions (Bandura, 1969, pp. 220-225), which may be externally applied, self-administered, or vicariously experienced (Bandura, 1969, pp. 233-241). Bandura's theory (1969, pp. 241-247, 255) emphasizes the emulation of the behavior of models possessing distinctive characteristics. The result is that these models eventually function as discriminative stimuli for identificatory responses toward unfamiliar models in different social situations. Bandura's theory of identificatory processes differs significantly from psychoanalytic theories of anaclitic and defensive or aggressive identification, and from Whiting's status-envy hypothesis of modeling stimuli and social power theories (Bandura, 1969, pp. 225-233). However, these latter theories will not be discussed here.

Motivation of the Socializee to Learn Content and Utilize It in Role Performance

Our previous discussion of the interactional processes through which socialization occurs has emphasized both the roles of external and internal sanctions, i.e., rewards and punishment imposed by significant others, and the internalization of dispositions and values as two major motivational forces enhancing the learning of role prescriptions and role behaviors (Aronfreed, 1969, pp. 270-292; Brim, 1966, pp. 11, 15-17; Elkin, 1976, pp. 358-359; Elkin and Handel, 1972, pp. 37-41; Ferguson, 1970, pp. 59-79; Kerckhoff, 1972, pp. 26-28; and Parke, 1970, pp. 81-108).

While there is some convergence of opinion among psychologists and sociologists that role learning and role enactment depend in part on the effectiveness of external and internal sanctions, the views of the learner taken by the psychologist and the sociologist lead to somewhat different interpretations of the function of reward and punishment in the socialization process (Goslin, 1969, p. 13). The psychologist appears to place greater emphasis upon the effects of reward and punishment in facilitating desired behavioral responses, upon the establishment of the link between the stimulus and the response, and upon the process through which external reward and punishment become internalized over time. The strength of the sanction imposed is important to the psychologist, whether the sanctions are positive or negative; so is the timing of the sanctions with respect to the learner's acts, the frequency and consistency with which the sanctions are imposed, and the form which the sanctions take, i.e., whether they are mediated by verbal and symbolic processes or involve direct physical impact, and whether they are experienced directly or are experienced vicariously through observation of outcomes for others (Goslin, 1969, pp. 14-16).

Psychologists have provided experimental evidence that extremely strong negative sanctions result in the acquiring of response dispositions that are accompanied by high performance motivation and high resistance to extinction. However, there is further evidence that very strong punishment inhibits the ability of the learner to make necessary subtle discriminations among stimuli, resulting in a decrease in the individual's motivation to perform. Mild sanctions have been found to permit full concentration on the relevant stimuli but may be ineffective in promoting high motivation to perform. It is reported that both positive and negative sanctions can be equally effective in enabling the learner to discriminate appropriate from inappropriate behavioral cues. Further, it has been found that rapid acquisition of desired responses by the learner results from close timing of reward or punishment with respect to the learner's act. More frequent and consistent sanctions are believed to make it easier for the learner to discriminate appropriate from inappropriate role behaviors. For some kinds of learning, however, partial reinforcement results in stronger response acquisition because sanctions are random in probability of occurrence but consistent in nature (Goslin, 1969, pp. 14-16; Parke, 1970, pp. 81-108; 1972, pp. 264-283).

In contrast to psychologists, the sociologist views the occurrence of rewards and punishments as providing the learner with cues that enable him to consciously evaluate the adequacy of his role performance and modify his behavior accordingly (Goslin, 1969, p. 13). Sanctions are viewed as an integral part of the role negotiation process with differential outcomes resulting from the distribution and redistribution of sanctioning power (Goslin, 1969, p. 16).

It is generally held that in situations characterized by the imposition of external rewards or punishment for inappropriate role performance, both learning and motivation are likely to be a function of the type of rewards and punishments present. In contrast, when imposition of external sanctions is low, both learning and motivation are likely to be the result of internalized dispositions, i.e., values and motives (Goslin, 1969, p. 14).

Aronfreed (1969, p. 264) defines the concept of internalization as referring "to the child's adoption of social norms or roles as its own, and to the resulting control of its behavior by the most complex mediational functions of cognitive and verbal processes." From Aronfreed's perspective, internalization of values and motives or development of conscience is accomplished through direct training and through observational learning (Aronfreed, 1969, pp. 270-304). Goslin (1969, pp. 16-17) summarizes findings from several studies supporting the notion that internalization is powerfully influenced by the immediacy, availability, and intensity of discriminative cues (rewards and punishments).

The process of acquisition or internalization of values and motives has been studied from several perspectives. The cognitive-developmental perspectives represented by the works of Piaget and Kohlberg trace the acquisition of values through successive stages (Kohlberg, 1969, pp. 347-480; Kohlberg and Kramer, 1972, pp. 336-361; Maccoby, 1968, pp. 229-239; Piaget, 1948). The social learning perspective emanating from the work of Bandura and Walters emphasizes the acquisition of self-control through modeling, direct reinforcement, and reinforcement patterns and disciplinary techniques (Bandura, 1969, pp. 213-262; Bandura and Walters, 1968, pp. 189-191; Maccoby, 1968, pp. 240-262). The psychoanalytic perspective represented by Freud emphasized the mechanisms of defensive and anaclitic identification as underlying the development of an inner conscience (Hoffman, 1963, pp. 295-318).

In contrast, Meadian role theorists emphasize the development of the self as the principal outcome of socialization, which makes internal or self-regulation of behavior possible. This capacity for self-regulation develops as a result of interaction with significant others who present themselves as authoritative role models utilizing positive and negative sanctions to encourage the internalization of appropriate values and norms (Brim, 1966, pp. 11, 15-17; Elkin, 1976, pp. 358-359; Elkin and Handel, 1972, pp. 49-53). It will be recalled that development of the self involves the ability of the individual to take the role of the other, thus enabling the person to act toward himself in much the same way that he acts toward other people. "Self-control refers to behavior that is redirected in the light of the manner in which it is imagined to appear from the standpoint of other people who are involved in a cooperative task" (Shibutani, 1968, p. 381). This capacity to form self-images or take the role of the other makes possible the control of the impulsive *I* which is inhibited by the *Me* or the generalized other, making self-criticism and self-control possible. Thus, from a Meadian role perspective, individuals are viewed as internalizing social controls over their own behavior by developing selves (Heiss, 1976, pp. 10-11; Hewitt, 1976, pp. 55-56, 60-61, 82-92; Mead, 1934, pp. 155, 162, 178, 186-192, 210-211, 254-255; Shibutani, 1968, pp. 379-381).

Outcomes of the Socialization Process as Specified by Society

It is the purpose of socialization to assist members of a society to acquire the knowledge, skills, and dispositions that will enable them to function as able members of the society (Brim, 1966, p. 3; Elkin and Handel, 1972, p. 10, Kerckhoff, 1972, pp. 34-35). Thus, a particular society specifies a socialization process wherein certain requirements, demands, and expectations—which serve as functional requisites for the continuance of that society —are made of its members. The socialized individual is expected to achieve established standards of the society with respect to physical development, skills and capacities, emotional expression, intellectual and conative activity, and patterning of relations with significant other (Brim, 1966, pp. 4-8; Inkeles, 1968, p. 75). Additionally, the society is primarily concerned with the acquisition of those characteristics having particular relevance for the performance of adult social roles that the individual will enact with respect to his status position within that society (Brim, 1966, pp. 4-7; Goslin, 1969, p. 10, Inkeles, 1968, p. 77).

The societally expected outcomes of socialization are also determined by the society's rules governing access to particular statuses and roles. Roles are either *ascribed* on the basis of such characteristics as social class, ethnic group membership, religion, and gender, or *achieved* on the basis of educational or occupational background (Elkin and Handel, 1972, p. 34; Hewitt, 1976, pp. 93-95; Inkeles, 1968, p. 78). Accordingly, society specifies criteria and procedures that differentiate among children of various social classes, ethnicity, religious affiliation, and sex-role identification, resulting in different sequences of experiences and ultimately different socialization outcomes (Elkin and Handel, 1972, pp. 34-37).

Society makes demands upon the individual member on three different levels of generality: those requirements common to any society, those characteristic of a particular society or cultural tradition, and those demanded of individuals belonging to certain subgroups or strata of the society (Inkeles, 1968, p. 78). Inkeles (1968, p. 79-83) summarizes the eight functional requisites for continuance of a particular society as developed by Levy (1952). These requisites for societal functioning include: (1) provision for an adequate physiologic relationship to the environment through individual acquisition of relevant information, skills, and techniques permitting physical survival and procreation; (2) *role differentiation* and *role assignment*, which facilitate the individual's development of his own sense of identity and the similarity and distinctiveness of his own identity from that of others, particularly with respect to gender and age; (3) a "shared, learned, symbolic mode of communication" accomplished through interaction with significant others; (4) "a shared cognitive orientation"; (5) a shared set of goals that have been articulated by the society, including values, needs, and motives; (6) regulations with respect to the means chosen to attain the designated goals, with additional emphasis upon the attainment of the *social self*; (7) regulations with respect to affective modes of expression or functioning; and (8) effective social control of deviant and disruptive forms of behavior through the utilization of sanctions (Inkeles, 1968, pp. 79-83).

Corresponding to these eight functional requisites developed by Levy (1952), Inkeles proposes eight elements of the personal system resulting from adequate socialization. These include motor and information skills; a personal identity or development of a self-system; language skills that are accompanied by cognitive content and development; the development of attitudes, opinions, and idea systems; the development of values; the development of the ego accompanying development of the self-system; modes of affective functioning; and finally, moral modes of functioning (Inkeles, 1968, p. 83).

In addition to the functional requisites common to any society, distinctive socialization demands or requirements are specified by particular societies and particular social statuses. These requirements may involve specific demands and personality traits for individuals who would occupy certain statuses in the society. The terms used for stating the requirements may be highly idiosyncratic and variable and they may be applied with varying levels of generality and degrees of precision. However, it is apparent that there are several recurrent themes in the socialization requirements expected by different societies and of different positions (Inkeles, 1968, p. 87).

In less complex societies, it is expected that individuals will learn through the process of socialization to be reasonably responsive to both the social order and to the requirements of others with whom they have immediate contact, thus demonstrating some degree of social conformity. Secondly, it is expected that the individual will acquire those skills that will enable him to orient himself in space and time, and to his physical setting, as well as to perform those requirements specific to particular statuses within the society. The knowledge and skills previously enumerated by Inkeles (1968, p. 83) include motor and mental skills; specialized knowledge appropriate to the individual's status; certain ways of thinking about the world that are organized into distinctive idea systems; development of a set of goals and/or values that guide the individual's actions; beliefs that are appropriate to attaining the goals; development of a self-concept that serves as the basis for social relations with others; development of a pattern of organizational and psychic functioning that facilitates moral functioning; and the development of a particular "cognitive, conative, and affective style" (Brim, 1966, pp. 8-11; Goslin, 1969, pp. 10-11; Inkeles, 1968, pp. 83-88; Kerckhoff, 1972, pp. 52-59).

Society also expects that the socialization process will develop individuals with characteristics that are common to others within the society, as well as other characteristics that distinguish particular individuals because they are more closely aligned with the social statuses and roles which the individuals occupy (Inkeles, 1968, p. 89).

In more complex societies it is anticipated that individuals will exhibit reasonable conformity to the society's social order, that they will acquire the knowledge the skills that will permit them to physically care for themselves, and that they will acquire those role prescriptions and role behaviors specific to the particular statuses occupied (Inkeles, 1968, p. 89). It is generally the case that society provides its members with a definition of the goals and means for attaining these goals through either tradition or expert advice (Inkeles, 1968, p. 90). Society is seen to influence the socialization process through direct instruction, which may involve formal or written systems of expectations, through explicit training, through the use of sanctions, and through retraining processes (Inkeles, 1968, pp. 93-102).

According to Elkin and Handel (1972, p. 32), the two most basic results sought through the process of socialization are a motivated commitment to continued responsible participation in society and that kind of competence that the society accepts as appropriate. These two anticipated results include: the expectation that the individual will recognize and accept the legitimate claims made upon him because of his position within the social structure; that the individual will function within the communication and emotional expression limits defined by the society as appropriate for varying situations; that the individual will accept the responsibilities associated with his respective roles; and that the individual will develop those competencies appropriate to the statuses and roles assumed (Elkin and Handel, 1972, pp. 29-30). It is anticipated that the socialization process will assist every individual to find his appropriate adult status within the society and to enact his role within the society with the particular type of commitment and competence appropriate to it (Elkin and Handel, 1972, p. 33).

In summary, it is the expectation of Meadian role theorists that the outcomes of socialization will include those acquired skills facilitating role acquisition and role performance, i.e., language acquisition and language facility, development of the capacity to take the role of the other, the development of the self, and the development of interpersonal competence and presentation of self. Equally important are the development of physical and cognitive skills, the learning of role negotiation, and the internalization of motives and values (Brim, 1966, pp. 9-11; Goslin, 1969, pp. 10-11; Heiss, 1976, pp. 6-16; Kerckhoff, 1972, pp. 34-35).

Individual Differences
In Socialization Outcomes or Role Performance

While the general purpose of the socialization process is to prepare its members to perform those adult social roles attached to specific statuses within the society, individual differences in outcomes and role performance may be attributable to the specificity of requirements common to a society, to the particular cultural or subcultural tradition to which the individual belongs, and finally to the particular statuses and roles to which the individual, by virtue of his position within the society, is allowed access (Elkin and Handel, 1972, p. 34; Hewitt, 1976, pp. 93-95; Inkeles, 1968, p. 78).

The importance of subcultures for socialization is emphasized by Elkin and Handel (1972, pp. 67-70). The child is seen as being socialized into a particular segment of the larger society and not into the society as a whole. Through the process of socialization within this subculture, the child learns the mores of that particular segment of society and not necessarily the knowledge, skills, dispositions, outlook, or assumptions shared by the larger society. The fact that the child is socialized within a subculture may subsequently limit his ability to function in the larger society, where values, beliefs, assumptions, and ways of life may differ significantly from the specific sector of society of which he is a member. The importance of the subculture to socialization is further emphasized by the fact that the individual's adult status within the society is in part determined by the sector of society of which his family is a member. The child's primary role models come from within the subculture to which he belongs. Thus the child's self— which is formed through interaction with significant others within his subculture—may limit his language facility, role-taking ability, development of the self, self-presentation and interpersonal competence, and his role performance in the larger society.

Brim (1960, pp. 127-128) sets forth a theory of personality in which he attributes interindividual differences in adult social role performance to variations in the individual's knowledge, ability, and motivation to meet role demands. These three result from the type of social structure in which the individual has been involved, as well as from the cultural and parental idiosyncratic variation in role performance to which he has been exposed.

Brim, in order to differentiate the variables important to the study of personality development as role learning, contrasts his theory to traditional clinical and sociopsychologic personality theories. Researchers interested in traditional personality theories seek to discover the antecedents for individual's high or low scores on various general traits. The dependent variable in these theories is interindividual differences in general traits, i.e., high, medium, or low scores for such characteristics as dependency, achievement, dominance, submissiveness, or aggressiveness. At this general trait level the focus is upon the consistency for the core of personality of an individual in almost every setting. In the traditional model, motivation is the single

TABLE 1

TRADITIONAL MODEL OF PERSONALITY THEORIES		
Independent Variables	Intervening Variables	Dependent Variables
Socialization practices	Motivation	Interindividual differences in general traits

After Brim, 1960.

intervening variable. Behavioral variation is explained post hoc by the high or low strength of one or another of the individual's motives. Socialization processes or practices that determine the individual's prior learning constitute the independent variable (Brim, 1960, pp. 132-133, 144-145; Zigler and Child, 1973, pp. 75-144) (Table 1).

In contrast to traditional personality theories, Brim (1960, pp. 131-143) proposes that the dependent variables are indeed interindividual differences in some characteristics, i.e., motives, ideas, behavior, or effects of action, but occurring within situational or role contexts. Brim's variables include: (1) specification of traits within a role context, (2) behavior variation resulting from the person with whom the individual interacts, and (3) the number of episodes in which role behavior is prescribed in ongoing interactions between individuals. Since Brim defines personality in terms of learned roles and role components, his focus is upon variation in role performance in response to situational demands rather than upon consistency or conformity of response in different situations. The focus is upon the variation within roles rather than between roles. Socialization is viewed as successful if it prepares individuals to respond to a variety of situational demands with the appropriate amount of a given role-characteristic. Socialization accomplishes this end by increasing the individual's repertoire of behavior through extension of the range and complexity of responses which the individual can enact, by freeing the individual from a learned series of stereotyped responses, by providing the individual with the ability to discriminate among social situations, and by increasing the number of motives which can be utilized (Brim, 1960, pp. 137-138). Socialization is viewed as unsuccessful if an individual has a consistency of behavioral response in face of variations in his situation.

While personality is viewed in Brim's theory as the learned repertoire of roles, self is viewed as a composite of several selves. Each self consists of a repertoire of self-perceptions which is specific both to one or another major role and to the expectations of one or another significant other (Brim, 1960, pp. 141, 143).

The intervening variables in Brim's model seek to explain individual differences in behavior in specific situations by conceptualizing what is learned through the process of socialization, i.e., roles or role demands (role prescriptions, social norms) which encompass both behaviors and values. While traditional personality theorists have explained variation in behavior by using motivation as the intervening explanatory variable, Brim sees three intervening variables as crucial to the explanation of individual differences in behavioral performance. These variables are: awareness and knowledge of the role demands, ability to fulfill the role demands, and motivation to meet the role demands. Thus, major sources of variation between individuals within roles may be the result of (1) ignorance of expectations or role prescriptions or inadequate knowledge, (2) inability on the part of the individual to perform or behave in the expected way because of genetic inadequacies, physical handicaps, or failures in training and learning for specific roles, and (3) lack of or diminished motivation to meet behavioral expectations because of variation in or failure of earlier socialization processes (Brim, 1960, pp. 143-147).

The independent variables in Brim's model seek to explain how differences in role learning occur and identify the variation sources in role learning. Brim identifies specific independent variables: social structural aspects, and cultural content and idiosyncratic differences in parental role performance (Table 2). Social structural aspects refer to the network of related statuses in which the individual can be involved, examples of which include the presence or absence of father, of siblings of the same or opposite sex, and of peers. Brim views the social structure as regulating to a large

TABLE 2

BRIM'S MODEL OF PERSONALITY DEVELOPMENT		
Independent Variables	Intervening Variables	Dependent Variables

Social structural
  aspects
 	
Cultural content and
  idiosyncratic
  parental role
  performance
	Role demands:
	  knowledge
	  of, ability
	  to meet,
	  and motiva-
	  tion to meet
		Interindividual differences
		  within roles as ex-
		  pressed within situa-
		  tional contexts

After Brim, 1960.

degree those aspects of the culture to which an individual can be exposed and, consequently, those which he can learn. If certain statuses are absent or societal rules prohibit access to specific statuses, role learning relative to these respective statuses is deficient. Brim assumes that role learning occurs in rather large response units and through actual interactions with individuals occupying specific statuses within the society. These assumptions raise questions regarding whether roles can be learned vicariously, whether the parent can make up for the absence of important statuses to which the child lacks exposure, and whether deficiencies of early role learning can be remedied through interaction in adulthood with persons in statuses to which the child had no exposure during his earlier years (Brim, 1960, pp. 147-151).

Research relevant to some of the social structural aspects has been done under the rubric of (1) father absence, (2) family size and family composition, (3) ordinal position, (4) absence of siblings or peers, and (5) working mothers.[3]

The second independent variable, cultural content and idiosyncratic differences in parent role performance, has generally been studied under the rubric of child-rearing practices. With respect to cultural content, Brim emphasizes that the content of socialization, i.e., role learning, will vary considerably according to the culture or particular subculture to which the individual belongs. Cultures and subcultures may differ significantly in their conceptions of desirable adult role performance, in the particular ends sought through the socialization process, in the means utilized to attain the desired socialization outcomes, and the idiosyncratic differences resulting from parental variation in role performance to which the child is exposed.

Research relevant to cultural content has been reviewed under the topics of (1) the effect of mother-infant interactions on subsequent personality and (2) the effects of variations in child-rearing practices in subcultural groups and the effects of between-parent variation in role performance.[4]

Although some findings are contradictory, social class differences in child-rearing practices seem to be of particular significance in accounting for individual differences in socialization outcomes and role performance.[5] However, there seems to be some consensus that the parent-child relationship in which love-oriented techniques (such as the use of praise, explanatory techniques, or withdrawal of love) are used rather than power-assertive techniques (such as physical punishment, expressive responses, or verbal threats) produces different effects on children's behavior in several ways. The use of love-oriented techniques is more likely to result in greater development of moral commitments, higher levels of achievement motivation, clearer and more favorable self-images, greater social sensitivity or role-taking and role-playing abilities, and greater language facility and cognitive development (Becker, 1964, pp. 169-208; 1972, pp. 29-72; Kerckhoff, 1972, pp. 52-57; Kohn and Schooler, 1972, pp. 223-249).

These outcomes are more likely to be observed in middle-class families: where love-oriented techniques are used more frequently; where occupational conditions that emphasize the manipulation of interpersonal relations, ideas, and symbols foster self-direction, and affirm that getting ahead is dependent upon the individual's own actions; where parents value self-direction and freedom of opportunity; where elaborated language and more complex cognitive structure result in greater language facility and increased cognitive ability; and where the parent-child relationship emphasizes the child's development of motives, self-control, and internal qualities of consideration, curiosity, and initiative (Kerckhoff, 1972, pp. 44-59; Kohn, 1963, pp. 471-480; 1969; Kohn and Schooler, 1972, pp. 223-249).

In contrast, the use of power-assertive techniques tends to mediate against the development of moral commitments and fosters low achievement motivation, low self-esteem, and low social sensitivity as a result of a greater emphasis on compliance. These outcomes are more likely to be observed in lower-class families: where power-assertive techniques are more frequently used; where occupational conditions that emphasize the manipulation of things, emphasize direct supervision, and affirm that getting ahead is achieved through collective action; where parents value conformity to external prescriptions, orderliness, and security; where restricted language and simple cognitive structure result in restricted language facility and cognitive ability; and where the parent-child relationship emphasizes traditional values of order, authority, cleanliness, obedience, and respectfulness (Kerckhoff,

1972, pp. 44-59; Kohn, 1963, pp. 471-480; 1969; Kohn and Schooler, 1972, pp. 223-249).

The outcome for the person of lower-class origin is likely to be inadequate early socialization, poor academic performance in elementary school, rejection of academic values in high school, and attainment of a lower level of education. The result is that the individual attains a lower adult status within society (Kerckhoff, 1972, p. 102).

SOCIALIZATION AS A CONTINUOUS AND CUMULATIVE PROCESS

Role Learning as a Continuous and Cumulative Process

It is a basic premise of Meadian role theorists that socialization for roles or role learning is a continuous and cumulative process that corresponds to the sequence of age-sex-statuses of the life cycle.[6] It is clear that socialization for roles begins in infancy and early childhood[7] with the acquisition of language or verbal skills, with the development of role-taking ability, and with the development of self, interpersonal competence, motivation, and moral values. However, the learning of specific role demands—the knowledge, abilities, and motivation to enact role behaviors and values—continues as the individual moves through the sequence of age-sex-statuses that correspond to the stages of the life cycle: (1) adolescence, (2) adulthood, (3) marriage and parenthood, and (4) middle and old age.[8]

With the exception of old age and, for some theorists, adolescence, each of these important age-sex-statuses is distinguished by three important properties of role transitions: rites of passage, social gains, and role continuity (Rosow, 1974, pp. 16-21). Rites of passage, which may be either public or private rituals or ceremonies such as initiations or graduations, facilitate formal status changes by publicly signaling the individual's change in status, by publicly and socially redefining the individual's role expectations, and by publicly assisting the individual to assume the new status through fostering isolation of the individual from his former group memberships and supports (Rosow, 1974, pp. 16, 124).

In addition, for the average individual, movement from a status of lower responsibility and prerogatives to one of a higher status of responsibility is accompanied by an increase in net social gains: increased prerogatives and rewards, larger spheres of decision making, larger numbers of people over whom he has authority, smaller numbers of persons who have authority

over him, and greater social recognition. Those gains of rewards and prerogatives—which are specifically age-related, i.e., specifically associated with role
transitions from one stage of the life cycle to the next—are fundamentally a
function of the individual's greater social maturity and competence in meeting increased social responsibilities (Rosow, 1974, pp. 16-19).

Finally, with some exceptions, status succession is accompanied
by role continuity, i.e., role demands (prescriptions and expectations relative
to behavior and values) of the previous stage prepare the individual for the
responsibilities and prerogatives associated with the next status or position
that he assumes. Thus, the individual experiences no major inconsistencies,
reversals, or unlearning of previously learned role demands but rather undergoes a coherent preparation and developmental extension of basic role
prescriptions from one age level to the next (Rosow, 1974, pp. 19-21).

Socialization for roles or role learning is further facilitated: by
minimizing previous status advantages and emphasizing similarities among
peer groups; by decreasing rewards for conformity to previous role prescriptions and reinforcing expectations associated with the newly assumed
statuses; by clarifying for the individual those responsibilities accompanying
the status change; by providing opportunities for rehearsal of future roles and
thus cultivating the skills, techniques, and insights of the new status, increasing the individual's commitment to the role prescriptions attached to the new
status, and changing the self-image that the individual associates with the new
status; and by providing opportunities for successful role performance of the
newly adopted status (Rosow, 1974, pp. 128-137).

In contrast, the transition to old age is marked by occasional
rites of passage, such as retirement dinners; social losses rather than gains:
declining responsibilities, increasing dependency, alienation from significant
social roles through widowhood and retirement, declining income, and increasing illness and physical handicaps; and finally, sharp role discontinuity
involving no anticipatory socialization for such losses and no formal role
prescriptions (Riley et. al., 1969, pp. 951-982; Rosow, 1974, pp. 22-27,
121-137).

Differences Between Childhood
and Adult Socialization

Our previous discussion has established the fact that there is need for socialization after childhood into roles not previously learned. From Brim's perspective, childhood and adult socialization differ in three principal ways:
(1) adult socialization is limited by the socialization that occurred during
childhood, (2) the content of socialization is different, and (3) the relationships

between and among socializing agents are different (Brim, 1966, pp. 21-39; 1968a, pp. 555-561).

ADULT SOCIALIZATION

Adult socialization may be limited by both the biologic capacities of the individual and the effects of earlier learning or lack of that learning. Biologic restrictions frequently limit or preclude adequate socialization at an earlier stage of development or at a subsequent time when the individual with limited capacities is unable to meet the role demands of a position or status requiring a higher level of role performance (Brim, 1966, pp. 20-21; 1968a, p. 558; Elkin and Handel, 1972, pp. 14-18).

Because early learning usually occurs under conditions of partial reinforcement within the primary group, the family, it is usually characterized by a particular tenacity and durability. When this learning conflicts with the needs of the adult learner, later learning is much more difficult to achieve. In contrast, when earlier learning provides a strong basis for adult learning, it facilitates the process of learning new roles. Where conditions have not fostered the learning of essential content (i.e., language acquisition and facility, role-taking ability, development of the self, interpersonal competence, motivation, and moral values, and role learning), learning as a subsequent time may be impossible, particularly if learning is found to depend upon the acquisition of particular knowledge, skills, and dispostions during certain "critical periods" of development (Brim, 1966, pp. 21-24; 1968a, pp. 557-558).

SOCIALIZATION CONTENT CHANGES

Brim (1966, 1968a) proposes that there are five major types of socialization content changes that distinguish adult socialization from childhood socialization. These changes include shifts to (1) an adult concern with the learning of new overt role behaviors versus a childhood socialization purpose of learning the societal values and motives, (2) a synthesis of material previously learned versus the acquisition of new material, (3) a concern with realism as opposed to a childhood concern with idealism, (4) learning how to mediate conflicts between and among role expectations versus the acquisition of role prescriptions themselves, and finally (5), a concern with the learning of role-specific expectations versus a childhood concern with the learning of the general role demands of the society (Brim, 1966, pp. 24-33; 1968a, pp. 559-561).

Overt Behavior Versus Values and Motives.   As previously noted in the discussion of Brim's model of personality as a learned repertoire of roles (P. 58, above), the intervening variables that Brim used to explain individual differences in behavior in specific situations centered upon the learning of role demands encompassing both behavior and values. With respect to this model, Brim proposes that the individual must have knowledge of the role demands (behavior and values) expected of him, have the ability to carry out these role demands and, finally, be motivated to fulfill the role demands. Brim uses this model to create a paradigm that distinguishes between the content of adult and childhood socialization. As the individual moves through the life cycle, the emphasis shifts from concern with motivation to concern with ability, and finally to concern with knowledge. Simultaneously, there is a shift from concern with values to a concern with behavior (Brim, 1960, pp. 127-159; 1966, pp. 25-26).

During childhood socialization the highest priority is given to the acquisition of motives and values, while adult socialization is usually most concerned with the acquisition of knowledge and behavior specific to a particular status. It is assumed that through childhood socialization the individual has been prepared with respect to the knowledge of values to be pursued in different roles and the motivation to pursue these values through socially appropriate means. Thus, adult socialization focuses upon the learning of behaviors appropriate to the acquisition of a specific role rather than upon either acquisition of motives or basic values (Brim, 1966, pp. 25-27; 1968a, p. 559; Kerckhoff, 1972, pp. 34-36).

Society uses at least two major solutions to the problems of the inadequately socialized adult. One solution consists of the anticipatory screening of candidates for a particular position in an adult organization with regard to their possessing the motives and values appropriate to that position and role within the organization. In the second solution, overt concern with the individual's motivation or value system is foregone. Society, which is represented by the organization seeking individuals to fill statuses within its structure, accepts the conformity to the behaviorial expectations as evidence of adequate socialization (Brim, 1966, pp. 27-28; 1968a, p. 559; Rosow, 1965, pp. 35-45).

Synthesis of old material versus acquisition of new.   As noted previously in this chapter, childhood socialization as viewed by Brim focuses upon developing within the individual a repertoire of behavioral responses that enables the learner to discriminate and utilize appropriate amounts of any given characteristic in response to a variety of situational demands. The focus of adult socialization shifts then, to a synthesizing of previously learned responses into new combinations and forms, rather than to the learning of wholly new complexes of appropriate responses. When necessary, new fragments of behavioral responses may be integrated with previously learned responses in order to meet complex situational demands (Brim, 1966, p. 28; 1968a, p. 559).

Realism versus Idealism.   The transformation of childhood idealism into adult realism involves two aspects: the learning of the informal status structure of the society and the learning associated with distinguishing between ideal role expectations and those which the individual is actually expected to enact in particular roles. During the period of childhood socialization, emphasis is placed upon the child's learning of the formal status structure of the society and the role prescriptions attached to these various positions. During this period the child is shielded from contact with the informal societal structure or at least is not formally instructed about informal status differentiations. Once the formal status structure has been legitimized for the child, later learning must include the realistic aspects of the informal status structure that facilitate the effective work of the formal system.

While childhood socialization has attempted to inculcate ideal role prescriptions that serve to strengthen and perpetuate the ideals of the society, upon maturation the individual must also learn to differentiate the ideal from the real role expectations of the society. For the individual this means taking part in society according to realistic expectations, rather than conformity to previously learned ideal norms (Brim, 1966, pp. 28-29; 1968a, pp. 559-560).

Intrarole and interrole conflict resolution.   With passage through the various stages of the life cycle, the individual frequently meets conflicting demands that must be resolved. These may be *intrarole* conflicts, of which there are two types: those in which expectations for role performance differ among two or more individuals, or those in which there is a conflict within the individual with respect to different aspects of a role; or they may be *interrole* conflicts, in which there exist conflicts between two or more individuals with respect to two different roles or conflict within the individual with respect to the performance of two different roles. Since the child has had little or no exposure to such conflicts during childhood socialization, the individual attaining adulthood must learn methods of conflict resolution. Brim, citing Linton and Becker, suggests that conflicts may be resolved by: (1) avoiding the conflict situation, (2) withdrawing from the conflict, (3) scheduling conflicting demands in a temporal sequence that results in the disappearance of conflict, or (4) compromising with conflicting demands. Brim suggests a further method of conflict resolution that he designates as learning to employ "metaprescriptions," which dictate solutions to conflicts that arise from role demands on one's time and loyalties (Brim, 1966, pp. 29-31; 1968a, p. 560).

Specificity versus generality.   The general purpose of the socialization process is to prepare individuals with the general knowledge, skills, and dispositions that will enable them to function as able members of their societies. As the individual matures and assumes particular roles within the status structure of the society, the role prescriptions attached to these positions become much more specific in directing the individual's behavioral responses. It has been previously noted (p. 60) that value systems are associated with particular social classes within a society. With upward social mobility, the individual is faced with a legitmate need for resocialization to the role prescriptions of the newly assumed status. There may also be occasion for resocialization which results from movement of an individual from one subculture or culture to another, which necessarily has different role expectations (Brim, 1966, pp. 31-32; 1968a, pp. 560-561).

CHANGES IN RELATIONSHIPS
WITH SOCIALIZING AGENTS

Childhood and adult socialization differ significantly with respect to the relationships of the individual to the socializing agents or agencies. Brim describes three types of changes in relationships during the transition to adult status: changes in (1) the formality of the relationship, (2) the power or support in the relationship, and (3) the group context in which the individual is being socialized (Brim, 1966, pp. 33-39; 1968a, pp. 558-559).

Formality of the relationship. Brim identifies two ways in which the relationship of the individual to socializing agents may become formalized: (1) the role of learner is clearly specified or (2) the agency or organization in which the individual is being socialized has either a formal or informal organizational structure. These two aspects of formality yield a fourfold classification scheme in which the individual may be socialized. In the first case, the organization is formal and the role of the learner is clearly specified. Under this circumstance learning occurs within a well-defined role through formal instruction or training. An example of such a condition might be the "on-the-job training" socializee or the newly inducted military recruit.

In the second case, the organization would be formal, but the role of the learner is not clearly specified. Under these circumstances the outcomes of the learning process depend greatly upon the individual's abilities to observe and obtain needed information through trial-and-error learning. This situation characterizes much of adult socialization.

In the third instance, the socialization agency is an informal group, but the role of the learner is clearly specified and prescribed. Under these circumstances, the learner's role is well defined; the rights and duties of the socializee are specified and serve to regulate the process through which learning occurs; and the informal group provided opportunities for the learner to be supervised and guided in learning the appropriate responses, while at the same time giving occasions for practice in which the individual is protected from punishment because of failure. This situation is characteristic of child-hood socialization which occurs within the primary group of the family.

In the fourth instance, the agency is informal and the role of the learner is unspecified. This particular situation is exemplified by such situations as peer group socialization; socialization of a child into a new neighbor-hood; or socialization of the adult into a new social class, a new community status, or a wider family circle through marriage (Brim, 1966, pp. 34-35).

Power and Support in Relationships. Brim, citing Straus, characterizes relationships along two major dimensions: degree of authority or power and degree of affectivity. Much of childhood socialization occurs in the context of high affectivity and high power on high support. It is under these conditions that children acquire deep-seated parental and cultural motives and values. Much of adult socialization by contrast occurs under conditions of low power and low affectivity, and thus is not conducive to the inculcation of motives and values (Brim, 1966, pp. 35-37).

Group context of the Person Being Socialized. Brim, citing Wheeler (1966, pp. 60-66), describes two further dimensions of group con-text: (1) where learning occurs on either an individual or collective basis and (2) where learning follows either a serial or disjunctive pattern. These two dimensions result in a four fold typology descriptive of socialization settings. The individual-disjunctive pattern is characteristic of the first or oldest child in the family or the first occupant of a newly created job. The collective-disjunctive pattern is characteristic of a group of individuals attending a summer training institute or a group of visiting scholars attending a foreign country. The individual-serial pattern is characteristic of the new occupant of a job which was previously occupied by another person, while the collective-serial pattern is characteristic of schools and universities where groups of individuals move together as a collectivity through the system (Wheeler, 1966, pp. 60-62; Brim, 1966, pp. 37-39).

DEVIANCE AND RESOCIALIZATION

Types of Deviance

Deviance is defined by Brim (1968a, p. 561) "as failure to conform to the expectations of other persons." From this perspective what is considered to be deviant behavior or values will be determined by both the cultural or subcultural tradition to which the individual belongs and the particular statuses and roles which the individual holds as a member of the particular society. Thus, what may be defined as deviance in one societal group may be seen as conformity in another (Brim, 1966, p. 39; 1968a, p. 561).

As noted in our previous discussion of individual differences in socialization outcomes, Brim (1960, pp. 127-159) identified social structural aspects, cultural content and idiosyncratic parental role performance, ignorance of expectations or role prescriptions, inability of the individual to meet role demands, and lack of motivation to meet role demands as explanatory variables for individual differences in role learning. The three latter variables were also used by Brim (1966, 1968) to delineate six types of deviance. Thus, an individual may be seen by his reference group as being deviant because of: (1) ignorance of the behavior that is expected in a particular situation, (2) ignorance of the values or ends to be sought, (3) inability to meet behavioral expectations because of biologic limitations, (4) inability to internalize particular values because of perceived punishing effects, (5) lack of motivation to fulfill behavioral expectations, or (6) lack of motivation to pursue appropriate values. These six simple types of deviance may also form the basis for more complex deviant actions that involve both values and behavior (Brim, 1966, pp. 40-41; 1968a, p. 561).

Excluding biologic limitations, Brim (1968a, p. 561) identifies two major causes of these deviations. One cause is seen to be ineffective socialization of the individual with respect to particular statuses and roles in a society that is relatively unchanging. The second cause is believed to occur when the adequately socialized individual experiences rapid social changes within the society that leave him relatively unprepared to enact new role demands.

Blake and Davis (1964, pp. 468-482) identify sources of both unintentionally deviant behavior and deviant motivation as outcomes of physical and environmental conditions, intrarole and interrole conflicts, temporal incompatibilities between statuses, restricted access to approved means of reaching societal goals, a state of relative deprivation, the pursuit of illegitimate goals, and failure to pursue legitimate goals. Blake and Davis suggest that internalization of norms, desire for approval, anticipation of formal punishment, anticipation of nonreward, and lack of opportunity for deviant behavior all act as inhibitors of deviance.

Resocialization as a Mode
of Control For Deviance

The particular modes of control used to deal with deviance reflect the theories, assumptions, and beliefs about human nature held by a particular society, group, or individual. In some societies and subcultural groups, methods involving isolation of the individual from others or severe punishment are used. In other societies or groups, resocialization is viewed as the most positive and effective mode of control over deviant behavior and values.

In these latter deviation of the individuals motivation and values is held to be the most serious form of deviance, since the individual does not share or may even reject the values and the means of the society. Deviance resulting from ignorance or inability to meet role demands is generally more acceptable in our society. However, there is a tendency to attribute all deviance to the motivation component. This results in placing the blame for deviance and the burden of proof that motives are pure upon the individual rather than upon the society. Because the society may mistakenly fail to accept that ignorance or inability to perform may be the causes of deviance, any punishment administered may result in the individual's complete rejection of the values of the society. In this instance, the modes of control used by the society do not result in resocialization of the individual but in the individual's alienation (Brim, 1966, pp. 42-44; 1968a, p. 561).

Resocialization would be more effective if modes of control were directed toward correcting the source of the individual's deviance. If the deviance was determined to stem from ignorance of particular role prescriptions and expectations, education would seem the most appropriate method of resocialization. If the deviance was found to result from the individual's inability to meet role demands, resocialization aimed at dealing with the individual's deficiencies would result in more effective resolution of the problem. If the deviance was attributable to deficiencies in motivation, a systematically planned program of reorientation of the individual to appropriate means and goals through the use of reward and punishment might be the most effective mode of resocialization (Brim, 1966, pp. 42-44; 1968a, p. 561).

Developmental and Resocialization Settings

Wheeler (1966, pp. 68-99) differentiates developmental socialization and resocialization systems along several dimensions: organizational goals, composition of the recruit population, interaction rates, role differentiation and formation of subcultures, the setting and the external environment, the social climate, and movement through the structure.

Developmental and resocialization agencies differ with respect to the specificity or generality of organization goals. Wheeler, citing Bidwell, distinguishes two types of socialization that may occur within an agency: role socialization and status socialization. Role socialization is defined as "the training and preparation for performance of specific tasks" and status socialization as "a broader pattern of training designed to prepare the recruit to occupy a generalized status in life with its associated life styles" (Wheeler, 1966, p. 70). In developmental socialization settings, both role and status socialization are sought concurrently. In resocialization settings, vocational or educational programs aimed at teaching the recruit specific skills (role socialization) may be in conflict with the individual's participation in counseling, guidance, spiritual, or moral training sessions (status socialization) (Wheeler, 1966, pp. 69-72).

Developmental and resocialization agencies are also seen as differing significantly in the composition of their recruit population. In the developmental setting—in a school for example—students are usually of similar age and marital status, but they may differ in gender and socioeconomic status. Thus, in this setting gender and social class are seen as broad organizing elements. In contrast, resocialization settings such as prisons are usually single-gender institutions, vary widely in the age of the inmates, have a high proportion of lower social class recruits, and have a large proportion of inmates who are either married or divorced. In this and other similar settings, great variations in age and marital status of the recruits are characteristic (Wheeler, 1966, pp. 72-73).

Socialization settings also differ with respect to the opportunity for the recruits to interact with staff. In some developmental and resocialization settings, the individual is isolated and has little contact with the socializing agents. In other settings there is freedom to interact with others. The amount of contact or interaction that does occur between the recruit and socializing agent is often a function of the social ecology of the organization. Thus, in both developmental and resocialization settings, interaction patterns may be determined by the ratio of recruit to socializing agent. The location of recruits within the setting will also determine the access they have to the socializing agents (Wheeler, 1966, pp. 73-75).

Organization goals, variance in group composition, and interaction rates influence the development of subcultures and informal social roles among the recruits in both settings (Wheeler, 1966, pp. 75-79). With respect to the setting's relationship to the external environment, ties may or may not be found between the developmental or resocialization setting and the external community, there may or may not be a transfer of knowledge from the community into the organization, and the organization may or may not have a motivational impact upon its recruits (Wheeler, 1966, pp. 79-81).

Developmental and resocialization agencies are also distinguished by the "social climate" or overall "feeling tone" of the setting. For example, some colleges and universities have developed traditions, values, and norms that clearly differentiate them from other institutions of higher learning. In contrast, resocialization settings such as prisons are seldom distinguished from one another by their distinctive qualities. In great part, the emotional tone of the organization is often the result of the positive or negative relations that exist between the staff and recruits in either developmental or resocialization settings (Wheeler, 1966, pp. 81-83).

Finally, the factor of procession or movement of individuals through the setting is of particular importance in distinguishing between developmental and resocialization settings. Developmental socialization settings are usually significantly different from resocialization settings with respect to several factors: anticipatory socialization, entry procedures, the amount and sources of knowledge about recruits, the fate of role failures, the length of stay, exit procedures, the organization's control over the recruit's later career, and the sequencing of socialization experiences (Wheeler, 1966, pp. 83-99).

Conclusion

It has been the purpose of this chapter to delineate the nature of childhood and adult socialization and resocialization from a role perspective. Socialization for roles begins in infancy and is a continuous and cumulative process that has significant implications for the development of individuals entering the various health professions.

NOTES

[1] See the following references: Brim (1966, pp. 9-15), Cooley (1968, pp. 87-91), Cottrell (1969, pp. 543-570), Elkin and Handel (1972, pp. 18-26, 37-41), Gergen (1971), Heiss (1976, pp. 8-12), Hewitt (1976, pp. 50-53, 55-56, 59-104), Kerckhoff (1972, pp. 22-31), Mead (1934, pp. 135-226; 1968, pp. 51-59; 1970, pp. 537-545), Turner (1968b, pp. 93-106).

[2] See the following references: (1) operant learning: Brim (1958, p. 1), Goslin 1969, p. 12), Kerckhoff (1972, pp. 20-24); (2) direct instruction: Elkin (1976, p. 359), Heiss (1976, pp. 6-7, 12-14), Kerckhoff (1972, pp. 20-21); (3) observational learning: Elkin and Handel (1972, p. 50), Elkin (1976, p. 360), Heiss (1976, pp. 7, 14); (4) imitation: Brim (1966, p. 10), Elkin (1976, p. 360), Flanders (1968, pp. 316-337), Hartup and Coates (1970, pp. 109-142), Heiss (1976, p. 14); (5) role-taking: Brim (1966, p. 11), Coutu (1951), Elkin and Handel (1972, p. 52), Heiss (1976, pp. 6-8, 12-14), Hewitt (1976, pp. 53-56, 112-124), Kerckhoff (1972, pp. 32, 57), Mead (1934, pp. 158-173), Turner (1956); (6) role-playing: Brim (1966, pp. 11-12), Elkin (1976, pp. 360-361), Elkin and Handel (1972, pp. 50-52), Mead (1934, pp. 160-161); (7) modeling: Brim (1966, p. 10), Elkin and Handel (1972, p. 50), Heiss (1976, p. 14), Inkeles (1968, pp. 121-123), Kerckhoff (1972, p. 32); (8) trial and error: Brim (1966,

p. 11), Elkin and Handel (1972, pp. 41-42), Heiss (1976, p. 7); (9) identification: Elkin (1976, p. 361); and (10) role negotiation: Goslin (1969, pp. 7-10).

[3] See the following references: (1) father absence: Biller (1972, pp. 407-433), Campbell (1964, pp. 289-322), Hetherington and Deur (1972, pp. 303-319), Kagan (1964, pp. 137-167), Yarrow (1964, pp. 89-136); (2) family size and family composition: Clausen (1966, pp. 1-53); (3) ordinal position: Bragg and Allen (1970, pp. 371-382), Clausen (1966, pp. 1-53), Sampson (1972, pp. 86-122); (4) absence of siblings or peers: Brim (1958, pp. 1-16), Campbell (1964, pp. 289-322); and (5) working mothers: Hoffman (1963), Nye and Hoffman (1963, Siegal (1963, pp. 513-542), Stolz (1960, 749-782), and Yarrow (1964, pp. 116-117).

[4] See the following references: (1) effects of mother-infant interactions: Ainsworth (1972, pp. 395-406), Caldwell (1964, pp. 9-87), Davis (1976, pp. 297-306), Palmer (1969, pp. 25-55), Rheingold (1969, pp. 779-790), Streissguth and Bee (1972, pp. 158-183), and Yarrow (1964, pp. 89-136); (2) effects of varying child-rearing practices: Becker (1964, pp. 169-208), Becker (1972, pp. 29-72), Elkin and Handel (1972, pp. 64-95), Kerckhoff (1972), and Kohn and Schooler (1972, pp. 223-249).

[5] See the following references: Becker (1964, pp. 169-208; 1972, pp. 29-72), Bronfenbrenner (1958, pp. 400-425), Caldwell (1964, pp. 67-75), Elkin and Handel (1972, pp. 70-82), Kerckhoff (1972), Kohn (1959, pp. 337-351; 1963, pp. 471-480), Kohn and Schooler (1972, pp. 223-249), Sewell (1961, pp. 340-356; 1970, pp. 572-574), Zigler and Child (1969, pp. 483-501; 1973, pp. 37-74).

[6] See the following references: Brim (1966, pp. 3, 8-12, 18; 1968b, p. 184), Clausen (1968c, pp. 133-138), Elkin and Handel (1972, p. 142), Gordon (1972, pp. 65-105), Inkeles (1969, pp. 620-632), Rosow (1974, pp. 14-15).

[7] See the following references: Brim (1960, pp. 127-159), Clausen (1968c, pp. 130-181), Davis (1976, pp. 297-306), Elkin and Handel (1972, pp. 27-53), Inkeles (1968, pp. 73-129; 1969, pp. 615-624), Kerckhoff (1972, pp. 39-59), McCandless (1969, pp. 791-817), Rheingold (1969, pp. 779-790).

[8] See the following references: adolescence: Berger (1963, pp. 394-408), Cain (1964, pp. 272-309), Campbell (1969, pp. 821-859), Douvan and Gold (1966, pp. 469-528), Dragastin and Elder (1975), Elkin and Westley (1955, pp. 680-684) Matza (1964, pp. 191-216), Parsons (1942, pp. 604-616; 1962, pp. 97-123), Westley and Elkin (1957, pp. 243-249); adulthood: Brim (1966, pp. 1-50, 1968a, pp. 552-557; 1968b, pp. 182-226), Elkin and Handel (1972, pp. 149-158), Moore (1969, pp. 861-884), Rosow (1965, pp. 35-45); marriage and parenthood: Barry (1972, pp. 170-179), Christensen (1964), Elder (1972, pp. 312-335), Goodman (1976, pp. 116-126), Gove (1976, pp. 156-176), Hill and Aldous (1969, pp. 885-950), Hoffman (1976, pp. 177-196), Kiesler and Baral (1976, pp. 105-115), Komarovsky (1976, pp. 129-143), Ladner (1976, pp. 72-89), Lewis (1976, pp. 33-57), Rossi (1976, pp. 129-143), Teevan (1976, pp. 90-104); and middle and old age: Barry and Wingrove (1977), Hoffman (1970), Loether (1967), Riley and Foner (1968), Riley, Foner, Hess, and Toby (1969, pp. 951-982), Rosow (1974).

4

Role Stress
and Role Strain

MARGARET E. HARDY

When a social structure creates very difficult, conflicting, or impossible demands for occupants of positions within the structure, the general condition can be identified as one of role stress. As we shall see, role stress for one individual also results in ambiguous and discordant conditions for occupants of interdependent positions. Thus the social structure forms a vital part of the individual's environment; it is a major determinant of social behavior.

Role stress is located in the social structure; it is primarily external to the individual. It may generate role strain (subjective feelings of frustration, tension, or anxiety) in central and associated individuals. High levels of role strain may not only disrupt social interaction but prevent goal attainment. Role strain, however, may be managed by behaviors such as role bargaining or reduced social interaction to limit negative effects. Although such actions may minimize the strain for one person, these actions may interfere with the activities of interdependent role occupants and can even jeopardize the goals of the related organization. In crisis-oriented settings, such as health care organizations, the effect of this role strain may lead to a reduced quality of care and may even jeopardize lives. Furthermore, when role strain is prevalent, dissatisfied, tension-ridden health care workers may be drained of both energy and commitment to the organization and to professional values.

Since role stress and role strain are pervasive and potentially detrimental social conditions, it is important that health professionals have a sound understanding of these phenomena. It is only when research is integrated with theory that practioners have a sound scientific base from which they may operate. Hence, in this chapter, minimal use will be made of descriptive accounts or literary opinion about role stress and role strain.

Guided by the belief that activities of health professionals must be based upon sound knowledge of the phenomena they confront in their roles, I have developed this chapter in the following manner. Basic concepts are defined and some well-established theoretical frameworks are identified. These frameworks are then integrated with role *theory* on the premise that this approach will further the reader's understanding. Next, role stress, role strain, and related processes are discussed. Heavy emphasis is placed on research related to role stress and role strain in order to identify empirically types of role stress, characteristics of role strain, and the relationship between role stress and role strain. Finally, strategies used to resolve role strain, conditions that alter the effects of role strain, and the effects of role strain on work performance are also examined.

DEFINITIONS AND ASSUMPTIONS

The general discussion of theory, the evolving nature of concepts, and empirical generalizations presented in Chapter 1 are highly relevant to this chapter. Some of the earliest studies in the social sciences in the field of role were on role problems such as role conflict and lack of clarity in roles. The concepts used to describe role problems have been constantly evolving. In general, the literature of role theory is difficult to analyze because of the diversity in the definitions of concepts studied and the wide variety of researchers' academic backgrounds. This difficulty perhaps is more acute in the area of role stress where role problems command the attention of scientists in both basic and applied fields. While such diversity compounds the complexity of role theory, it certainly adds to the richness of the literature and the generalizability of findings.

General Definitions

In this chapter attention is focused on a social unit. A *social unit* is two or more persons engaged in a transaction, productive social exchange, or role relationship. The discussion generally will focus on a dyad or simple two-person role relationship in which there is an occupant of a focal position and an occupant of a counter position.

Norms are rules that either prescribe or proscribe behavior. Norms are expectations, standards, or guidelines that suggest what a person "ought," "should," or "must" as well as "ought not," "should not," or "must not" do, think, or feel. Adherence to norms is positively sanctioned while violations are negatively sanctioned. Behavior is not simply compliance with external sanctions; it is strongly influenced by the internalization of norms. This internalization of norms is manifested by moral outrage at the misbehavior of others and by guilt following a personal transgression.

Negative sanctions are punishments for violations of norms. These punishments include criticism, disapproval, and ostracism; they are delivered either actually or symbolically by the group.

Positive sanctions are rewards or reinforcing acts for adherence to norms. These are social rewards, such as social approval, liking, praise, and support; they are delivered either actually or symbolically by the group.

Sanctions, both positive and negative, are used to modify behavior and to maximize adherence to prevailing group norms or prescriptions. Although sanctions are generally external, they may be self imposed. The degree and type of sanctioning depends upon the visibility of an act and the extent to which it is valued. A nurse, for example, would be more severely sanctioned for narcotic abuse than for unpolished shoes.

Social structures are positions and patterns of behavior woven into systematic and relatively enduring relationships. The structure partially determines the availability of social goals, the means for attaining these goals, and the type and extent of sanctions permissible and employed.

A *position* (status or office) is a location in a social structure. Occupants of positions are collective categories of persons who differ from the general public in some specific shared attribute or behavior. The basis for the differentiation depends upon the interest of the researcher. For example, groups may be differentiated on the basis of age, race, occupation, or some other characteristic such as staff nurse, head nurse and supervisor.

The term *role* has had exceptionally diverse use. It has been used to indicate prescriptions, descriptions, evaluations, and actions as well as refer to overt and covert processes, to refer to self, and to refer to other (Thomas and Biddle, 1966, p. 29). The term is commonly used in the literature to refer to both the expected and the actual behaviors associated with a position. In this chapter the more specific referents employed with role, such as role sender or role incumbent, will be utilized for the sake of clarity:

> *Role occupant* (role incumbent) is a person who holds a position within the social structure.

Role expectations are position-specific norms that identify the attitudes, behaviors, and cognitions that are required and antici-pated for a role occupant.

Role performance (role behavior or role enactment) is differ-entiated behavior or action relevant to a specific position.

A *focal position* is the position under consideration or study, while *actor* is the occupant of this position.

Role sender (role partner, counter-role occupant) is a person occupying an interdependent position with the occupant of the focal position and holding role expectations for the occupant. Role senders may enact the same role as the incumbent, for example, staff nurse with staff nurse. Role senders may enact reciprocal roles, for example, staff nurse with head nurse.

A *role set* is the constellation of relationships with the role partners of a particular position (Merton, 1957, p. 369). A role set is comprised of all of an actor's role senders.

Role stress is a social structural condition in which role obliga-tions are vague, irritating, difficult, conflicting, or impossible to meet.

Role strain is the subjective state of distress experienced by a role occupant when exposed to role stress.

The following concepts from the social exchange framework are used to further the understanding of the dynamics of role stress and role strain:

A *social exchange* is a transaction in which role occupants con-tribute different behaviors such that their final product is differ-ent from that available from any of their individual behaviors.

A *resource* is the set of attributes such as education, experience, and skill that a role occupant possesses that is of value to his role senders.

An *output* is the joint product resulting from the transaction of two or more actors.

An *outcome* is the set of rewards an actor receives from a social exchange. The nature of such rewards may be social, such as praise and approval; personal, such as a feeling of pride and self confidence; or material, such as a prize, money, or income.

Assumptions

Role theorists have described conditions that make role enactment difficult and that adversely affect role occupants. The stress-strain analogy and the frameworks of social systems, social exchange, and mastery will be utilized in this chapter to aid in the understanding of these conditions.

An underlying assumption made in employing the terms *role stress* and *role strain* is that a stress-strain analogy can be utilized to examine role problems and their consequences. An appraisal of the literature on stress makes it apparent that the term has been used often and in different ways by physicists, biologists, and social scientists. Stress has been used to describe conditions producing stress reactions, that is, the sequence of events beginning with cause (stressor) and ending with a stress response. It has also been used to describe a general field of study (McGrath, 1970).

In the biologic sciences, the social sciences, and in the health-related literature, the term *stress* is used vaguely and inconsistently. However, it has been used with precision and consistency in the fields of physics and engineering where it originated. In these fields, stress refers to an external force that produces a deformation or strain. Strain is a temporary or permanent alteration in the structure of the object subjected to stress. Although the use of the engineering analogy has been criticized because it ignores the function of perception and cognition (Kahn, 1970), some writers have conceptualized stress in such a way that the major focus is not on cognitive processes (Kuhn, 1974: Mechanic, 1970; Miller, 1972). One of these theoretical approaches, which in part avoids the question of the importance of individual perception and cognition, is general systems theory. In this interdisciplinary framework (Berrien, 1968; Buckley, 1968; Kuhn, 1974; Miller, 1972), stress (Kuhn, 1974; Miller, 1971, 1972) and strain (Miller, 1971, 1972) have been defined in a manner compatible with the engineering analogy (Kuhn, 1974; Miller, 1972). Drawing upon both the engineering analogy and general systems theory, one may define *stress* as an external force that disturbs the internal stability or steady state of a system. The resulting disturbance may be termed *strain*. The use of the engineering

and systems theory analogies for the study of disturbances in role relationships is valuable because they make use of well-established analogies and of
concepts applicable to many situations.

The general stress-strain formulation is that a problematic social
condition (stress) leads to an individual internal response (strain). The subjective response of the individual is termed strain; stress refers to the demands
or external pressures. If the problematic condition is one of conflicting, confusing, irritating, or impossible role demands, the condition is *role stress*. If
the role occupant exposed to these demands experiences tension or frustration, this is a condition of *role strain*.

Another assumption that will be utilized in this chapter is that
role relationshps may be studied as social transactions within a framework
of social exchange. The social exchange framework (Blau, 1964; Emerson,
1969; Homans, 1974; Thibault and Kelley, 1959) makes use of concepts from
economics and operant psychology to analyze social interactions. Thus,
interaction is analyzed in terms of rewards (positive aspects), costs (negative
aspects), equity (sense of fairness), and outcomes. As in role theory, the
basic unit of analysis is a social unit consisting of two or more persons. The
relationship is conceptualized as a social exchange.

The social exchange framework, in addition to introducing
some new and useful concepts, provides a basis for evaluating dynamic
coping methods—such as bargaining—utilized by persons confronted with
role problems. The linking of role theory to the social exchange framework
increases the descriptive, explanatory, and predictive capabilities available for
the study of social interactions.

Another basic assumption employed in this chapter is that man
does not attempt to eliminate all tension and anxiety but rather may actively
seek some level of tension. This is in keeping with literature on mastery,
competence (Smith, 1968; Weinstein, 1970), effectance motivation (White,
1959), and self-actualization (Allport, 1955; Maslow, 1954). This approach
suggests that man is predisposed to actualize his own potential while interacting effectively with his social environment. Socialization may be viewed
as facilitating self-actualization, facilitating interpersonal competence, and
facilitating competence in role relationships. Clearly, the terms *mastery* and
competence imply that role problems or role stress are conditions that will
be approached as problems requiring solutions. Mastery has been proposed as
an essential concept for the analysis of stress (Howard and Scott, 1965).

GENERAL CONDITIONS CONTRIBUTING TO ROLE STRAIN

Role stress—including role conflict, role ambiguity, role incongruity, and role
overload—is probably more prevalent today than ever before. It is reasonable

to assume that such prevailing social conditions as inadequate adult social-ization, rapid change in social organizations, and accelerated technology contribute to more numerous and extensive role stresses and strains today than in the past. These conditions will be discussed next.

Socialization Deficits

Socialization (see chap. 3) is a complex process directed at the acquisition of appropriate attitudes, cognitions, emotions, values, motivations, skills, knowledge, and social patterns necessary to cope with the physical, cultural, and social environment. Socialization is a continuous process occurring from birth to death. Although persons enter and pass through the adult world with some anticipatory socialization, this socialization is not sufficient to meet the demands of adult roles. A lack of adequate socialization for roles and status changes also occurs for those in the health professions. Medical and nursing students, for example, expend considerable time and energy develop-ing the knowledge, skills, and attitudes deemed necessary for the acquisition of their professional roles. (Becker, Geer, Hughes, and Strauss, 1961; Olesen and Whittaker 1968). However, their basic professional socialization has been found inadequate in preparing students for moving into the work force (Kramer, 1969, 1970). The self-sustaining and self-actualizing process of socialization is for health professionals, as for all adults, continuous.

Within the health profession, explicit anticipatory socialization seldom occurs after the initial professional socialization period. Continuing education programs available for health professionals offer informational updates but rarely address the problems associated with changes in position or status. Movement into a new social position such as from staff nurse to assistant head nurse is likely to be associated with feelings of uncertainty and role ambiguity. By failing to sufficiently socialize the professional who is moving into new social positions, the health care system builds in role stress to a certain extent and thus contributes to role strain. It is uncommon to find nursing supervisors, clinical nurse specialists, members of interdisciplinary health teams, or assistant professors in the health professions, for example, being processed through formal programs that will increase their professional and interprofessional competence prior to their occupancy of higher levels or new positions within the health care system.

Transition into new positions or roles would probably be asso-ciated with less role strain for these new incumbents, as well as for their co-workers, if the incumbents-to-be were provided with programs designed to facilitate modification and expansion of exisiting attitudes, knowledge, values, and behaviors appropriate for their new roles. Role transition might then occur with greater ease and with a greater probability of successful performance. Unfortunately, individuals moving into many positions in the health care field must rely almost entirely upon their basic education experience, intuition, and on-the-job orientation. Assuming this is the typical pattern, the higher ranking and less traditional positions in the health care system are probably occupied by persons who have received minimal specific preparation for these positions. These individuals are expected to meet new role obligations in positions with expanded role sets within relatively complicated social networks. To the extent that socialization for roles is deficient, role problems and strain are likely to be prevalent.

Increased Rate of Social Change in Organizations

An important general condition contributing to the proliferation and significance of role problems is the rapidity with which social organizations are developing and changing. In the political system, for example, rapid changes are occuring in the size and structure of subsystems. Decentralization is occuring in some areas through, for example, the creation of mini-city halls; while centralization, such as regional planning, is occuring in others. The net result is rapid expansion and a proliferation of social positions and enlargement of the system's goals and activities. These kinds of changes can be seen and felt in all areas of daily living.

Significant expansion and changes can be seen in health-related occupations and professions, as well as in the utilization and delivery of health care services (Andersen and Anderson, 1967). As health care organizations, professions, and occupations expand, social networks become more complex and role expectations are altered. Under such conditions a role occupant tends to accrue more and different obligations, while at the same time the number of persons in his role set grows. Traditional health care workers, such as nurses, have not only acquired new responsibilities but are accountable to more persons within the system. It is not unreasonable to assume that as such organizational growth and change take place, individuals in the system will tend to focus their attention on their own responsibilities and their interaction with members of their role set. They may well lose sight of the goals of the total organization and the part they play within it. The health care worker in a rapidly expanding system may become less aware of some subsystems within that organization and only minimally aware of interfacing with other health care groups. To the extent that this occurs and energies and activities are restricted to one's own role set, it is likely that role problems and role strain will increase.

Advances in Technology

Another important factor, the rapid advancement of technology, contributes to the creation of role problems and contributes its own unique social difficulties. In industry, for example, self-regulating and self-monitoring machinery is now frequently replacing individual workers. This technologic trend affects individuals through such activities as automated check cashing and computerized billing methods. Although technology has greatly eased some aspects of life, contending with such problems as computer errors causes considerable depersonalization and frustration.

Technical advancement is very evident in the health care settings as computers, new machinery, and mechnical devices become firmly established parts of the health care environment. Existing roles must be altered to include utilization and monitoring of this equipment and a host of new positions created to maintain and operate the equipment. Although technologic advances presumably contribute to patient health and welfare, it is likely that these very advances also augment role problems for health care workers as expectations expand and the number of role partners increases.

ROLE STRESS

The term *role stress* has had only limited use in the social science literature, whereas the term *role strain* has been used much more frequently. The literature does, however, identify sources of role strain by utilizing a variety of labels and definitions. Through introduction of a general concept of role stress, numerous role problems discussed in the literature may all be seen as specific types of role stress. Role problems may be grouped into six general areas: role ambiguity, role conflict, role incongruity, role overload, role incompetence, and role overqualification. Each of these will now be discussed.

Role Ambiguity

The social science literature suggests that participants in social systems may not entirely agree on which norms are relevant for some positions. The norms may be vague, ill-defined, or unclear. Disagreements on role expectations are generally associated with a lack of clarity in role expectations rather than conflicting role expectations. To the extent that ambiguous conditions prevail, the role performance of actors may be idiosyncratic, while sanctions may be inconsistent and may be haphazardly applied.

Studies of *role ambiguity* suggest that the condition is prevalent and occurs in many different social positions (Table 1, pp. 84-85). Although these studies use a variety of terms and definitions for this role stress, the definitions have a consistent central theme of vagueness, uncertainty, and lack of actor agreement on role expectations. These studies generally examine role ambiguity associated with one position from the perspective of the occupant of a focal position in interaction with members of his role set.

Role Conflict

Role conflict is a condition in which existing role expectations are contradictory or mutually exclusive. This condition also has been studied in a variety of settings and found a significant problem (Table 2, pp. 86-87). The studies, although defining the prevailing problematic condition in differing ways, all examine the existence of clear but competing role expectations. An example of conflicting role expectations would be associated with the position of nursing supervisor; there is an expectation that as a nurse and a woman the supervisor will be supportive and show deference, but that as a supervisor she will demonstrate strong, innovative leadership.

Role Incongruity

A source of difficulty in fulfilling role obligations may arise when a role occupant finds that expectations for his role performance run counter to his self-perception, disposition, attitudes, and values. This type of role stress, termed *role incongruity*, has also been the object of studies (Table 3, p. 88). The specific term *role incongruity* is not utilized in all the studies, but the general condition examined is one of incongruity. Role incongruity would exist, for example, for any health care worker whose central view of himself is as being altruistic but who occupies an administrative position that focuses on budget, coordinating activities of others, and record keeping.

Role incongruity may commonly occur when individuals undergo role transitions involving a significant modification in attitudes and values. Such may be the case in socialization into one of the professions. The socialization process that enables an individual to make a significant role transition has been found to create conflict between the individual's values and those of the profession. Instances of this have been studied with novices (Martin and Katz, 1961) and student nurses (Davis and Olesen, 1963) as both become exposed to the values of their chosen profession.

Role Overload

Another source of difficulty in fulfilling role demands occurs when an actor is confronted with excessive demands. Although able to perform each role demand competently, the actor is unable to carry out all of his role obligations in the time available. This condition has been investigated in relatively few studies (Table 4 p. 89). Lack of available time is a distinct impediment to complete fulfillment of role demands in each of these studies. Although the reported investigations of this problem are few, role overload does appear to be a significant type of role stress. The recency of its appearance in the literature and the limited number of studies conducted do not necessarily indicate that this is a new problem. It may, however, be one type of role stress that is more prevalent in highly industrialized societies; it may occur primarily in higher level positions or in positions that link one or more systems.

Role Incompetence
and Role Overqualification

Two types of role stress that have received minimal attention are *role incompetence* and *role overqualification*. Role incompetence exists whenever a role occupant's resources are inadequate relative to the demands of his position. Role overqualification, on the other hand, exists whenever a role occupant's resources are in excess of those required for his position. Role overqualification might be expected to be present when jobs are highly routine, job mobility is prevalent, or interdisciplinary positions are created. In any system, strain may be produced by a lack or by an excess of some aspect of that system's input or output (Miller, 1971). Therefore, the conditions of role incompetence or role overqualification may produce strain for both the actor and for those in his role set.

Role incompetence, for example, might exist for a nurse who has been out of the work force for 20 years and reenters nursing. She would be aware she lacked sufficient skill and the necessary expertise for patient care. An uncertainty in her ability to provide sound care would be a source of anxiety for the nurse, the patient, and for members of each of their role sets.

Role overqualification may exist when a staff nurse clinician, who earlier had a career in nursing administration, is faced with a situation in which patient care is impaired as a result of poor management by the head nurse. The staff nurse clinician might attempt to improve the quality of patient care by suggesting improved management techniques. The implementation of these techniques may gain little support from both the head

TABLE 1

ROLE AMBIGUITY: DEFINITIONS AND SUBJECTS STUDIED BY DIFFERENT INVESTIGATORS

Investigator	Subjects Studied	Definition of Role Ambiguity*
Arndt and Laeger (1970)	Directors of nursing service	Vague or unclear role demands
Beehr (1976)	Male wage earners	Uncertainty about role expectations
Bible and McComas (1963)	Teachers	Lack of congruity or consensus on role demands
Ben-David (1958)	Physicians	Disagreement on role expectations
Borgotta (1961)	Military personnel	Lack of congruity or consensus on role expectations
Caplan and Jones (1975)	College professors	Unclear role expectations
Cogswell (1967)	Paraplegics	Vague or unclear role demands
Davis (1954)	Military personnel	Lack of congruity or consensus on role expectations
Hall (1954)	Military personnel	Lack of congruity or consensus on role expectations
Hardy (1976)	Hospital nurses	Lack of clarity in role demands

84

Author	Sample	Definition
Johnson and Stinson (1975)	Military and civilian personnel	Lack of clarity about role demands
Kahn et al. (1964)	Male wage earners	Lack of information about position
Komarovsky (1946)	College women	Vague or unclear role demands
Lennard and Bernstein (1966)	Physicians and patients	Dissimilarity in role expectations
Lyons (1971)	Hospital nurses	Role sender's expectations unclear
Miles (1975)	Professional-level employees	Lack of clarity in role expectations and predictability of outcomes
Overall and Aronson (1966)	Physicians and patients	Dissimilarity in expectations for physician
Palola (1962)	College students	Discrepancy between performance and expectations
Snoek (1966)	School superintendents	Lack of information about position
Smith (1957)	College students	Lack of information about position
Wardwell (1955)	Chiropractors	Vague or unclear role demands

*The definitions provided by the different authors have been paraphrased here.

TABLE 2

ROLE CONFLICT: DEFINITIONS AND SUBJECTS STUDIED BY DIFFERENT INVESTIGATORS

Investigator	Subjects Studied	Definition of Role Conflict*
Arndt and Laeger (1970)	Directors of nursing service	Conflicting role demands
Becker et al. (1961)	Medical students and faculty	Different role expectations
Bidwell (1961)	Professionals in army	Inconsistent role demands
Burchard (1954)	Military chaplains	Conflicting role demands
Corwin (1961)	Hospital nurses	Disparity between role norms and behavior
Getzel and Guba (1954)	Military personnel	Contradictory role demands
Gross et al. (1958)	School boards and superintendents	Conflicting role demands
Goss (1961)	Physicians	Lack of congruence in norms
Gullahorn (1954)	Union members	Incompatible role demands
Hardy (1976)	Hospital nurses	Disagreement over role demands

Jacobson (1958)	Family members	Disparity in attitudes
Jacobson et al. (1951)	Union members	Discrepancies in norms
Johnson and Stinson (1976)	Military and civilian personnel	Disagreement over role expectations
Killian (1966)	Families and community	Competing values
Kahn et al. (1964)	Male wage earners	Different role expectations
Kramer (1968, 1969)	Hospital nurses	Disparity between role norms and behavior
Miles (1975)	Professional-levels employees	Incongruity in role expectations
Scott (1969)	Social workers	Incompatible role expectations
Simmons (1968)	First-line supervisors	Conflicting role expectations
Smith (1965)	Head nurses and nursing educators	Discrepancies in role expectation
Wilenski (1956)	Labor union members	Conflicting role demands

*The definitions provided by the different authors have been paraphrased here.

TABLE 3

ROLE INCONGRUITY: DEFINITIONS AND SUBJECTS STUDIED BY DIFFERENT INVESTIGATORS

Investigator	Subjects Studied	Definition of Role Incongruity*
Backman and Secord (1968)	College students	Demands of role incompatible with self-concept
Beckhouse (1969)	College students	Role expectations run counter to individual disposition, attitudes, and values
Borgotta (1955)	Military personnel	Lack of congruence between role demands and personality
Davis and Olesen (1963)	Student nurses	Norms in new role conflict with occupant's values
Hardy (1976)	Hospital nurses	Personal values conflict with role demands
Johnson and Stinson (1975)	Military and civilian personnel	Need for achievement and independence and their effects on role conflict and ambiguity
Lyons (1971)	Hospital nurses	Need for clarity and its effect on role ambiguity
Martin and Katz (1961)	Novices	Norms in new role conflict with occupant's values

*The definitions provided by the different authors have been paraphrased here.

88

TABLE 4

ROLE OVERLOAD: DEFINITIONS AND SUBJECTS STUDIED BY DIFFERENT INVESTIGATORS

Investigator	Subjects Studied	Definition of Role Overload*
Arndt and Laeger (1970)	Directors of nursing	Too heavy a workload
Hardy (1971)	Male college students	Lack of time to meet role demands
Hardy (1976)	Hospital nurses	Lack of time to carry out role obligations
Caplan and Jones (1975)	University professors	The amount of work to be completed in a given amount of time is too much
Kahn et al. (1964)	Male wage earners	Impossible to meet role demands within given time
Sales (1969)	Chartered accountants	Incapable of meeting role obligations in allotted time
Snoek (1966)	School superintendents	Role demands exceed worker's capacity

*The definitions provided by the different authors have been paraphrased here.

nurse and her co-workers with the result that quality patient care is not provided. The staff nurse clinician may be very frustrated at her inability to take advantage of optimal management techniques to advance the quality of patient care and her co-workers may well feel inadequate.

With the rapid expansion of knowledge and technology along with increasing job mobility and interdisciplinary approaches to health problems, role incompetence and role overqualification are likely to become increasingly significant types of role stress.

Structural Location of Role Stress

The studies cited in Tables 1-4 identify different types of role stress and different structural sources of role stress. An examination of role conflict may be helpful in illustrating how role stress may result from different social structural pressures. A similar examination could be made with each of the other types of role stress.

Conflicting role expectations may come from one's reference groups (Becker et al., 1971; Bidwell, 1961; Gross et al., 1968). This has been found to be the case for such professional groups as physicians (Goss, 1961), college professors (Gouldner, 1958), scientists (Kornhauser, 1962), nurses (Kramer, 1968), and social workers (Scott, 1969). The student nurse, for example, may be confronted with conflicting expectations from her faculty and from her family. Her faculty will probably expect that she will give top priority to nursing. Her family may, on the other hand, expect her to value marriage and child rearing more highly than her career. Thus, the two reference groups have different values and expect different behaviors.

Another source of conflicting role expectations is one's role set (Arndt and Laeger, 1970; Bidwell, 1961; Burchard, 1954; Goss 1961; Kahn et al., 1964). Various role senders may hold conflicting role expectation for the role occupant. Positions that are located at the boundary of an organization or positions that link one system to another would be subjected to relatively high role stress. This condition would exist for a community health nurse when she finds that the nursing supervisor, a staff nurse, the agency's physician, the school psychologist, and the patient's family do not agree on how she should work with a particular adolescent.

Role conflict may also exist when a person occupies multiple positions (Burchard, 1954; Getzels and Guba, 1954; Gullahorn, 1956; Kahn et al., 1964). This interpositional conflict arises when the actor occupies one position that has one set of role expectations, such as staff nurse, and another position that has another set of role expectations, such as church member. For example, with the legalization of abortion, a nurse faced with the professional expectation that supportive care be given to patients who receive abortions might find this activity in direct opposition to the tenets held by her church.

Nor is role conflict limited to occupancy of multiple positions. It may exist with occupancy of a single position (Goss, 1961; Becker et al., 1964). Here the role expectations the role occupant himself holds are incompatible. Such intrapositional conflict may be present, for example, for social workers who are expected to be active in professional organizations yet not permitted to attend professional meetings held during work hours.

Role conflict has been identified as a significant problem in a variety of settings. Although the sources of role conflict may differ, the essential feature of this type of role stress is always present: the role occupant is confronted with role expectations that are mutually exclusive and thus are impossible to carry out.

Role Stress: Resource or System Deficits

Role stress has been introduced as a general concept encompassing those conditions in which role demands are difficult or impossible to meet. Six types of role stress have been identified. Four of these—role ambiguity, incongruity, conflict, and overload—have been investigated in a variety of settings, including dyads, small groups, organizations, and socialization settings. Two other types of role stress—role incompetence and overqualification—have not yet been systematically researched.

Role stress is more prevalent in some roles and positions than in others. It is likely to be more common in those positions located at the boundary of a system or between systems. It is also likely to be relatively more common in emerging roles and during position shifts. If the trends of increasing social change, technologic advancement, and growing bureaucracy continue and if there continues to be a lack of formal socialization for position changes, then it can be assumed that most types of role stress will become more prevalent. The relative significance of the individual's characteristics and the characteristics of the system in creating the stress may remain unclear.

Role stress may be associated with vague or impossible demands from the social structure and/or with resource excesses or deficits of role occupants. It is difficult to differentiate the part that the social structure plays from the part that the actor's resource level plays in creating role stress. The same set of inappropriate role behaviors may be viewed in two ways. On one hand, the behaviors may be seen as the result of resource deficits of a role occupant. On the other hand, these same behaviors may be seen as the effect of the system in either failing to select individuals with appropriate resources or failing to provide adequate socialization for the development of resources.

Although role incompetence, incongruity, and overqualification may be primarily considered as a role occupant's inadequate or inappropriate resources, they may also be viewed, in part, as a function of the social system. Similarly, role ambiguity, conflict, and overload have all been identified as conditions in which role demands are difficult or impossible to meet. These role problems appear to develop within the social structure and to be present regardless of who occupies the positions. Nevertheless, they too may represent some degree of resource deficit. Role conflict and overload could be compounded by an actor's lack of skill in handling role demands, in establishing priorities, and in allocating time wisely.

The difficulties inherent in the condition of role ambiguity could be attributed to poor discriminatory powers on the part of role occupants rather than to unclear or inadequate information coming from counter-role occupants. For example, there may also be an inability to adequately deploy the available resources, either because environmental demands really cannot be met or because they are defined in a manner that precludes a satisfactory solution. In should now be clear that role stress may result from the characteristics of the social structure, the resources of role incumbents, or a combination of these.

Role Strain: A Subjective State

The term role stress, while a relatively new concept, has been defined and extensively discussed by Goode (1960). His definition of role strain—as felt difficulty in fulfilling role obligations—clearly refers to the subjective nature of role strain. Other terms—including anxiety, tension, frustration, apathy, and futility—have been used to describe this state. Role strain, as a subjective response to role problems, has been to some subject research. (Arndt and Laeger, 1971; Evan, 1962, Hardy, 1971, 1976; Snoek, 1966). Other studies, which do not use the term role strain, describe conditions that are synonymous with Goode's definition. For instance, the anxiety condition arising in response to incompatibility between an organization's norms and professional norms of workers has been referred to as a condition of strain (Blau, 1961) and role deprivation (Corwin, 1961; Kramer, 1974). Elsewhere, strain has been used to refer to the tension developed when a role occupant's behavior does not conform to the expectations of the other role occupant (Blau and Scott, 1962; Lennard and Bernstein, 1966). Strain has also been used to refer to the condition of anxiety and indecision that occurs when one's role expectations are unclear (Wardwell, 1955).

Thus far, various sources of role strain have been identified. These include conflicting expectations, overload, and ambiguity (Snoek, 1966, p. 371); insecurity in occupancy of a position, conflict, ambiguity, and time pressure (Mitchell, 1958, pp. 212-223); and role uncertainty, role disparity, and role incompatibility (Palola, 1962, pp. 72-76).

Relationship
Between Role Stress and Role Strain

It is postulated here that role strain is the subjective response to role stress. Empirically, emotional and personal responses have been found to be associated with role stress, suggesting that role stress is a precursor of role strain.

Role ambiguity and lack of role clarity have been related to tension (Kahn et al., 1964; Lyons, 1971; Wardwell, 1955), anxiety and perceived threat (Caplan and Jones, 1975; Hamner and Tosi, 1974), futility (Kahn et al., 1964), frustration in meeting role obligations (Hardy, 1976), and job dissatisfaction (Beehr, 1976; Kahn et al., 1964; Kramer, 1968; Hardy, 1976; Hamner and Tosi, 1974). Role conflict has been found to be related to tension (House and Rizzo, 1972; Kahn et al., 1964; Wolfe and Snock, 1962), anxiety (House and Rizzo, 1972; Tosi, 1971), and job dissatisfaction (Gross et al., 1968; Hardy, 1976; Kramer 1974; Tosi, 1971). Role incongruity has been associated with frustration, role strain, and job dissatisfaction (Hardy, 1976).

Role overload has also been correlated with subjective responses, including role strain (Hardy, 1976), tension (Kahn et al., 1964), anxiety (Caplan and Jones, 1975), and various physiologic indicators of stress (Caplan and Jones, 1975; Sales, 1969).

Assuming adverse personal and emotional responses are indicators of role strain, one can see from the studies cited that there is strong empirical support for the contention that role strain is associated with role stress. It should be noted that in most of these studies the significant correlations between specific role problems and emotional or personal responses are interpreted as causal. However, the generalization that role stress creates role strain must be made cautiously pending more definitive studies.

RESOLUTION OF ROLE STRAIN

The general formulation in this chapter is that problematic situations such as role stress induce an internal response, role strain. The individual subjected to stress will attempt to utilize personal resources and problem-solving processes to manage the environment and reduce role strain. If the negative experience —strain—is not reduced, there is reason to assume that other adaptive responses may be employed. Since the role theory literature *per se* does not fully explicate techniques for strain reduction, additional processes derived from the social exchange literature will be described in order to demonstrate the broad range of strain-reducing strategies available. The strain-reducing strategies may range from simple problem-solving methods, through various bargaining techniques, to symbolic interaction strategies. These adaptive processes will be explored next and related to the role theory concepts with which they are entwined.

Problem-Solving Response

An actor or role occupant, faced with an ambiguous situation, may proceed to deal with the "problem," but not necessarily at a fully conscious level. First, he might appraise the situation in order to identify the various facets and the available lines of action and their probable consequences. On the basis of the alternatives available, probable outcomes, and personal values and motivation, the actor would select a line of action. He would then mobilize the resources necessary to act.

As a consequence of this role enactment and from subsequent information or feedback, the actor would then evaluate the behavior. If found to be unfavorable, he might then take steps to modify the decision-performance sequence. Modification might involve reformulation of the problem, identification of additional or different lines of action, or mobilization of other resources. It should be noted that even when a problem-solving attempt is successful, a time gap may exist between the identification of the problem and its acceptance as being solved.

During the period when resources are being mobilized, subjective tension is experienced. This tension may be dissipated when it becomes apparent that the problem is or can be successfully managed. It should also be noted that the entire problem-solving response may be experienced symbolically; that is, an anticipation of failure or success in coping can respectively induce or reduce the strain. If the problem is not solved or if it becomes apparent that no solution is available, tension will remain high and must itself be handled. Unresolved tension may be managed by intrapersonal adaptive techniques or by role bargaining and symbolic interaction strategies.

Role-Bargaining Responses

Role bargaining has been identified as an actor's allocation of some bearable portion of his total available resources (Goode, 1960). Role bargaining is defined here as a process of negotiation, involving two or more actors, on acceptable role behaviors to be enacted by the parties involved. There is a considerable range in the explicitness of the bargaining process. In some situations, role bargaining involves open communication to reach agreement, while in other cases the process is less explicit with one role occupant as the prime decider and the counter-role occupants indicating acceptance or rejection of the solution only by their ensuing behavior.

The resolution of role strain is a complicated process that can, hopefully, be clarified by future studies. A promising new direction in the social sciences is the examination of social behavior in terms of transactions or exchanges. This approach leads to a consideration of the relative costs and rewards associated with actors' social structure, resources, and outcomes. It further leads to a consideration of role relationships as dynamic processes where actors engage with varying degrees of awareness in role bargaining. Social exchanges and the bargaining processes will now be discussed in further detail.

Role relationships may be examined as transactions or *social exchanges* in which role occupants are aware of the resources (skill, experience, education) they contribute to the transaction, the costs (role strain, anxiety, frustration, tension) they bear in the transaction, and the outcomes or rewards (social approval, feeling of self-worth, monetary gains) they gain from the transaction.

The social psychologic research literature suggests that people prefer to maintain a sense of equity or fairness in their social relationships (Adams, 1965; Blau, 1964; Homans, 1974). Role incumbents would thus not be expected to endure excessively costly role relationships nor sustain relationships where the rewards far outweigh the costs. Rather, they would be expected to bargain for equitable relationships or to eliminate from the various positions they occupy those in which they experience a strong sense of inequity. Furthermore, persons might be expected to develop a hierarchy of positions ranging from the most to the least equitable and rewarding. The least equitable and rewarding positions would receive the least commitment and presumably they would be the most expendable. Thus, role occupants would aim to achieve a set of positions that taken together are relatively equitable and rewarding.

SELECTING POSITIONS

All actors have a degree of freedom in selecting or rejecting some positions they could occupy. However, some positions, particularly those associated with gender, age, and race, cannot be discarded. Other positions once occupied, such as parent and wager earner, are relatively obligatory positions and cannot easily be abandoned. A factor that significantly influences the decision to eliminate a position is the degree of dependence upon that position. Positions representing considerable commitment on the part of an actor are also less readily eliminated, whereas positions with relatively low commitment, such as those in voluntary organizations, can be more easily dismissed. For example, a nurse who accumulates 10 years of college education and 15 years of experience in nursing has made a major career commitment. Developing a career in an unrelated field would involve a major position change and with it a significant degree of role strain. The same nurse might easily give up her involvement in a local choral group if a conflict arises.

RESOURCE ALLOCATION

Actors can decide to what degree they will allocate their resources to the social positions they do hold. One person, wishing to excel in a particular career, may expend far more time and energy in career-related enterprises than in family-related enterprises; another person, who gives priority to the family, may make the opposite choice. In each position they occupy, role occupants can overtly or covertly negotiate with their role partners concerning the allocation of their available resources. This negotiation over inputs into a role relationship centers around the issues of whether a relationship will occur, when it will occur, and what it will entail. The negotiation over deployment of resources may involve a variety of strategies. If an actor decides a relationship is feasible, he may modify his role through the processes of role-taking and role-making. In addition he may determine his performance in a role relationship by controlling his availability, accessability, and visibility. An actor may further influence the nature of his relationships through self-presentation (Goffman, 1959), altercasting (Weinstein and Deutschberger, 1968), and ingratiation (Jones, 1968).

Role-Taking and Role-Making. These two techniques, described in symbolic interaction theory, may be utilized in the process of role bargaining. Role-taking and role-making are discussed by Turner (1956) as means of creating and modifying one's concept of his own role and his concept of the role of other. Role-taking is the process of imputing purpose and motive to other. This projection of oneself into the situation of another, including imagining how one would feel in the other person's position, will reflect, with varying degrees of accuracy, the motives and feelings of the other. The process of role-taking, which may be viewed as being synonymous with empathy, is necessary for skillful interaction and successful role bargaining. Having imputed a purpose to other's behavior, the actor modifies his own behavior to sustain or to alter other's behavior.

Role-making emphasizes the interpretation of one's own role prescriptions and emphasizes the positive process of creating and modifying one's own role. Role prescriptions are generally not rigidly defined but rather are loosely outlined. To some degree they are open to individual interpretation, with selective emphasis and selective lines of action. The development of an acceptable role enactment occurs through a process of interaction. In this process both actor and other present behaviors interpreted by each as appropriate for his own position in a subtle and complex process of role bargaining.

A social worker, for example, may negotiate her role by de-emphasizing some behaviors and emphasizing others. She may find individual counseling relatively unrewarding and take the option of spending relatively less time directly with clients and more time arranging for client placement or performing other tasks involving interacting with staff and other health care givers. She will meticulously carry out these activities. Her role performance may be positively sanctioned by members of her role set even though it involves relatively little care to clients. If she receives such santioning, then her role bargain is settled; the social worker will likely have redefined her role so that she perceives client placement as an important part of her role expectations.

In another example, a physician may negotiate her role obligations to delegate some of the less desirable activities and simply omit others. For instance, talking with patients' families may be delegated to nurses and specific patient teaching and counseling may be entirely omitted. These delegated and omitted role behaviors may be defined by the physician as not being essential to her primary role.

The processes of role-taking and role-making are influenced by an actor's definition of his role. Redefining or cognitive restructuring of one's role is a method of resolving conflict. This technique has not been specifically investigated for occupants of a single position, but it has been examined for occupants of multiple positions. Role restructuring may be a typical response in multiple-position occupancy (Bidwell, 1961; Getzels and Guba, 1954; Gross et al., 1958) or in roles characterized by strong cross pressures (Bar-Yosef and Schild, 1966). In health care organizations, the nature of the compromises and the degree of role restructuring would affect the health care given to clients.

Controlling the Availability of Resources.   A role occupant may influence role relationships by controlling availability, accessibility, and visibility to role senders. One health care worker, a director, may manage his role obligations by presenting himself as a busy individual occupying many positions and appearing to be highly involved in each. By presenting himself as a scarce resource in high demand, the actor may convey the message to his counter-role occupants that he should not be expected to carry out all normal role obligations. Thus, it may be acceptable that the busy director might miss or be late for meetings, while other staff members do not have this same freedom. A physician may establish a tradition of being difficult for staff nurses to locate. A nursing director may utilize her secretary to judiciously schedule contacts with members of her role set and a professor may maintain low visibility by being absent from the office or building when not lecturing. By attempting to control one's accessibility, availability, and visibility, an actor attempts to influence the nature of his role relationships. In essence, an actor negotiates the availability of his resources.

If an actor limits the extent to which he is available to his role senders, he is partially withdrawing from his role relationship. Partial withdrawal and avoidance are adaptive techniques often found in association with the presence of role stress (Bidwell, 1961; Kahn et al., 1964; Weitz, 1956). These two responses may be detrimental to both the actor's role performance and to the role performance of members of his role set. Partial withdrawal from interaction with role senders creates difficulty in coordinating activity and in performance. The conditions of partial withdrawal have been discussed in terms of role distance (Coser, 1966; Merton, 1957) and partial withdrawal has been viewed as one way of resolving ambivalence (Coser, 1966, p. 175) and avoiding role conflict (Kahn et al., 1964; Wolfe and Snoek, 1962). Coser makes a distinction between withdrawing from a status one plans eventually to abandon and withdrawing in order to better maintain status (Coser 1966, p. 184). This latter type of withdrawal may facilitate carrying out role obligations, but there do not seem to be empirical studies suggesting that the mechanism is successful. In fact, several studies (Kahn et al., 1964; Overall and Aronson, 1966; Wardwell, 1955; Weitz, 1956) indicate that partial withdrawal reduces the actor's level of performance. Thus, the use of this mechanism in health care organizations would probably adversely influence the health care given to clients.

Selective Presentation of Self.   In selective presentation of self (Goffman, 1959), the actor conveys to others an image or identity he wishes to assume in a situation. In assuming the identity, the actor also indicates the resources he possesses. If the performance is skillful, others will not question the presented identity nor its associated resources. The actor's performance both presents and sustains his claim; if he succeeds, others interact with him accordingly. This self-presentation involves proficient use of dress, demeanor, and conduct. For example, a person in a white lab coat with a concerned expression walking purposefully down the corridor of a hospital and carrying a stethescope will probably be perceived by others as a physician. This same person, attired in a white dress and cap and walking down the same hallway, would probably be perceived as a nurse. By the act of selective presentation to others, an individual makes a claim to a certain identity and to the resources associated with that identity. An individual's presentation exerts a social pressure on others to support his identity claim.

Altercasting.   Another interactional tactic similar to presentation of self is altercasting (Weinstein and Deutschberger, 1963). The focus here is on influencing the behavior of a counter-role occupant rather than on portraying and thereby establishing an identity by the actor. The compliant behavior produced by successful altercasting advances the actor's preferences and goals by influencing the resource allocation of other. For example, when a physician interacts with a nurse as if the nurse were his handmaiden, the physician is engaged in altercasting. The nurse may or may not act in a manner to support the physician's conception. If the altercasting is successful, the nurse will indeed behave toward the physician as if she were his hand-maiden rather than a co-worker.

Ingratiation.   Ingratiation strategies are employed to increase one's attractiveness in the eyes of others in the hope of augmenting one's own rewards (Jones, 1964). This strategy may be employed in role bargaining to enhance the value of one's own resources. An occupant of a focal position may complement and conform to opinions of his role partner in the hope that he will seem similar, likeable, and intelligent. Being liked by one's role partner increases the significance of an actor's resources and the probability that the role partner will provide help and rewards.

Coalition.   Bargainers may combine their resources or form a coalition to achieve a common outcome against a competing party. Caplow, 1968; Gamson, 1961; Tedeschi, Schlenker and Bonoma, 1973). Likewise, role incumbents experiencing similar problems may pool their resources to eliminate or neutralize role strain.

The study of group resolution of role strain has received only brief attention (Bar-Yosef and Schild, 1966; Becker et al., 1961; Blau and Scott, 1962). These studies have shown that when confronted with cross-pressures, role occupants reduce the impact of pressure by creating mechanisms for collective decision making or altered divisions of labor.

Two studies indicate that group responses can reduce the effect of external pressures (Becker et al., 1961; Blau and Scott, 1962). Other studies indicate that role strain experienced within one position may be responded to by the group (Davis and Olesen, 1963; Olesen and Whittaker, 1968). These and other studies (Goldman, 1966; Kahn, et al., 1964; Perry and Wynne, 1959) suggest that conflict may be resolved by restructuring roles or by joint action within the group. The conditions that increase or decrease the likelihood of utilizing such methods of resolution have not yet been identified, nor have the subsequent effects on group performance been analyzed.

CONDITIONS INFLUENCING
THE ROLE-BARGAINING RESPONSE

As a dynamic and flexible feature of role relationships, role bargaining may occur in the initial phase of a relationship and may be repeated as circumstances change. When two people interact with each other they will probably both engage in role-taking, role-making, and selective presentation of self; both may altercast and both may use some form of ingratiation. The extent to which lines of action, resources, roles, and the identities presented by each and imputed to the other are agreed upon or found acceptable is negotiable. In order to continue a role relationship, the two parties must come to some form of agreement on each other's claims. Furthermore, they must agree on when the relationship will occur and on acceptable role behaviors and resources. This bargaining process may be influenced by a variety of conditions. These conditions, discussed in the following sections, have been identified in social psychologic studies of bargaining and negotiation—and they appear to be highly relevant to role bargaining.

The Presence of Others. It is not equally mandatory that all role expectations be met. Personal and internalized professional values, as well as the type, strength, and availability of sanctions within a system are major determinants of which role behaviors are negotiable. The presence of other individuals, audiences, and reference groups plays a major part in defining the values, norms, and sanctions to be taken into account by a role occupant. If the other is a reference group, the additional social influences of loyalty and commitment to the group would be expected to operate. If the third party is nonsignificant or neutral, the social influence of this audience on the actor may be much less strong.

The presence of groups important to an actor brings into play the actor's self-esteem and need for social approval and therefore may significantly influence bargaining. It has been found that concessions in a bargaining situation may be associated with loss of self-esteem and loss of face (Deutsch and Krauss, 1962; Stevens, 1963). In summarizing a variety of experimental bargaining studies, Rubin and Brown (1975) concluded that audiences of significant others are likely to generate strong feelings of loyalty, commitment, and advocacy of the preferred position of bargainers; at the same time such audiences are likely to reduce the number of perceived alternatives. This would suggest that an actor confronted with conflicting bureaucratic and professional expectations will, if professional ties are dominant, resist the bureaucratic demands and remain strongly committed to professional norms. Special note should be made of the possibility that, even though reference groups may only be present symbolically, their impact on an actor may be very strong. This would be the case, for example, when a nurse representative negotiates with an administrator for improved working conditions. Although she is only one person engaged in a transaction with an administrator, the wishes and values of the group she represents will significantly influence her actions.

Effect of a Neutral Party. Intervention by a neutral third party can facilitate the reduction of conflict in bargaining situations (Krauss and Deutsch, 1966; Meeker and Shure, 1969; Pruitt and Johnson, 1970). The third party may facilitate agreement by minimizing both irrationality and costs to each party and aid in the identification of additional resources and alternative solutions. In addition, the presence of the third party may legitimize the removal of negotiations from public scrutiny, thus saving face for both negotiating parties while still enforcing social norms.

Communication Patterns. Communication patterns have been identified as important for the perception and resolution of role stress (Kahn et al., 1964; Wolfe and Snoek, 1962). The degree of openness in communication may depend on the issue at stake, the intensity of the conflict, and the behavior of the involved parties. For bargainers to reach agreement, not only must channels of communication be available, but the parties must use these channels and demonstrate a sense of openness and trust. Deutsch and Krauss (1960) found that the higher the intensity of a conflict, the less effective was the bargaining, regardless of the communication channels available. Several other studies of bargaining indicate that a relative increase in bargaining effectiveness occurs when open and free communication exists (Bixenstine and Douglass, 1967; Deutsch, 1958; Martin, 1966; Terhune, 1968). These findings suggest that, for role bargaining to be successful, role incumbents must be readily available to each other, be able to freely communicate, and actually communicate. Thus, two health care professionals who respect each other and work in the same neighborhood clinic may more readily resolve their role conflicts than would two professionals located in different agencies.

Among the communications that bargainers may exchange are threats and promises associated with compliance. An actor must assess the credibility of the other bargainer's stance, as well as the projected costs and rewards. In general, bargainers comply more frequently when greater cost is associated with noncompliance (Tedeschi, Bonoma, and Brown, 1971). Also, bargainers are more compliant to an accommodative than to an exploitative stance, since the accomodative bargainer provides positive incentive for compliance (Schlenker, Bonoma, Tedeschi, and Pivnick, 1970).

Rank and Power of Bargainer.   A variety of factors—including social structure, environmental conditions, and personal characteristics—has been considered to affect the outcome of bargaining. One factor that may be particularly relevant is the degree of legitimate power or rank held by a bargainer. Faley and Tedeschi (1971) found that low-ranking bargainers are more compliant than high-ranking bargainers and that the latter are more resistant to threats from their low-ranking adversaries. In their review of bargaining studies and power, Rubin and Brown (1975, p. 199) found that a common level of power among bargainers facilitates bargaining. They also reported that conditions of unequal power results in a tendency to exploit the less powerful bargainers. In applying these findings to a health care setting, one would expect that relatively low ranking health care workers would bargain more effectively with each other than with those of higher rank. Thus, a staff nurse may role bargain effectively with other staff nurses or with nurses aides, but in negotiating with a nursing supervisor or staff physician her bargaining might be less effective and she would tend to be more compliant and more open to exploitation.

Behavioral Disposition of Bargainer.   Individual differences in values, beliefs, and behavioral dispositions would be expected to influence both the extent to which an actor engages in bargaining and the effectiveness of the bargaining efforts. The literature examining the effects of individual differences in bargainers is extensive and will not be reviewed in detail here; however, some general characteristics will be noted.

Persons who think abstractly or demonstrate cognitive complexity as opposed to those who think in more concrete terms or demonstrate less cognitive complexity have been found to be relatively more cooperative in bargaining situations (Leff, 1969; Phelan and Richardson, 1969).

The need for achievement affiliation and power have been found to affect the conditions of bargaining. Persons with a high need to achieve and a high need for power tend to behave competitively, while those with a high need for affiliation tend to behave cooperatively when bargaining (Terhune, 1968). In summarizing studies in this field, Rubin and Brown (1976, p. 181) suggest that persons with a high need to achieve behave competitively, while persons with a high need for affiliation and power respond to the expected or actual behavior of their opponent: if the opponent is cooperative, they are cooperative; but if the opponent is competitive, they are competitive. Further, those with a high need for affiliation and power are sensitive to the behavior of opponents, but only those with a high need for power use this behavior as a source of information about their opponent; this information, in turn, is used for the purposes of exploitation.

Other studies of behavioral dispositions and studies of such attributes as age, race, gender, intelligence, and social rank all suggest that differences in backgrounds of individual bargainers are important determinants of both the approach to bargaining and the bargaining outcome.

In some of the literature on social interaction (including social exchange theory, symbolic interaction theory, role theory, and theory derived from studies of bargaining in conflict situations), interaction is conceptualized as a dynamic process. This literature depicts interaction as a process in which lines of action are open to interpretation and modification. The bargaining model implicit in both the social exchange and the symbolic interaction formulations assumes that behavior is goal directed and that individuals selectively engage in lines of actions that will further these goals. The theory and research relevant to role bargaining and the growing body of bargaining research suggest that roles may be perceived as opportunity structures in which actors actively negotiate by utilizing resources to their advantage.

Conditions Influencing
the General Response to Role Strain

In addition to the implications for role bargaining derived from bargaining studies, there are a number of factors that have been found which alter the manner in which individuals respond to role strain. The major factors to be considered are the actor's resources, the structural location of the target of stress, and the characteristics of the structure.

RESOURCES OF THE ROLE OCCUPANT

A role incumbent's resources are not only valued by his role partners, but they influence his role strain and his response to strain. A review of studies of role stress and strain indicates that personality variables (Mishler, 1953; Stouffer and Toby, 1949), educational level (Bar-Yosef and Schild, 1966), status incongruity (Grief and MacDonald, 1973), race (Rich, 1975), age, aspiration level, and length of employment (Kahn et al., 1964), values (Martin and Katz, 1961), and behavioral dispostion (Kahn et al., 1964; Lyons, 1971) are factors influencing both the perception of role strain and the response to it. It should be noted that many of these factors were identified earlier as influencing the process of bargaining.

Actors who occupy similar positions within a social system may experience different degrees of strain if their resource levels are dissimilar.

For example, a nurse with a masters degree and five years of teaching experience is likely to perceive fewer environmental stressors in a new teaching position than a nurse with a bachelors degree and no teaching experience. A speech therapist who has a high need to achieve may be more vulnerable to an increased work load than a co-worker who has a relatively low need to achieve.

STRUCTURAL LOCATION
OF THE TARGET OF STRESS

An additional important factor bearing on the response to stress is the structural location of the target of the stress. The response will be significantly affected by whether the target of the stress occupies a single position or several positions. If role strain arises from the incompatible demands of several positions occupied by a single actor, the actor may be able to manipulate his role structure to manage the stress. There is evidence that role strain arising from multiple-position occupancy is resolved by subordinating one or more roles (Burchard, 1954; Getzels and Guba, 1954). By making some roles subordinate to others, a person decreases the relative significance of the associated role expectations. If, on the other hand, the strain arises from incompatible demands associated with a single position, the role occupant has less freedom to manage stress. The difference between intrapositional and interpositional role stress is illustrated in the following. A nurse researcher may have difficulty resolving demands for sufficient research that is also at a high level of quality, since there may be a point at which these demands are mutually exclusive. She may, however, experience less difficulty reducing the strain associated with the competing demands for her time in the positions of mother and researcher. A subordination of one of the positions—the position of mother through the use of day care facilities, for instance—reduces the strain experienced with those positions. In order to resolve intrapositional role strain, an actor may attempt to establish a priority in the role demands within one role, although this technique is likely to be less satisfactory than when it is used by the occupant of multiple positions. Conflict associated with a single position can result in a very high tension level (Gross et al., 1958; Kahn et al., 1964).

CHARACTERISTICS OF THE SOCIAL STRUCTURE

The social structure plays a major part in producing and sustaining conditions of role strain. The communication network, affective network, normative structure, power structure, and interaction network all modify the impact of role stress and the response to role strain. The social structure may influence the extent to which the environment is identified as stressful.

In addition, the nature of the subjective experience, the availability of responses, the consequences of such responses, and the feedback available to evaluate performance are all factors influencing strain. Furthermore, the social structure may itself create stressful positions. Some research has been conducted on this important area. For instance, it has been found that the presence of others is an important factor in defining an ambiguous situation as threatening or nonthreatening (Schacter and Singer, 1963) and that the presence of friends may reduce the perception of environmental events as threatening (Gerard and Rabbie, 1961). Other research suggests that existing norms may define which resources are available (Roy, 1952) and what adaptive responses may be used.

The choice of adaptive response may be influenced by the perceived legitimacy of norms and by perceived sanctions and values (Ehrlich et al., 1962; Getzels and Guba, 1954; Gross et al., 1958; 1962; Snoek, 1966). Other social factors that can influence the response to stress are: visibility of the role occupant in an organization (Coser, 1966; Kahn et al., 1964; Wolf and Snoek, 1962), dependence on a role (Kahn et al., 1964), rank or social status of both role occupant and role senders (Kahn et al., 1964; Simmons, 1968; Wolfe and Snoek, 1962), patterns of interaction and communication in a group (Kahn et al., 1964), group cohesion (Blau and Scott, 1962), and an actor's reference groups (Bidwell, 1961; Goss, 1961; Gullahorn, 1956).

EFFECT OF ROLE STRESS AND ROLE STRAIN ON WORK PERFORMANCE

Of major concern is the impact that role strain in a focal position has on the output or productivity of role relationships. In discussing this question, possible effects will first be considered and then pertinent research findings reviewed. Since few studies of role strain consider output or level of productivity as dependent variables, these must often be inferred from the available data.

If the role occupant experiences difficulty in meeting role obligations, then his input and output levels will probably change. For instance, his inputs (energy level or concentration) may increase. As a result, the level of his performance (also an input) may then be adequate or it may still be less than adequate in terms of the relative outputs and outcomes of the relationship. In any case, the continued presence of role strain for the actor is likely to impact on the counter-role occupant and result in an increased use of resources by one or both actors. Thus, role strain generally will impact on the relationship.

Consider a situation of two interdependent actors, a community health nurse and a social worker working in the home of a family with an alcoholic member. If the nurse observes that her input in the form of home visits and counseling is increasing, although not necessarily observable to the social worker, the nurse may face role ambiguity and role overload and consider the escalating cost of the associated role strain excessive. In subsequent interactions the nurse might seek less costly roles and transfer a greater proportion of her efforts to roles where the outcomes are more in accord with her input. Such a response would become evident in terms of decreased level of performance in the role relationship with the social worker. The alteration in the role performance by the nurse will in the long run have an effect on the inputs required by the social worker, who would be required to invest greater inputs to maintain the relationship. The social worker may decide that such an increased input would be undesirable, and she might even reduce her inputs—perhaps expending more of her resources on other role activities with higher outcomes. The net result would be a decline in productivity (output) of the nurse-social worker relationship. Since this relationship is focused on client care, the client would ultimately receive a reduced level of health care.

Studies of the Effects of Role Stress and Strain: Productivity

There are only a few studies that have directly examined the effect of role stress and role strain on the productivity of social relationships. These studies examine the effects of role stress; it is assumed that role strain is the intervening variable. Role incongruity (Borgatta, 1961; Smelser, 1961), role ambiguity (Greene and Organ, 1973; Smith, 1957), role conflict (Greene and Organ 1973), and role overload (Hardy, 1971) have all been found to be associated with relatively low levels of productivity or job performance. Results from other studies indirectly indicate that role performance is adversely affected by the presence of role strain. Teachers perform with greater efficiency when role consensus exists among their role senders (Bible and McComas, 1963). Also, for individuals in the military, conflicts between a teacher role and officer role result in a reduction in the efficiency of performance of at least one of these positions (Getzels and Guba, 1954). These studies clearly indicate that certain types of role stress can be detrimental to role enactment.

Studies of Indirect Effects
of Role Stress and Strain: Partial Withdrawal

Partial withdrawal is one response to role strain. It has been found, for example, that resolution of role conflict in multiple-position occupancy occurs by establishing one role as dominant (Bidwell, 1961; Burchard, 1954; Gouldner, 1957; Gross et al., 1958). A resolution of this type implies that some subordinate roles will be performed less adequately, if at all. In the example discussed earlier, both the nurse and social worker were providing less than optimal care in the specific transaction involving the two of them, but each could have redirected her energies into transactions involving other role partners. Partial withdrawal from a role relationship presumably would adversely affect the quality of work.

The impact of partial withdrawal is likely to be strongest where there is high interdependency between role partners. Kahn et al. (1964, p. 222) noted that a strong interdependency is conducive to the development of intense inner conflicts, low satisfaction, and a sense of futility. As a result, occupants of focal positions having strong interdependency might exhibit psychologic withdrawal that would be reflected in a weakening of interpersonal bonds. Furthermore, it was noted that partial withdrawal from interaction does not necessarily eliminate strain. These investigators found that a relatively low degree of communication (i.e., a partial withdrawal) is associated with a high probability of conflict. Thus, attempts to avoid stress in role relationships by withdrawal can create the very conditions the role occupant is trying to avoid, i.e., further role conflict. In highly interdependent relationships, resolution by partial withdrawal may not be permitted by role partners (Kahn et al., 1964, p. 222). For example, partial withdrawal of an assistant head nurse from interaction with the head nurse may ultimately increase role strain because of the inherent strong interdependency of these two positions. Because of the this interdependency the head nurse may insist on resolving the conflict in ways other than by partial withdrawal.

Decreased Conformity to Norms

Decreased conformity to norms may occur in response to role strain. It has been reported that persons who identify strongly with groups outside of the work situation exhibit more limited conformity to their work organization (Gouldner, 1957). Role strain has been found to be associated with a reduction in conformity (Beckhouse, 1969; Kahn and Wolfe, 1962) and a decrease in risk taking (Beckhouse, 1969; Mitchell, 1958). Information from these studies makes it apparent that role strain is associated with decreased conformity to organizational norms. Kahn and Wolfe (1962, p. 120) suggest this is expensive to organizations. From the perspective of the organization, conformity is desirable since it is associated with predictability of performance and dependable output.

Nonconformity to role demands could, however, be a successful means of coping with role strain. Role occupants either individually or in concert develop successful methods that both reduce role strain and facilitate the functioning of the organization. These methods may not conform with the normative structure but may produce an effective alteration of the role structure; the development of new roles can decrease both the presence and effects of strain. For instance, the development of such roles as clinical nurse specialist, intensive care unit nurse, and nurse practioner was contrary to prevailing norms; such developments, however, may have been a means of reducing strain associated with the existing traditional nursing positions. Although role strain is usually considered to be undesirable, it can ultimately lead to higher levels of functioning. This perspective, however, has not yet been explored in detail.

SUMMARY

When the social structure is a source of vague, difficult, or conflicting role expectations, role occupants may experience tension, frustration, and anxiety. The condition exerted by the social structure is role stress; the subjective response experienced by the individual is role strain. The stress-strain analogy along with role theory, social exchange theory, and social systems theory have been utilized to examine the types of stress and the responses available to resolve role strain. Role ambiguity, role incongruity, role conflict, and role overload are types of role stress identified in empirical studies, while role incompetence and role overqualification are types of role stress that have not as yet been systematically researched. Research on role strain has been reviewed and the relationship between role stress and role strain described.

In this chapter a thesis is developed that role occupants initially attempt to reduce role strain through problem solving. If the environmental stress is not successfully eliminated or substantially reduced, other adaptive strategies such as role bargaining are then utilized. In addition, characteristics of the social structure and of role occupants that may influence both the response to stress and the resolution of role strain were examined. Research findings were presented that indicate directly or indirectly that role strain adversely affects individuals and organizations and jeopardizes the quality of performance and the productivity of both. The presence of role stress and role strain in the health care system is illustrated throughout the chapter and highlights the relevance of role issues for the health professional.

5

Organizations, Professional Autonomy, and Roles

MARY E. CONWAY

Organizations can be thought of as social entities that have been fashioned to serve human purposes. While it is evident that organizations differ in terms of goals, decision-making processes, and the bases of their authority, they also have many features in common. For example, all organizations have a discernible administrative hierarchy, a more or less complex division of labor, specified procedures for decision making and a domain within which they market their product or service. In order for individuals to understand how they *fit* into organizations and how functional roles are developed, it may be helpful to examine in some detail those aspects of organizational life that are particularly salient for understanding the roles of professional workers in contemporary organizations. In keeping with the organizing framework of this book—the roles of health professionals—theoretical concepts will be illustrated with appropriate examples drawn from health care settings.

The plan for this chapter is to examine organizations from a systems perspective. The systems perspective offers a unifying concept within which one may examine any number of subsystems; in this particular text it is the subsystem of roles that is of interest. The health professional is trained to perform certain functions that are considered unique—that is, these functions distinguish the sphere of action of health professionals from those of other professionals. Yet, within an organization, the role behaviors of the health professional together with the behaviors of all other persons within the organization form a social system (Katz and Kahn, 1966, p. 37) and a given role can be considered the "set of system states and actions of a subsystem, of an organization, including its interactions with other systems or nonsystem elements" (Kuhn, 1974, p. 298).

Understanding the nature of systems may help the professional cope more adequately with some of the problems that confront him as he attempts to perform his role. For example, Kuhn's (1974) definition of role as a set of system states serves as a reminder that the actions of the individual are not independent but relate to the actions of others and to the state of other subsystems of the organization at any one point in time. Or, still another way of viewing one's relationship to an organization is to understand that one is involved in a series of *transactions* that are part of the exchange of energy that characterize the system's goal directedness.

ORGANIZATIONS AS SYSTEMS

A formal organization is both a subsystem of a larger system and a composite of additional subsystems that interact toward some goal. The larger system is the institutional system that includes law, government, religion, finance, and education. Subsystems of the organization itself consist of those that deal with maintenance, production, decision making, and technology, to name but a few. For purposes of analysis, organizations can then be viewed as located at one level in a multilevel systems hierarchy. In addition, as systems, organizations are bounded entities having interrelated component parts through which matter, energy, and information are transmitted in the form of inputs, throughputs, outputs, and feedback.

Definitions

Input. Any information, matter, or energy entering the system across its boundary from the environment.

Output. Any information, matter, or energy leaving the system across the boundary of the system to the environment.

Feedback. Return of information as an input when the system after a series of interactions has deviated from its preset internal state. Feedback is called "negative feedback" when it acts to return the system to a steady state.

Equilibrium. That state in which components of the system continue to interact while at least one variable remains within a specified range (Kuhn, 1974, p. 27).

In the social system model, examples of inputs that relate to hospitals include patients, specialized personnel at both professional and technical levels, knowledge, the sophisticated technologies that are applied in diagnosis and treatment, and the financial resources required to sustain all of these. Examples of throughputs include the activities that facilitate a patient's progress toward wellness. Among the outputs of this system are the patients who are treated, improvements in technology, knowledge about disease and its treatment, trained workers, and, in some instances, the provision of technical assistance to other health settings. Examples of this latter output might include the social worker who assists another hospital to organize its social services department, or the director of nursing who offers consultation to his/her counterpart in another setting, or the medical records librarian who helps organize the record keeping system in another hospital so that it can meet accreditation standards.

The following is an example of feedback. A situation might occur in which a number of patients who were admitted to have surgery have not fully completed all of the necessary preoperative diagnostic tests by the day their surgery was scheduled. The intended operations must be cancelled. This information results in a reordering of work schedules for the radiology and laboratory departments so that all patients admitted with the designation "preoperative" are scheduled to have their tests completed within 12 hours of admission. Nonpreoperative patients, except for emergencies, are given second priority. Thus, the state of the system is "corrected."

While information is considered essential to all living systems, the amount of information available to a system is distributed differentially according to the level of the system. That is, those systems at higher levels within a hierarchy of systems presumably have more information available to them and, further, a small amount of matter or energy at the higher level triggers a large amount of activity of other components in the system, thus making available more energy (Buckley, 1967).

If Buckley's assumption holds with respect to a sociocultural systems hierarchy, we can conclude that less information is available at the level of the individual and more is available at the level of the institution. By the same reasoning we can conclude that a small input of matter or energy at the institutional level should have a considerable impact on individuals. (Figure 1 suggests this relationship.)

From a systems perspective, organizations are frequently

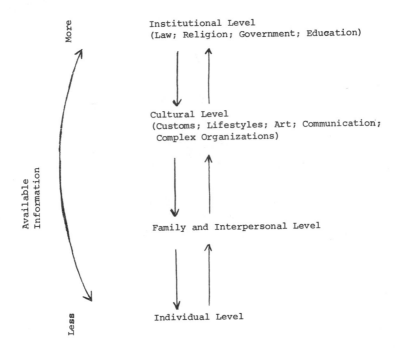

FIGURE 1. Information as a differential aspect of a sociocultural systems hierarchy.

described as relatively open or closed. Those organizations that attempt to exert strong control over their environments are characterized as *closed*; those that do not attempt such stringent control are characterized as *open*. This is much more a theoretical consideration than a pragmatic one; it is doubtful that any organization can exert a significant amount of control over its external environment given the interrelatedness of such factors as fluctuation in market demands, externally imposed controls (e.g., governmental), rapid developments in technology, and the immediate availability of new knowledge. At least one theorist has proposed that organizations aim for *bounded rationality*—a condition of limited rather than total control (Thompson, 1967). Essentially, bounded rationality is the attempt to exert reasonable control over both the task (internal) environment and the external environment in order to achieve the goal of maximizing profit. It assumes the possibility of some unintended events occurring during the course of the organization's progress toward its goals. Further, such controls as the organization does attempt are directed specifically toward protecting the task environment (Thompson, 1967).

PROBLEMS COMMON TO SOCIAL SYSTEMS

There are a number of problems common to social systems. Etzioni (1975, p. 141) conceptualizes four so-called universal functional problems. These include the system's need to: (1) control the environment, (2) secure its goals, (3) maintain solidarity among units of the system, and (4) preserve the system's values. Decisions relating to all of these are of extreme importance to an organization. The better the decision making, the more successful an organization is likely to be in achieving its goals. The ground rules for decision making are generally known to those who are responsible for making decisions at various levels within the organization. For instance, a ground rule might be that decisions are to be made that will yield the greatest profit in the short run; another might be to make decisions that will yield the greatest profit in the long run; still another might be to choose decisions that will sustain the organization's reputation in the market. In the case of a hospital, for instance, decisions that are likely to gain approval of the community will be made at least they will if the organization wishes to maintain one of its important resources: good will.

At a more abstract level, decision making can be defined as the outcome of a series of transactions engaged in by all relevant role occupants at the various levels of the system (Kuhn, 1974, p. 307). This definition of decision making assumes that all persons involved are in agreement as to the goals of the organization; one person or group may have to "give up" something during the process of arriving at the decision, while others may reciprocate by yielding on some other respect of the process.

Efficiency

Efficiency is a criterion by which organizations are often assessed. Organizations are characterized as efficient when they make progress toward their goals with a minimum of waste and a maximum of output (Katz and Kahn, 1966; Simon, 1957; Thompson, 1967). In addition, efficiency has been defined as the production of a given effect with the least cost (Rushing, 1974), production of the greatest result given a specific amount of resources (Thompson, 1967), and the ability to exploit resources—that is, obtain the greatest number of positive inputs from the environment (Yuchtman and Seashore, 1967).

Skilled labor is an example of one of the most important of the resources that an organization depends on. If the organization is to be efficient, each worker in the organization must be placed in that job for which he is best trained or suited by temperament. Limiting the number of workers employed precisely to that number that will produce the desired number of units of output would also be considered efficient. Another view of efficiency relates the organization's bargaining position to its resources. Seashore and Yuchtman (1972, p. 902) state the following proposition: "The highest level of organizational effectiveness is reached when the organization maximizes its bargaining position and optimizes its resource procurement." It is possible for an organization to have more *potential* for efficiency in its operations than is being used. For example, a receptionist in the radiology department of a hospital who, while on the job, has learned how to process films but who, however remains employed as a receptionist is operating at less than full potential and the department, therefore, could be considered not to be maximizing its potential for efficiency.

For purposes of assessing efficiency, we can characterize organizations in energy terms as having both "energic inputs" and "energic outputs" (Katz and Kahn, 1966). Energic by definition includes both people and materials. Katz and Kahn, using a system's perspective, suggest assessing the efficiency of an organization by examining the ratio of energic output to energic input. Presumably, in their view, if the total cost of people and materials far exceeds the value of net profit of the output, the organization is considered to be nonefficient. There are a number of factors that can cause low efficiency. Among them are inadequate information, a high ratio of production cost to unit output, inadequate supervision, physical location of the organization (i.e., boundaries at too great a distance from its market or the source of its raw materials), and repeated errors in forecasting market conditions. This is by no means an exhaustive list.

An additional condition that can be both a cause and consequence of lowered efficiency, and one that merits discussion here, is that of *goal displacement*. Goal displacement occurs when the means (bureaucratic symbols or status, for example) for achieving the goals of an organization take on more importance than the goals themselves (Merton, 1968, p. 256) or they are substituted for the ends (Etzioni, 1964). The most serious form of goal displacement—and a potentially destructive one—occurs when the organization actually reverses the priorities given to its goals and its means and commits its resources to the means (Etzioni, 1964, p. 10). Health care agencies are no exception to the rule in this regard, and examples of goal displacement are common occurrences. One example relates to the problem of the access of clients to the sources of care. For example, the screening procedures of an agency that have been instituted to help ensure that clients applying for assistance will get the services they need sometimes have the effect of excluding from those services the individuals who need them most.

The mother whose infant needs an immunization may be denied this service at her neighborhood health center because her income is judged to be slightly higher than the income level that the agency has set as the qualifying level. At the same time, the mother may not have enough money for transportation to a health center that is at some distance from her home. Overly rigid adherence to guidelines in this instance represents an extreme case of goal displacement. A different example of the same phenomenon is the employee who never comes to a decision of his own making because he is so concerned with following the "rules." Merton (1968) refers to this phenomenon as "trained incapacity." While rules of procedure are necessary for the orderly functioning of an organization and in addition serve to routinize work conditions so that the worker does not have to "think out" the simple actions that are to be performed repeatedly, the rules should serve as "enablers" toward the provision of a service or the processing of a product. While the structure of a large organization in general fosters adherence to rules, there are times when some workers become so involved with application of those rules that this occupies their entire attention. When workers in a service organization such as a health care facility become concerned with rules to this extent, the client becomes "invisible." He is in effect depersonalized—transformed into the status of an object to be acted upon rather than a person to be assisted (Freidson, 1966).

Rationality

The complex organizations of the post industrial era are structured according to what is called the *rational* model (Perrow, 1970; Simon, 1959). The term *rational* implies that all of the resources required for accomplishing an organization's goals (i.e., produce its product or service) have been identified and are brought into the production effort in sufficient quantity and at appropriate points in the production process in a way that maximizes goal attainment. Two further assumptions of the rational model are that excessive amounts of input are avoided and that random occurrences are controlled to the extent possible. Those resources needed by all organizations include capital, raw materials, technology, and people. Within health care organizations resources take the form of complex technologies, such as brain and soft-tissue scanners, autoanalyzers, and heart by-pass machines; the specialized technicians who operate these machines; and the professional personnel who make the determinations for the employment of such technologies or evaluate the outcomes of their use. There is disagreement, however, as to how valid the rational model is for use in attempting to study the behavior of organizations. It has been pointed out that the assumptions of the model fail to consider that organizations are subject to environmental influences (Thompson, 1967), that the principles of rationality do not stand the test of empirical research (March and Simon, 1958), and that decision making rests more on the structure of the organization—itself a product of a chain of decisions—than on strict rationality (Sofer, 1972, p. 174).

Of course, random or unanticipated events do occur from time to time in the life of an organization despite attempts on the part of the organization to protect itself from them. A potentially serious disruptive occurrence in a hospital, for example, would be the breakdown of the heart-lung machine on the day that open heart surgery is scheduled. The hospital would presumably have taken precautions against such an event by having a stand-by machine, or by having an experienced repair technician available to repair the problem. Similarly, the hospital would very likely have at least two or more experienced technicians to operate the machines so that in the event one became unavailable, the other would take over. Other more general kinds of disruptions to an organization's rational order are such events as fire, theft, strikes of workers, and depression of the market in which the organization's product is sold. While organizations take steps to protect themselves from these sources of disruption, obviously, they cannot protect themselves completely. The community health agency operates on the rationality principle when it makes decisions regarding the mix of health professionals it will employ. Such agencies provide a variety of services to their clients, including on-site ambulatory care and, in some instances, care for home-bound persons. The demographic characteristics of the population served may vary from agency to agency; for example, one agency may serve a relatively lower income, older population while another may serve a younger, middle-income population in which children comprise a large percentage of those receiving health services. In deciding what type and how many professionals (or paraprofessionals) it will employ, an agency takes these demographic variables into account. In addition it considers such other variables as its specified goals, its commitment to the community, the major health problems of the population to be served, the incomes to be returned via third-party payments such as Medicaid, and the incomes to be realized through direct payment by clients.

Let us take employment of nurses as an example of application of the rationality principle within such an agency. Professional nurses (holders of the B.S. degree) generally comprise the largest share of professional workers in a community health agency. In addition, some agencies employ nurse clinical specialists. These latter are nurses with additional training beyond the baccalaureate degree who specialize in a specified area such as maternal-child health or mental health nursing. If the population to be served by the specified agency is young, highly mobile, and in a middle-income bracket, it might be a rational decision to employ at least one maternal-child health clinical specialist. The specialist, it should be pointed out, will command a higher salary than the generalist nurse. In attempting to make a decision, the agency director considers the additional need of the target population for guidance in nutrition and food purchasing. Given that such a need exists, it would be desirable to employ a nutritionist in addition to the clinical specialist. However, rationality demands that the agency attempt to balance—at least in its planning—the possible payoff to be achieved if it employs both of these health specialists, one of them, or neither. Given that each could provide needed services, the agency may have to compromise by hiring one but not both, after considering its total anticipated income.

Further complicating the decision process for the agency director is the fact that estimates of income may be imprecise. A large proportion of the community health agency's income is derived from third-party payers such as Medicare (Title XVIII) and Medicaid (Title XIX) and reimbursement rates are subject to change on short notice. In addition, services generally are provided to clients before client eligibility for services is approved by the third party's fiscal intermediary. Those claims that are denied represent income lost. Altogether, absolute rationality in this particular decision process is unattainable.

Inadequacies of the Rational Model

Although the rational model offers insight into how organizations cope with their tasks and achieve their goals, it provides less than an adequate explanation for some aspects of organization behavior. Why, for example, when past experience is evaluated and inputs are known, provided in sufficient amounts, and processed with little untoward interruption do some organizations find the market less than receptive to their product? Or, why does a service agency suddenly find that a competitor can provide essentially the same service as a cost so much lower that the first agency is forced into bankruptcy? Has rational planning failed? Part of the answer lies in the fact that knowledge is expanding so rapidly that an organization can comprehend only a limited amount of it at any one time and, further, of that which is comprehended, only a fraction can be integrated into the system's environment within a given period of time. Another part of the answer lies in the fact that over time the external environment becomes increasingly important to the focal organization; and if the analogy to living systems holds, an organization's continued survival depends upon the extent to which it can adapt to the changing contingencies in its environment (Terreberry, 1968). Although the rational model describes the kinds of interchange an organization may have with its external environment and accounts for its dependence upon the environment for both resources and disposal of its product, it gives less attention to the influence on the focal organization of the actions of all other organizations within the same environment.

An additional explanation as to why rational planning as traditionally practiced may fail in the present unstable, rapidly changing socio-technologic environment is that reliance on past performance as one variable in forecasting the future—an integral feature of the rational model—is increasingly inappropriate. The past is too unlike the present in terms of significant variables (nuclear energy, for example, being one such variable). In addition to reducing the reliance on the past in predicting the future, there are difficulties inherent in using the present conditions as data with which make future predictions. This difficulty has been identified as the principle of equifinality (Bertalanffy, 1950); that is, systems at the same initial state may reach different end points. Also, the principle of equifinality suggests that systems that are at different initial stages may reach similar end points through a variety of developmental paths. The increasing complexity and rapidly accelerating change of living systems are, perhaps, increasing our awareness of shortcomings of the rational model.

In summary, although we can anticipate that organizations will continue to plan for the future using all available indicators and relevant data, it is apparent that the achievement of their goals is likely to depend more on their ability to *respond to changing conditions* within their given environments than on the construction of elaborate plans for an uncertain future. Further, it seems a safe assumption that those organizations that are able to apprehend information quickly and to incorporate it, while at the same time maintaining sufficient flexibility to respond to unanticipated events within their external environments, will be more likely than others to maximize their goals.

THE DIVISION OF LABOR

A functional division of labor is crucial to the goal achievement of an organization whether the goal is a product or a service. Essentially, goal achievement is related to how efficiently workers perform their individual jobs. In turn, worker efficiency is closely related to the degree of order and stability that is maintained within the work environment. Frequent reassignment of work content within jobs or a high rate of worker turnover within an organization are threats to stability of the organization and, in addition, may contribute to such deleterious effects as worker uncertainty and lowered morale. Both types of changes can and often do result in decreased work performance—both qualitatively and quantitatively.

Given that the division of labor is crucial to organization outcomes, it cannot be left to chance. It is deliberately planned (Etzioni, 1964; Simon, 1965). In role terminology it is appropriate to speak of the division of labor as role differentiation and specialization. That is, roles encompassing specific functions necessary to the accomplishment of the organization's work are identified and persons qualified by training or experience are assigned to these roles. In general, it is fair to say that the requisite skills and responsibilities associated with roles at each level of the system's hierarchy are considered crucial to the goal achievement of an organization (Conway, 1974).

For any number of reasons, it not infrequently happens that a worker with the appropriate qualifications for a particular role is unavailable and it becomes necessary to substitute an unqualified individual either temporarily or for an extended period. In the unlikely event that the substitute individual learns the job requirements quickly and performs capably, all is well. The more likely occurrence, however, is that the work will be performed less than competently, and in the case of the manufacture of a product, the product may be damaged or, at the least, slow in production. The consequences can be equally grave, although of a different order, in the human service sector.

While in the profit sector, the absence of qualified workers can result in a reduced profit margin, in the nonprofit sector—a hospital, for example—absence of qualified workers can be life threatening for patients. Even if not life threatening, either poor performance by hospital personnel or the absence of an essential service, for whatever reasons, is likely to be reflected in lowered quality of care. If such lowered performance persists over an extended period of time, the hospital's reputation will also suffer. Just as the profit-making corporation depends upon its consumer market for survival, so the hospital depends upon consumer evaluation of its service. To the extent that the hospital's reputation is diminished, it is highly probable that it will lose at least a portion of the financial input necessary to sustain its continued operation at a cost-effective level. Voluntary community organizations such as social service agencies have even more to "lose" than the hospital if their reputations are diminished by reason of inadequate or callous rendering of service. Clients generally can avoid use of a social service agency without endangering their lives, but they cannot avoid using the hospital in the event of a sufficiently grave illness.

Management of Order

As we have indicated earlier, order is important to organizations and, in recognition of this fact, the management of order is generally a full-time occupation for a specified number of personnel within each organization. Generally speaking, order is enhanced to some extent if the expectations of the occupants of various role positions are congruent with the expectations of other members of their role set (Gross et al., 1966; Merton, 1968, p. 44) and if nearly all subscribe to the organization's goals—at least insofar as they hold similar perceptions of what the goals may be.

Organizations that employ a large number of professionals—as opposed to those composed of a predominately skilled labor force—depend upon the voluntary compliance of their employees to maintain order. This is not to suggest that skilled laborers are more inclined to noncompliance but to emphasize a traditional distinction that is made between the orientation of professionals versus other classes of workers. For professionals the ethic of a service orientation and the salience of the professional organization as a reference group have influenced the means by which professionals have sought to achieve their goals within organizations. Historically, these means have largely been the kind of negotiation that precludes the strike as an acceptable weapon for gaining employee demands. By contrast, technical workers and skilled laborers have sought to win improvements in their working conditions through negotiations in which the strike remains the ultimate weapon for enforcing their demands. The earlier distinction between these two general classes of workers no longer obtains in a strict sense, since all wokers have increasingly come to view themselves as professionals. At the same time, professionals such as physicians, nurses, and teachers have turned to the strike as a means of last resort in attempting to achieve their demands. The demands made by professionals in health care institutions tend to deal not only with work conditions per se and monetary issues but with work conditions that adversely affect the quality of their work and, in turn, the quality of care delivered to clients.

Types of Control

The norms that guide behavior in social situations and the sanctions that are applied to enforce these norms are powerful entities of control. The management officials of organizations recognize the potential that both hold for the behavior of employees and encourage their application.

Order within organizations in terms of employee behavior is the rule rather than the exception. This situation exists partly because it is in the interests of both employers and workers to maintain order, that is, to comply with the rules. Unpredictable work situations and work disruptions are costly for both labor and management in terms of time, energy, and effectiveness. Prudence dictates that organizations take precautions to ensure the maintenance of order among the workers in the event that voluntary compliance is not forthcoming. To this end certain controls are applied—some consistently and others as the need arises. Control may be of two general types: *coercive* and *normative* (Etzioni, 1964). Coercive control is the securing of compliance by force, or the threat of force, where compliance would not occur otherwise. Prisons and mental hospitals, for example, rely on this type of control. Normative control derives from an appeal—implied or explicit—to employees to comply with the organization's rules and policies because that is the reasonable and desirable thing to do.

Normative control is *implicit* when a policy directive from an officer of the organization is published and employees act in accordance with the new policy; it is *explicit* when such a policy directive is formulated and a rationale is appended explaining why it is important that workers conform to the policy. In the latter instance, the explanation is attached as an added inducement to compliance. Normative controls consist of such actions as appeals for cooperation and pep talks; additionally, rewards such as citations for meritorious performance may be given from time to time. Annual award days are a feature of many organizations that employ normative controls. Finally, in the event of occasional failure of a worker to perform at an established standard, punishment is rarely meted out, at least not overtly, where normative control is in effect. Punishment may ensue, however, in the form of failure to grant vacation to an employee who is entitled to such vacation at the specific date he requests.

LEGITIMACY

As we have noted in the preceding discussion of types of control, a majority of workers apparently comply with the rules and policies of the work setting because they perceive that it is the appropriate thing to do. For professionals the acceptance and adoption of appropriate rules and policies governing behavior occur primarily during socialization into the profession. Employees' acceptance of compliance as appropriate behavior is linked to their perception of the *legitimacy* of management of an organization. In other words, when the authority of those who make the rules is viewed by workers as being properly vested, they are more likely to comply voluntarily with the rules of the work place. Legitimacy is an important attribute to an organization and one that cannot easily be acquired. The value of this attribute is apparent when the owner of a business he is selling puts a price on the "good will" that he lists as one of the assets of the firm. The following proposition can be stated with respect to the relationship existing between compliance and legitimacy: compliance on the part of members (employees) of an organization will vary positively with the degree of legitimacy ascribed to the authority structure by the members. It could be argued that while individuals are likely to adhere closely to the rules of their employment setting, they are less likely to be constrained by the rules of those social or religious organizations in which they hold membership. However, on closer inspection it would seem that this proposition needs to be qualified to take into account time and involvement. Those individuals who become increasingly involved in the activities of these affiliate organizations gradually tend to conform more closely to the rules and policies which govern the membership group. Further, it seems likely that this type of conformance takes place without conscious awareness on the part of the individuals concerned (Katz and Kahn, 1966).

TYPES OF AUTHORITY

The classic typology of authority is the one developed by the German sociologist Max Weber. Weber described three types of authority: traditional, rational-legal, and charismatic (Parsons, 1961). Only the rational-legal type will be discussed here since it is characteristic of modern organizations. In fact, the bureaucratic structure of complex organizations is viewed by some as the embodiment of the rational-legal authority. In the bureaucratic structure the authority to give orders and force compliance is lodged in the particular office rather than in the incumbent of the office. Thus, the authority is "rational" in that it is impersonally constituted and directed toward the goals of the organization as opposed to those of the individual. Of particular interest within the context of professional roles in organizations is the conclusion of one critique of the Weberian model. Satow (1975) holds that Weber failed to account for yet another type of authority: the *value-rational* type. Value-rational as defined by Satow is obedience given to an ideology or set of ideologic norms rather than to an impersonally constituted set of so-called legal norms. Satow goes on to explain that Weber did not distinguish between those organizations in which the dominant mode of action is based on the *rationally derived purposes* of the organization and those in which the dominant mode of action is based upon *commitment to an ideology*. The assumption is, of course, that professionals are committed first to the goals of their profession and second to the goals of the organization. The notion of a value-rational type of authority does not appear to contradict Weber's essential idea, but it does add to our understanding of the apparent ease with which a majority of professionals are able to function within organizations while maintaining a sense of professional identity.

MOTIVATION

An important problem for the modern organization is how to motivate workers to optimal efforts in the performance of their jobs. The routine nature of many jobs and the worker's distance from the product or service that is the end result of his efforts is often linked to worker apathy. The labor force in general enjoys a high standard of living, with many so-called blue collar workers owning a recreational dwelling as well as a year-round home. Hence, the higher wages that once provided an incentive for employees are no longer sufficient to encourage greater production; in fact, at least one theorist holds that the "dominance of non-monetary considerations" is more important in motivating workers (Caplow, 1965). Psychologic growth of the worker and the opportunity to participate in the decision making of the organization by workers at all levels are widely believed to be at least as important to workers as monetary considerations (Argyris, 1957; McGregor, 1957). The concept of motivation and theories of motivation have captured the attention of researchers in organization, as well as presidents and managers of all kinds of enterprises that depend upon human labor. To the extent that worker motivation is related to the rate of production or output of a profit-making organization—hence profit—even stockholders of corporations have an interest in motivation, theoretically, at least.

Theories of Motivation

MASLOW'S THEORY OF MOTIVATION

Motivation has been variously defined. One definition is simply that motivation is the propensity to take action toward a certain goal or goals. For purposes of analysis and comparison when attempting to apply motivation theory to organizations, theories can be categorized as either *content* or *process* oriented (Campbell et al., 1970). Content theories are those that focus on what it is in the individual's environment that sustains or extinguishes his behavior. Process theories are said to be those that explain the *how* of behavior. Nearly all prevailing theories of motivation draw on the work of Maslow, a pioneer in enlarging our understanding of the forces that prompt individuals to act as they do. Maslow has postulated five basic needs a person strives to satisfy: physiologic demands, safety, love, esteem, and self-actualization (Maslow, 1954). These needs are presumed to exist in a hierarchy that puts physiologic needs on the first level. According to Maslow's theory, as lower-order needs are met, the meeting of higher-order needs is attempted. The hierarchical order of these needs is not a constant one; for example, at one time the need for safety may be more important than the need for esteem. It would thus appear that Maslow's theory of motivation fits into the category of content theory.

EXPECTANCY THEORY

An additional theoretical model of motivation is expectancy theory (Vroom, 1964). Vroom's explanation of this theory holds that employees are faced with alternative choices for action in the work setting and that they select from among these alternatives on the basis of expected first- and second-level outcomes. The notion of *expectancy* in the theory is that the individual anticipates that a certain action will be followed by some reward that has value—a promotion or a raise in pay, for example. A further assumption of expectancy theory is that workers internalize some order of outcomes that they desire and that a value is attached to each. There is as yet little empirical evidence, if any, to support this theory. There is a problem of intersubjectivity within the model in that the concept Vroom defines as first-level *outcome* appears to be an *action* rather than an outcome. According to Vroom, an employee's increased productivity, for example (which Vroom would term a first-level outcome), is related to what is termed a second-level outcome, i.e., an increase in pay, or a reward for the increased productivity. It would seem that in more generally accepted semantic usage, the employee *acts* to increase his output and in so doing demonstrates an instrumental behavior. Vroom, however, reserves the word *instrumentality* for the link between what he calls first- and second-level outcomes.

EQUITY THEORY

The extent to which individuals are motivated to perform in the employment situation depends at least in part on whether they perceive themselves to be fairly rewarded with respect to their co-workers. Equity theory proposes that individuals assess the outcomes of their interactions with others in terms of the relationship between the contribution each makes to the interaction and the outcomes accruing to each from it. Such interactions can be viewed as exchanges. By definition any situation in which two persons act, communicate with each other, and find the interaction rewarding to both, can be called a social exchange (Homans, 1974, p. 53). Each exchange relationship involves both costs and rewards to the participants. Outcomes are the consequences of the interaction and may be either positive or negative. Positive outcomes are defined as rewards and negative outcomes as costs (Walster, et al., 1976, p. 3); the net gain or "reward" to an individual consists of the total outcome minus the cost incurred. Even in instances where one or the other participant in an exchange receives a net gain, he may perceive the gain as not worth the cost involved. It is important to note here that it is not objectively quantifiable outcomes as seen by an

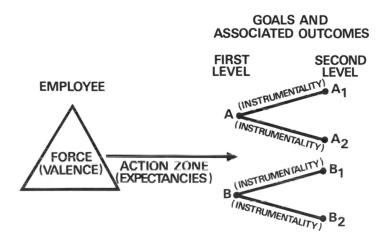

FIGURE 2. Vroom's theory of motivation (From Gibson et al., 1973; courtesy of Business Publications, Inc.)

observer that determine whether outcomes in an exchange are equal but rather the extent to which the participants perceive themselves rewarded or not rewarded relative to their costs.

An equitable relationship can be said to exist when both participants in an exchange perceive that the outcomes for each are roughly equivalent with respect to the amount each contributed to the exchange (Homans, 1974) or when a participant or an outside observer perceives that the participants are receiving relatively equal rewards from the exchange (Walster, et al., 1976, p. 2). Investigations conducted in a variety of work settings have found that individuals tend to behave equitably toward each other (Adams, 1965; Homans, 1961) and, further, that when inequitable situations arise the individuals involved attempt to restore equity (Adams and Jacobsen, 1964; Lawler, et al., 1968).

In the work setting, decisions regarding how rewards will be allocated are made on the basis of experience; that is, where the allocator (manager or president of the organization) believes that previous equitable allocations have brought about improved performance, he will tend to continue the practice (Lawler, 1971). Reports of research on the effects of equitable allocations are however, conflicting. Miller and Hamblin (1963) found that competition for rewards can disrupt a group's task activities, while Goode (1967) and Steiner (1972) noted that those who are less productive tend to become angry when rewards are given on the basis of merit alone.

Exceptions to the norm of equity in employment situations do occur as, for instance, when in an attempt to motivate less-productive workers, such workers are paid more than their inputs merit (Goodman and Friedman, 1968; Greenberg and Leventhal, 1973), or where workers of lesser ability than others produce as much as these others and are accordingly rated as more deserving and rewarded more (Taynor and Deaux, 1973; Weiner and Kukla, 1970).

While it is obvious that overreward for work is likely to be counterproductive to an organization in the long run, short-run benefits to the organization may justify the practice. And despite the fact that experimental and survey evidence to date suggest that workers tend to be motivated toward greater productivity when they perceive the rewards to be just, much remains unknown about what motivates individuals. An individual's perception of the intrinsic worth of his role or the reward he receives from the knowledge that he has helped a distressed individual by means of his special ability, whatever it may be, are examples of variables which preclude making accurate predictions about behavior where differing types of reward allocation are applied.

Another theory of motivation that draws on Maslow's need-hierarchy is that of Herzberg (1966). In this model a distinction is made between those taken-for-granted aspects of the work situation and the *recognition* aspects. Herzberg labels the former "hygiene" factors and the latter "motivators." His point is that the so-called hygiene factors are not likely to enhance a worker's loyalty to the organization or stimulate him to improve his performance. A major difference between Herzberg's conceptualization of motivation and Maslow's is that Maslow holds that any unfulfilled need can be a motivator, while Herzberg claims that only the higher-order needs are motivators (Gibson, et al, 1973). One can infer, for example, that some individuals derive satisfaction or gratification from the work they perform that is quite apart from the tangible reward of a wage. Further, it can be speculated that the amount of pleasure or gratification an individual derives from his membership in a work group is an influencing factor in determining whether that individual will adhere to the rules and norms governing his work situation. In addition, the greater the amount of gratification an individual derives relative to the amount of deprivation he experiences, the more likely it is that he will adhere to those behaviorial expectations that are normative for the particular group in which he finds himself.

One conception of the relationship between gratification and deprivation is that it represents a *balance* phenomenon. At some time, gratification and deprivation can be said to exist in about equal measure for an individual relative to this membership in the group, at least theoretically. When this theoretical balance occurs, it is presumed that a "total potential return" exists for the individual (Jackson, 1966). That is, the possibility exists for either more gratification or more deprivation. As group inter-action continues, feelings of approval or disapproval will be communicated to the individual. And, of course, the individual in turn is conveying those same kinds of feelings to the other members of the group with whom he is in contact. A number of organizations exert considerable efforts to enhance the affective "attachment" of their employees to the organization. Presum-ably this is to increase employee motivation. They encourage employees to participate in activities tangentially related to their work by providing a variety of leisure and educational programs that fall in the category of self-improvement. Etzioni refers to this propensity of organizations to engage their employees' off-the-job time as the attempt to *embrace* the individual (Etzioni, 1975). In those instances where an organization offers a large number of activities in which members participate more with each other than with outsiders, the scope of the organization is said to be broad. By contrast, an organization whose employees share in few non-job-related activities is said to be narrow in its scope (Etzioni, 1975). The trend at the present time is away from broad-scope organizations, large organizations preferring instead to build favorable community relationships where they are located. They do this through their support of those educational, cultural, and recreational activities already existing in the community. The now largely out-dated custom of insisting that medical interns and student nurses live in hospital-attached dormitories is an example of the attempt to embrace.

Organizations continue to encourage positive affective attach-ment on the part of employees. At the same time, however, they attempt to avoid the appearance of the manifest paternalism of the broad-scope activ-ities of earlier years.

AUTONOMY: A STRUCTURAL ASPECT OF HEALTH CARE

Organized autonomy

The problems of decision making, division of labor, maintenance of order, control and motivation are common to organizations in general. Organiza-tions that exist for the purpose of delivering health or welfare services are not exempt from these problems. Such organizations do differ, however, in at least one important respect from other organizations. This difference lies in the exercise—or potential exercise—of professional autonomy by those employees of the organization who occupy the additional status of professional practitioner, e.g., physician, nurse, or social worker. The members of one profession—medicine—exercise what amounts to near absolute autonomy within the health delivery sector. As members of the dominant professional group in health care, physicians have historically exerted effective control of both the activities and scope of practice of all other groups of health workers—professional and nonprofessional alike. The medical profession, as Freidson (1970) points out, represents an outstanding example of *organized autonomy*. That is, it is largely free from external control and, in addition, it controls or delimits the activities of nearly all other allied health professionals. This control stems not only from the dominant position of *each* member of the profession within the total hierarchy of health professionals but from the dominant position of the profession of medicine as an ideal-typical collectivity when measured against the other professions. In the area of legislation, for example, the official voice of the collectivity, the American Medical Association, is regularly heard, if not always followed, when new health legislation is under consideration. It is doubtful whether any other professional collectivity has had as much influence in shaping health legislation as has this one association.

Another important consequence of medical dominance has been the control of access to clients. Once an individual becomes his patient, the physician controls which providers, if any, of a health service shall assist in the care of the patient. In effect, once an individual seeks out a physician and accepts his prescribed treatment he becomes what amounts to the property of that physician. Professionals other than the physician who might be qualified to provide a needed health service can gain access to the patient only by the express permission or invitation of the physician. The physical therapist serves as a case in point. The therapist is well qualified by education and training to assess neuromuscular damage resulting from specific neurologic pathologies in a patient and to institute an appropriate treatment regimen intended to either restore function or retard the loss of function. Yet, in a majority of health care settings such treatment cannot be instituted without the physician's approval or explicit request for the service.

Control of access to clients is closely related to another kind of control: *control of information*. Physician control of the information given to clients was reasonable in an earlier era when the physician was both the sole provider of treatment and certainly the practitioner with the greatest amount of scientifically derived knowledge. However, this control of information is much less appropriate than it once was, given the state of modern health care practice and the knowledge possessed by consumers. Given the increasing professionalization of nursing together with the establishment of schools of allied health professions, there are now many practitioners in a variety of health care settings sufficiently knowledgeable to provide information of a technical nature to clients. Furthermore, clients tend to be well informed on a wide range of matters.

In a study conducted by the author (Conway, 1972) using an attitudinal response instrument, attitudes of a randomly selected sample of an urban population were elicited with respect to readiness to seek medical care. Five items describing conditions symptomatic of illness were used to measure this variable with responses scored on an "agree-disagree" continuum. When controlling for education (years of formal school attendance), an inverse relationship between education and readiness to seek care was found. That is, as expressed by respondents, the higher the level of education the less readiness was there to seek care ($r = -.25; p < .05$).

In general, the norm is that information of a technical nature relating to a patient's diagnosis (test results, for example) is not to be communicated to him except by his physician. To the extent that such information could be provided promptly and accurately to patients, that patients or clients would understand it, and that patients do pay for it, it is inappropriate to withhold such information. There are instances, of course, in which it is entirely appropriate and even preferable that the physician be the individual to give information to the patient about his diagnosis and treatment. Such instances would be those in which the relevant information is of a highly technical or esoteric nature and the questions that the patient is likely to pose would be beyond the scope of knowledge of any other health professional. The reluctance of the physician to relinquish control over the provision of information leads to what has been described by at least one authority as a conspiracy of silence against the patient (Freidson, 1970). Freidson also notes that there are instances when patients *could* be given relevant information but it is withheld even when it is clear that no physician's order or organization policy restricts such provision.

Quint's (1965) findings lend further support to Freidson's observation. In a study of 21 postmastectomy patients (with a diagnosis of cancer), Quint found that patients were not adequately informed about the relative success of their surgery or of its extent. Further, nurses were observed to use avoidance mechanisms such as frequent rotation of assignments to patients in order to limit opportunity for these patients to verbalize their concerns (Quint, 1965).

There are at least two reasons why the matter of control of information will continue to be a problem for some time to come. One of these is that the line of demarcation between what is and what is not legitimate medical practice is increasingly difficult to define as more paraprofessionals enter the field of health care and take on responsibilities that once belonged to the physician. The traditional rule of thumb that held that diagnosis and prescribing were functions reserved to physicians can no longer be relied on as an absolute. The term *diagnosis* is periodically submitted to reevaluation and redefinition as, for example, when a state's attorney general promulgates a revised defintion of the nursing practice act in that state.

Regardless of statutory definition, it is quite clear that in the coronary care unit of a hospital the registered nurse makes a diagnosis from the electrocardiogram pattern on a cardiac monitor, determines that a patient is defibrillating, and decides to apply electric shock to the heart muscle in an attempt to restore normal sinus rhythm.

A second reason for the control of information remaining a problem is the sheer rapidity of the rate of discovery and transmission of new knowledge. No one professional, regardless of his field, can comprehend or apply all the knowledge that is theoretically available, yet the consumer's demand to know—as soon as possible and as much as possible—can be expected to continue unabated.

Recent trends in the health care system may portend alterations in various kinds of control that impact on consumers. The inflationary spiral in the cost of health care, as well as increased response on the part of government to consumer pressures in the making of health care policy, have paved the way for a readiness to experiment with alternatives to the physician as sole provider of care in the delivery system (Brunetto and Birle, 1972; Levine, 1970). Also, there is a heightened awareness among the public that there exists a variety of trained professionals other than the physician who are qualified and able to provide primary care.

As these other professionals (and paraprofessionals) continue to be prepared through education programs to provide primary care to individuals, restriction of access to clients should lessen. There are, in fact, indications that such restriction has already lessened (Abdellah, 1976; Duncan et al., 1971; West, 1967). What seems likely to evolve in place of the present medically dominated system of health delivery is a model in which health care management will be shared by a team of professionals. The physician will retain control of health care when the client requires what is distinctly medical care; other health team members will direct the health team's activities when health *prevention* or health maintenance is required, or when teaching or counseling are needed. Within the *shared* model of health delivery and policy making, those practitioners who by their education and training are specialists in a particular area of health will be called upon to advise on the preparation and allocation of practitioners and the development of training programs that will assist the carrying out of federally mandated health policy priorities. For example, it is highly probable that health educators, nurses, social workers, and nutritionists will increasingly be enlisted to help develop programs aimed at combating such persistent social problems as drug abuse and alcoholism in pre-teen and teenage populations. In addition, continued monitoring and funding by the Federal government of health care services, together with consumer representation on Health Systems Agency Councils (HSAs), are likely to ensure continued movement toward shared professional control of health policy making and delivery.

Autonomy: A Professional Attribute

Thus far I have examined some aspects of what can be termed structural autonomy as it relates to the provision of health care. Let us now consider autonomy as it applies to individuals in their exercise of professional roles. Autonomy has been held by some to be a necessary condition for the optimal exercise of one's professional role (Goode, 1957; Moore, 1970). It has been variously defined as freedom on the part of the practitioner to make decisions without external pressure from clients or the members of one's profession (Hall, 1968); as the control over strategic aspects of work (Freidson, 1970); and as the freedom to practice one's profession in accordance with one's training (Engel, 1970). While at one time professionals such as physicians and lawyers commonly exercised what amounted to almost complete autonomy by reason of their relatively small numbers and their monopoly of esoteric knowledge, such is no longer the case. Indeed, it is difficult to find examples of professionals who practice entirely autonomously, at least within the construction of the above definitions.

In actual practice professional autonomy is relative rather than absolute. That is, the amount of autonomy a given professional possesses is constrained by both the social and professional milieu in which he acts. For example, both nurses and physicians possess autonomy by virtue of their being members of learned professions. Yet, it is readily apparent that physicians are more autonomous in their professional practice than are nurses. This is explained by a presumption about the physician's comprehensive command of expert knowledge in the diagnosis and treatment of illness, as well as by his legally protected right to diagnose—a right denied to other practitioners. Even the physician is not completely autonomous, however, as can readily be seen. The successful practice of his craft depends upon the cooperation of a number of other professionals, as well as upon the support of such services as clinical laboratories and x-ray facilities—all important adjuncts to the physician's diagnosis and treatment of the sick. Peer review acts as yet another limitation on the absolute autonomy of any professional. The consensus of one's peers about what is correct action in a given set of circumstances acts to define a normative structure that circumscribes the individual's actions. The recent imposition of a Federal review system (PSRO) further limits the options for individual decision on the part of physicians in the treatment or medical management of patients (P.L., 92-603, 1973).

Autonomy and Commitment to Organizational Norms

The relative strength or weakness of norms in the work setting may influence both the amount of autonomy an individual perceives himself to have and the amount he actualizes in his practice (Goode, 1966). For example, some organizations place a high value on shared decision making. If, for example, the administration of a public elementary school supports the idea of shared decision making relative to curriculum and the decision is made to adopt a given pedagogical style of teaching reading, the individual teacher will have little or no opportunity to experiment with a variety of teaching methods even though he has reason to believe a different method might be more beneficial for his students. Similarly, in group health care settings, such as Health Maintenance Organizations (HMOs), group norms rather than individual professional norms tend to govern medical judgments and treatment. One reason for this is that, in general, clients who subscribe to HMOs for their health care are likely to be seen in the course of their treatment by several health care providers. The types of diagnostic tests ordered and even the drugs prescribed for specific illnesses are more likely to be a matter of group consensus among the physicians in that setting than a matter of independent decisions. Within every organization there exist competing sets of norms and in the case of those organizations employing a large number of professionals, the norms of the profession represent one such set. Several studies of organizations have attempted to make the case that the existence of two sets of norms, i.e., the organization's and the profession's, are mutually exclusive and so are inevitably in conflict. In light of available evidence, this may be an overstated position (Kohn, 1971; Wilensky, 1964). It is precisely because organizations have particular goals requiring the expertise of professional workers that professionals tend to find the environment of such settings conducive to using their skills. In fact, the model of bureaucracy upon which organizations are constructed has much in common with the ideal model of the professions. That is, both place a high value on rationality, specialization of skills, and application of knowledge (Kast and Rosenzweig, 1970). While organization and professional norms tend to make mutual accommodation in the majority of settings, there are instances in which the professional's attachment to the norms of his profession may make for conflict. Several studies of organizations have found that some persons tend to act more on their perception of what the profession's ideals call for than what the organization's norms call for (Hall, 1968; Pavalko, 1971). Such persons have been described as *cosmopolitans*, while those who adhere more to the organization's norms have been termed *locals* (Gouldner, 1957).

The organization's need for routine is not readily apparent to the professional who is employed at a large organization, but it remains a constraining force nevertheless. The activities of professionals—who, it should be noted, account for only a fraction of the work force—must be meshed with the activities of all other workers in order to accomplish the work of the organization (Blau, 1956; Scott, 1966). The hospital-based nurse, for example, may be unable to give an individual patient the amount of attention she believes the patient's condition warrants if, in the judgment of management, the amount of time involved is too expensive when judged against competing demands for the nurse's expert skills.

In view of present patterns of multidisciplinary approaches to the delivery of health care and evidence that suggests that such patterns will increase, there seems to be a clear implication for health professionals as they develop their roles. One major task facing professionals who seek to maintain their autonomy is that of applying their specialized knowledge in the interest of clients in such a way that the rationality of their professional judgments supports, or at least articulates, the rationality of the organizations in which they find themselves. The decisions that the professional must make for his clients on a day-to-day basis call for his being able to make an accurate assessment of a number of key variables within the specific setting at any given point in time, and then base his decision for action on this assessment.

SUMMARY

In this chapter organizations have been examined using a systems framework to emphasize the fact that efforts to manage order, provide for a functional division of labor, and motivate workers are problems or tasks common to all so-called rational organizations. In addition, some problems unique to those organizations in which professionals form the largest single group of employees have been identified, highlighting autonomy as a structural variable in organizations that provide health care. Further, some consequences for health professionals, other than physicians, who perceive themselves as entitled to autonomy but who have difficulty actualizing it were discussed. Attention was called to the negative impact on consumers that the control exerted by one dominant professional group can have in restricting the access of other health professionals to clients.

6

Reference Groups and Professional Socialization

JEAN L.J. LUM

The concepts of reference group and socialization have always been central to role theory and the symbolic interactionist tradition. Reference groups provide the individual with the sources of values that he selects in guiding his behavior, especially in situations where a choice has to be made. In other words, reference groups are those groups whose perspectives constitute the frame of reference for the individual. When viewed as a perspective (Shibutani, 1955), the concept of reference group points more to a psychologic phenomenon than to an objectively existing group and may therefore refer to a cognitive organization of an individual's experience. A reference group thus becomes any collectivity, real or imagined, envied or despised, whose perspective is assumed by the individual.

Reference groups may be groups to which an individual belongs but not necessarily. In any case, they provide direction for the behavior of the individual concerned. In the enactment of their professional roles, the actions of health care professionals are strongly influenced by their perception of the norms and values of those groups in which they hold membership, or those groups to which they aspire.

Reference groups play a significant part in the socialization process. In this chapter these and related concepts are presented as a fruitful and useful perspective for understanding the process by which neophytes become health professionals.

137

REFERENCE GROUPS

The term reference group was first proposed by Hebert Hyman (1942) and was used to increase the understanding of how an individual forms a conception of his status or position in society. Hyman suggested that, since one's position in society is defined relative to that of others, a person's view of his status depends upon the particular group of people he compares himself with, i.e., his reference group. Reference groups were thus originally viewed as points of comparison in evaluating one's own status.

The concept of reference group did not come into general usage until Merton and Kitt (1950) published their widely known work on the utilization of the reference group idea as developed by Stouffer and his associates (1949) to account for the attitudes and feelings about willingness to go into combat of American soldiers during World War II. Three groups of soldiers were studied: (1) inexperienced soldiers in units composed wholly of their own kind, (2) inexperienced soldiers who were replacements in units otherwise composed of combat veterans, and (3) veteran soldiers. Combat veterans had a strong group code against any tendencies to glamorize combat or to express eagerness for combat. Comparisons of attitudes indicated that while 45 percent of the inexperienced men were ready to get into an actual battle zone, only 15 percent of the veterans felt the same way. In units otherwise composed of combat veterans, 28 percent of the inexperienced replacements expressed readiness for combat. Merton and Kitt interpreted these results as indicating some degree of assimilation by these soldiers of the attitudes held by the veterans. As the inexperienced replacements sought affiliation with the authoritative and prestigious group of veterans, they moved from civilianlike values toward the more tough-minded values of the veterans.

With the passage of time, the concept of reference group has acquired an increasingly broader meaning. It is now commonly used to refer to any group to which a person relates his attitudes or to any group that influences his attitudes. It denotes any group, collectivity, or person that an individual takes into account in some manner in the course of selecting a behavior from a set of alternatives, or in making a judgment about a problematic issue.

Based upon the above usage, Newcomb (1965), Sherif (1948), and Siegel and Siegel (1957) have developed a general theory of reference groups designed to take account of attitudes anchored in both membership and nonmembership groups. It is important to note that reference groups and membership groups are not necessarily identical: a reference group may be a membership or a nonmembership group. They are identical when an individual aspires to *maintain* membership in the group of which he is a part, and they are disparate when the group in which a person aspires to *attain* membership is one in which he is not a member. Thus, both membership and reference groups affect the attitudes held by the individual.

A reference group to which an individual does not yet belong can serve as a powerful influencing factor provided the person perceives that group to be one in which he would seek acceptance and approval. Such a group is said to have a *positive* influence on the individual. In other instances, and individual may be influenced by a group that he dislikes. In this case he is motivated to adopt attitudes and behaviors contrary to those of the group. In this situation, the group is a *negative* reference group. Individuals generally have multiple reference groups. However, their impact varies according to given situations. The effect of a reference group does depend on its salience at a given moment with regard to a particular problem at hand and with respect to the degree of attractiveness of the group to the individual.

In an experimental study on positive and negative referent *others* as sources of influence on helping behavior, Schwartz and Ames (1977) noted that observers of positive referents tend to behave in congruence with the information provided by the referents, while observers of negative referents tend to behave in opposition to the information the referents provided. Observers helped most when positive referents expressed favorable feelings and negative referents expressed unfavorable feelings.

TYPE AND FUNCTIONS OF REFERENCE GROUPS

Several types of reference groups are identified in the literature. These include normative groups, comparison groups, and audience groups. As will be seen, each of these groups serves different functions.

Normative Groups

Kelley (1965) describes normative groups as those groups, collectivities, or persons that provide a person with a guide to action by explicitly setting norms and values. The normative group makes its expectations known and assumes that the person will comply with these norms and values. For example, one's family, one's religious community, and one's nation may each constitute a person's normative group. The major characteristic of a normative group is that the person acts relative to norms and values that the group has espoused and brought to the person's attention. The group functions as a normative reference group for a person to the extent that his evaluation of himself and the group's evaluation of him are based upon the degree of his conformity to certain standards of behavior or attitude and to the extent that the delivery of rewards or punishments is determined by the results of these evaluations. Normative reference groups then become the sources and enforcers of standards. The normative functions are a part of a general reference group theory of goal setting and motivation.

Comparison Groups

Another type of reference group identified by Kelley (1965) is that of comparison groups. These are groups, collectivities, or persons that provide a person with standards or comparison points that he can use to make judgments and evaluations. Comparison groups in this instance set the standards themselves against which a person can evaluate himself and others. A group serves as a comparison reference group only when it is so perceived by an individual.

More recently, Kemper (1968) has elaborated on the concept of comparison groups and proposed four types. The first type is called the *equity group* and is used as a frame of reference for judging whether or not a person's situation or fate is fair or equitable. As an example, Merton's (1950) "married men in the army" employed as equity groups both married men *not* in the army and unmarried men *in* the army. According to culturally traditional standards of equity, the married men in the army perceived unfairness in the fact that not all married men were enduring the same fate and that they were forced to be in the same situation as unmarried men. An even more drastic comparison could have been made had the married soldier employed as their equity group unmarried men *not* in the army.

Kemper's second type of comparison group is referred to as the *legitimator group*. This is a group that an individual uses when a question arises as to the validity of his behaviors or opinions. For example, opinion leaders who set the *tone* for their social circles act as legitimators of attitudes and behaviors. In like manner, the Kinsey study sample can be assumed to have been a legitimator group for persons who previously considered their own sexual behavior as deviant. The knowledge that other people are doing the same thing as oneself serves to legitimate behaviors.

The *role model* is proposed as the third type of comparison group. The role model is generally viewed as an individual (rather than as a group) who possesses certain skills and displays techniques that the individual lacks and from whom, by observation and comparison with his own performance, the individual can learn. For example, a student may adopt his professor as a role model or a son may adopt his father as his role model.

The fourth type of comparison group is the *accommodator group*. As Kemper explains, this refers to a group or person that provides cues for a person's responses in cooperative or competitive situations. Behavior is accommodated or adjusted to the perceived behavior of the other. For example, in a cooperative situation there is a normative overtone to the behavior of the other. In competitive situations on the other hand, the other's behavior serves as a trigger for greater exertion for the individual. In both cases, however, the other is a referent and guide to the individual's behavior.

Audience Groups

An additional type of reference group cited in the literature is that of audience groups. In the ideal case, audience groups are said to demand neither normative nor value-validating behavior of the person for whom they serve as referents. With respect to this type of group, the individual is believed to attribute certain values to an audience group and to attempt to behave in accordance with those values. The individual is guided by what he understands to be the values of his audience. To this extent, the audience is like the normative group, but it differs in that an audience group does not even take notice of the individual while a normative group demands conformity to its norms and values. On the contrary, according to this theory, an individual must attract the attention of the audience.

Goffman (1958) has identified the audience as a group whose presumed interests *guide the actor in special ways*. In his introductory remarks in *The Presentation of Self in Everyday Life*, Goffman describes how Preedy, a vacationing Englishman, makes his appearance on the beach and calculates his performance to evoke a positive impression on the people on the beach who constitute his audience.

While the above discussion presents an analysis of the "ideal" types of reference groups, it does not presume that the types and functions are mutually exclusive within a given group. In other words, normative, comparison, and audience groups can coincide and often do. In addition, there may also be an overlap between these functions in the same group or person. This introductory discussion has been primarily analytical and has highlighted the richness of the reference group concept. The various conceptualizations are useful in accounting for the choices individuals make among apparent alternatives, in summarizing differential associations and loyalties, and in understanding the mechanism by which the socialization process is enhanced and facilitated.

REFERENCE GROUPS AND SOCIALIZATION

The preceding discussion on reference groups illustrates their value in guiding the opinion or action of the individual. In like manner, reference groups also serve to articulate individuals with significant social processes in society, especially that of socialization. Socialization refers to the "process by which individuals acquire the knowledge, skills, and dispositions that enable them to participate as more or less effective members of groups and the society" (Brim, 1966). It is primarily in interactional processes whereby a person's behaviors and attitudes are modified to conform to expectations of the group or groups to which he belongs or to which he aspires. Additionally, it is primarily by virtue of the normative function of reference groups that the norms and values are prescribed and espoused for a given group. Normative reference groups therefore play a significant part in the socialization process by providing an individual with a set of norms and values and a standard for the proper level of performance in a given role.

The comparison reference group, particularly a role model, is likewise relevant to the socialization process by providing assistance on how a role is to be performed. The availability of a role model facilitates the acquisition of an adequate level of role performance. Finally, it is Kemper's (1968) contention that it is the audience reference group, with its stated or imputed values, that encourages and motivates an individual to exert himself to bring his performance to an achievement level in the socialization process.

By definition, socialization entails social learning. In this sense, learning is contrasted with maturation, which is the unfolding of the potentialities of the organism occurring more or less automatically except in situations of marked deprivation. Social learning includes learning to behave, feel, and see the world in a similar manner as other persons occupying the same role position as oneself. Social or role learning also includes acquiring an understanding of the attitudes of occupants of counter positions and learning certain skills and techniques associated with the role.

An inherent aspect of the socialization process is that of social control. According to Janowitz (1975), social control refers to the capacity of a social group to regulate itself through conformity and adherence to group norms in order to maintain the social order or organization within a group. Norms are enforced by means of sanctions. Sanctions refer to those actions of others or of an individual himself that have the effect of rewarding conformity or punishing nonconformity to norms. Positive sanctions are rewarding to the individual while negative sanctions have the effect of punishing the individual.

Furthermore, where the source of the reward or punishment

rests in the behavior of others, external sanction is employed. An example of an external negative sanctioning is that of a mother punishing her child for an inappropriate behavior. Internal sanction is employed where the source of the reward or punishment lies within the individual. An example of an internal positive sanctioning is that of an individual rewarding himself for a job well done. Both role learning and adequate role performance during the socialization process depend, in part, on the effectiveness of these internal sanctions.

From a sociologic perspective, reward and punishment may also be viewed as a means of providing the learner with cues that enable him consciously to evaluate the adequacy of his performance and modify his behavior where necessary. Expectations on the part of individuals that reward and punishment for specified acts will be forthcoming serve as important energizers or inhibitors of behavior. Socialization implies that the individual is induced to conform willingly to the ways of the particular groups to which he belongs. Norms therefore become internalized standards. More emphasis is likely to be focused on internal as opposed to external sanctions (Shibutani, 1962, pp. 128-147). Hopefully, the group's values become the individual's values and are recognized as having legitimacy or validity.

Various factors that either facilitate or interfere with the socialization process have been identified in the social system. One important condition is the clarity and consensus with which roles and positions are perceived by occupants, aspirants, and counter-position occupants. Another important condition is the degree of compatibility of expectations within role sectors and within role sets. To some degree, role learning may be facilitated by learning that occurs before entry to a position. Socialization agents, such as teachers, also differ in both their capacity and their efforts to manage the socialization process. There is variation in faculty's ability to select recruits, in the amount of advance preparation they require of the recruit, and in the amount of time that intervenes between selection for an organization and actual participation in it. In addition, socialization agents differ in their capacity to control the sources and extent of prior knowledge the learner acquires about the profession he is to enter.

Anticipatory Socialization

Many elements of a role are learned prior to the time a person occupies a given position. This premature taking on of the behaviors and attitudes of an aspired-to reference group is termed anticipatory socialization (Wheeler, 1966). It is by virtue of a person's capacity for reflective thought through the manipulation of symbols that social situations and social roles can be acted out in the imagination. By adopting a role in play and in fantasy, persons can rehearse in advance the roles that they will play in the future.

For example, small children "playing house" are not merely imitating their parents; they are also rehearsing in advance the roles that they will play in the future. Their portrayal of their role is based on their perceptions of the routines and interactions of family life. Often they are given feedback from their playmates as to how they are performing. By means of reflective thinking a medical student envisions himself as a doctor confronted with difficult clinical decisions and imagines what demands will be placed on him and what expectations he will be asked to fulfill. Anticipatory socialization thus entails a variety of mental activities that includes daydreaming, forecasting future situations, and role rehearsing (Clausen, 1968). In essence, it requires of the individual some degree of self-socialization and role rehearsal, wherein he learns a new self identity. The individual has the ability to see himself in many different situations and to predict his action in them. However, the individual can only rehearse those roles or social situations that have been made known to him. Furthermore, the individual will tend to rehearse those roles that seem most desirable.

Additionally, learning a new role can also be facilitated by learning roles of a similar type. For example, first-aid techniques learned in Boy or Girl Scout groups can later be part of a nursing student's repertory of skills. Similarly, occupying a position that relates to another position provides a person with additional opportunities to gain acquaintance with the roles associated with that counter position. For example, a nursing student who has occupied the position of patient may have learned certain elements of the counter position, nurse. Many students find numerous opportunities for role rehearsal by working in related jobs prior to entering school for formal professional education. Olesen and Whittaker (1968) found that almost one-half (44 percent) of the nursing class they studied had prior experiences in hospital jobs such as aides, ward clerks, or volunteers. Another 23 percent had worked in blood banks, medical libraries, doctors' offices, or had nursed sick relatives at home.

Such prior experiences are common among young adults since formal education of the student professional occurs in late adolescence or early adulthood. Some socialization to a professional role frequently occurs for the individual prior to his entry into a professional school. Accordingly, most persons are thus introduced to a new institution or organization only after they have had time to think about and to tentatively develop their own perspective on the profession.

SOCIALIZATION IN THE HEALTH PROFESSIONS

The process of becoming a health professional is a process of both adult and occupational socialization. As in any other role or position, social forces and trends move the individual toward or away from his particular life goals. The decision to become a health professional is influenced by the individual's perceptions of positive and negative consequences that he weighs in some manner. People are differentially attracted to occupations by factors such as income, accessibility, and the fit of the job to their skills and their personalities. Unlike providing training for an occupation in general, the goal of professional training institutions is to inculcate into their aspirants the norms, values, and behaviors deemed imperative for survival of the occupation.

The Origin and Nature of Professions

In its early simplicity, society existed with few special services and therefore with few professional groups. By contrast, recent decades have seen an increase in the numbers of professionals that, as a proportion of the labor force, has exceeded that of all other categories of workers except clerical workers (Kerr, 1973). There has been a tremendous growth in new and emerging health professions and with this development, a consequent growth in professional education. Each profession has struggled with competing occupations and crafts; each has or is trying to secure greater legitimacy for itself in society; and each has sought to define professional territories and to bring about uniformity in practice and among practitioners. Finally, each attempts to define and meet the needs of new and changing clienteles. Examples include the role and function of the psychiatrist as contrasted with those of the psychologist, psychiatric social worker, and psychiatric nurse.

    The professions have developed as outgrowths of society's needs or desires for special services. Historically, professions arose when a group of men was recognized as having unusual abilities to assuage the hurts and calm the fears of others by mediating among and between them and the powers of the universe. Only those with special preparation and skills, such as the medicine man, could deal with these forces, for no lay person could command the power. Since the time of the medicine man, the professional person has been recognized as an individual possessing unusual but needed gifts. Because of these special competencies and society's need for them, society allows the professional person to have a monopoly in his particular occupation. Only those with the necessary skills and knowledge are permitted to practice. Over the years, more detailed descriptions and criteria have evolved to distinguish professions from other occupations. Briefly stated, professions are intellectual, learned, and practical; they have techniques that can be taught; their members are organized into associations; they are guided by altruism; and they deal with matters of great human urgency and significance (McGlothlin, 1964). In consideration of these special conditions, society continues to allow professions to have a monopoly over their specialized services. Under this monopoly, the profession controls the body of knowledge on which its practice rests; it controls the number and kind of persons who are allowed to practice; it regulates the number and kind of persons entering the profession, and it guides the education of these neophytes.

Characteristics of Professional Socialization

FORMAL AND INFORMAL EDUCATIONAL PROCESS

Of the many roles that the adult is called upon to perform, few exceed in importance the acquisition of the requisite skills, norms, values, and attitudes for occupations. All occupations that are called professions are entered in a similar way and require a long period of formal schooling. The number of years of schooling varies, but the sequence is fixed and follows the general pattern of high school (standard four years), college (varying from none to four years), and professional study (varying from one to four years). The medical and legal professional models illustrate the pattern of study most clearly. During or after completing the standard sequence required for admission to the profession, the candidate may either be required or may choose to engage in supervised practice. An internship program in a particular discipline illustrates this characteristic. In addition, the candidate may study in a particular area for certification as a specialist, such as is required during a surgical residency. Hughes (1973) has described this sequence as the fixed nature of American professional education.

The processes by which persons become professional are similar regardless of the specific profession. A profession requires not only formal education but also an informal, internalized system of ethics that guide the practice of the professional role. Therefore, while the knowledge acquisition necessary for achieving professional status varies, the process in common for all professions. These socialization procedures result in new images, expectations, skills, values, and norms related to how the person defines himself and to how others view him. There are both internal and external changes within the individual, in his role set, and in the interactions among all of these.

Students undergoing professional socialization are placed in subordinate role arrangements in relation to their teachers. This is not surprising since it is, after all, the faculty in whom the institution and the profession have invested the authority and responsibility to pace, order, and sanction the progress of neophytes in the profession. Faculty therefore establish entry criteria, develop curricula, structure learning experiences, and evaluate students as they progress through the program. However, at the same time, it is apparent that students do take an active part in shaping their own education and roles and even in influencing the faculty. Students in any professional school participate in their own education by making those choices necessary to meet faculty demands, to handle noninstitutional pressures, and to handle situations of their own creation.

EXPOSURE TO MULTIPLE AGENTS
OF SOCIALIZATION

At the same time, students are exposed to multiple agents of socialization. Some of the agents whom students encounter include clients, professional colleagues, other health professionals, and family and friends who occupy roles both within and outside the formal institutional structure. Students therefore have access to many sources of information about the profession in addition to the faculty. Information thus obtained is sometimes congruent to and sometimes discrepant from what students think of themselves or what the faculty want students to think of themselves. For example, Olesen and Whittaker found students with nurse relatives have a more negative image of nursing than the faculty would have preferred (1968, p. 98). The ability to place in perspective the views of those in other roles as sources of information and as ratifiers of a professional self is an important aspect of students' separation from the world of laymen. As indicated earlier, these multiple others influence students not only during their formal schooling but also before and after formal schooling. Socialization into the professional role may therefore be either facilitated or hindered depending upon the degree of congruity between the role expectations of these multiple agents, those of the faculty, and those held by the neophyte aspiring to the profession.

TRANSITION FROM ADOLESCENCE TO ADULTHOOD

An additional facet of professional socialization merits attention here. A large segment of professional education occurs for many students while they are making the transition from adolescence to adulthood and from layman to professional. For this reason these years of professional socialization may take on the additional dimensions of developmental socialization related to acquiring an adult role and a conception of self during resocialization from layman to professional. While these socialization procedures occur simultaneously, they do not necessarily proceed smoothly or harmoniously. The roles that an individual assumes in other spheres of his life may not blend comfortably with the roles in professional education. For example, a medical student who finds himself in the new roles of husband and father may discover that he does not have the time to devote to his wife and family because of his busy clinical schedule. Socialization during this period of an individual's life is thus multidimensional in that students simultaneously acquire new views of self along with new role behaviors.

HETEROGENEITY OF STUDENTS
AND SOCIALIZING AGENTS

While the process of socialization is similar for all aspirants to a profession, students cannot be viewed as entirely homogeneous upon entry into professional schools. Not every student starts from the same baseline with respect to his qualifications or the awareness he has of the profession and of the self as a professional. Furthermore, instructors may also differ on this. For example, there are differences for both students and instructors with respect to age, lifestyle, social class, marital status, and in outlook, all of which impact differently on the individual. The socialization process involves taking a heterogeneous group of students and changing them into a more homogeneous group with respect to the knowledge, values, attitudes, behaviors, and skills that they will have following socialization.

HAZING, RITUALISM,
AND MONOPOLY OF STUDENT'S TIME

Moore (1969) contends that in order to achieve maximum socialization some professional schools virtually sequester their trainees in situations that amount almost to "total institutions," setting them apart from normal social activity. Still other professional schools approximate such isolation by the sheer burden of work demanded of students through extended class, laboratory, study, and practice hours. Moore further contends, as support for his punishment-centered theory of socialization, that the initiate is often required to perform unpleasant and even hazardous tasks and duties in order to remain in good standing. It is his thesis that practices such as hazing or suffering have a definite function in the socialization into all occupations, and particularly into the professions. These practices are intended to emphasize strong attention to standards of competence and performance and to identify with the occupation as a collectivity. Some of these difficult tasks are commonly ritualized and to that extent are arbitrary. Marks of success are likewise ritualized. However, punishment is prolonged for neophytes in occupations high in the scale of professionalism. The neophyte professional in medicine, for example, is usually required to do the "dirty work" or the "scut work" of his profession until such time as he has proven himself worthy to enter into the professional community by demonstrating knowledge, competence, and adherence to appropriate norms. While greater freedom follows successful survival of trials, the persistent possibility of failure is a characteristic of most professional occupations. Moore (1969) suggests this is an important ingredient of continuing professional occupational commitment.

LEARNING A TECHNICAL LANGUAGE

Another feature of professional socialization is the learning of a technical language. Aside from facilitating precise technical communication, an esoteric vocabulary serves to identify those who belong in the group and to exclude those who do not. Thus it confirms occupational identity. Those who successfully learn the language and skills and survive the ordeals of punishment will emerge with an internalized professional commitment and identification with the collectivity. As long as the socializing system endures, the shared experiences of past suffering and success serve as a powerful bond for continued commitment and identification among and between the young and the elders within the professional collectivity.

PROFESSIONS IN A STATE OF FLUX

It has been observed that professional socialization proceeds at a more uneven pace and results in a less integrated professional self-image in those institutions that are in a state of flux and in those professions undergoing a transition in role definition. Olesen and Whittaker (1968) illustrate some of the problems faced by students confronted with such dilemmas. They found that the institutional climate impacted upon students. For example, the introduction of advanced ideas and avant-garde themes into a nursing program served to heighten previously existing strains among various faculty factions. In turn, faculty factionalism posed problems for the students in their relationships with their instructors. The differing nursing ideologies not only resulted in differential emphasis within the faculty culture and curriculum but also became the foci around which students could interact with faculty and around which the students gradually came to see different styles of nursing and different models of the nurse in contrast to an initially undifferentiated picture of nursing.

The impact of changing *role definitions* on socialization has received little study. Nursing, however, provides a classic example of a profession undergoing dynamic reconsideration of itself and its social role.

Conflicts in definition of and preparation for the nursing role are brought sharply into focus with the proliferation of such new categories as the expanded and extended roles of the nurse. The less-established and emerging health professions may be confronted with similar situations in their development. Unless there is consensus and clarity of the norms, values, and behaviors expected within the given profession, it will be increasingly difficult to socialize the neophyte into its ranks.

STUDENT CULTURE

Socialization in professional schools does not take place in formal classroom and clinical situations alone nor solely with professors. Without question, one of the most powerful mechanisms of professional socialization is informal interaction with fellow students. The peer group therefore serves as a potent reference group for the student in the development and acquisition of values and norms. Studies of medical and nursing schools in particular have pointed to the existence of student cultures. These cultures represent a rich life of interaction and shared understanding that develops among cohorts of students. Students collectively set the level and direction of their efforts to learn and hence exercise social control over the extent and direction of socialization. Students tend to develop perspectives incorporating such crucial elements as a definition of the situation in which they are involved, a statement of the goals they are trying to achieve, a set of ideas specifying what kinds of activities are expedient and proper, and a set of activities or practices congruent with all of these. The following discussion of student cultures will revolve around significant case studies of professional socialization in medicine and nursing.

In their classic study *Boys in White*, Becker et al. (1961) found that freshmen medical students at the Kansas University Medical School evolved their own set of goals, working agreements, and solutions that were sometimes in conflict with official definitions of the student role, e.g., when they were confronted with a common problem such as having to do more work than they could possibly handle. During the clinical years of medical education, students defined their situation as one in which the goal of learning what was necessary for the practice of medicine might be interfered with by the structure of the hospital and by the necessity of making a good impression on the faculty. These students developed new goals that were more specific than prior ones as they came in contact with clinical medicine. They learned to want clinical experience and to want the opportunity of exercising medical responsibility. They developed ideas about how they must deal with the faculty, with patients, and with each other. And they developed ways of cooperating among themselves to handle their work load, to deal with the problem of making a good impression on the faculty, and to get as much clinical experience and medical responsibility as possible. Under these existing circumstances, students tried out various solutions to problems encountered and those solutions that worked best were then used by all the students, provided it was possible for them to communicate their thoughts and discoveries to one another. As a result of shared goals and exposure to a body of crucial experiences and adversities, these medical students became a community of fate and of suffering, bound together by feelings of mutual cooperation, support, and solidarity.

Similarly, Olesen and Whittaker (1968) observed the existence of a student culture in their study of professional socialization among undergraduate nursing students at the University of California School of Nursing in San Francisco. *Studentmanship* describes a form of underground student behavior that played a prominent part in shaping interactional styles, operational values, and staunchly held attitudes among students. The term *studentmanship* closely approximates the *student culture* concept of Becker et al. By practicing the art of studentmanship, these undergraduates managed to exercise some control over the process of becoming a nurse and found solutions to the perpetual problems of how to get through school with the greatest comfort and least effort and how to preserve themselves as persons, while at the same time being a success and attaining the necessities for their future life. Students were found to develop norms on a wide range of activities with regard to scholastic achievement, methods of bargaining, *fronting* (how to make a good impression on the faculty), how to bolster a classmate in the eyes of the faculty, how to "psych out" the faculty, how best to look attentive in a classroom, and how to behave appropriately "nursely" on a ward.

Olesen and Whittaker found for some students, however, that there was a self-established pressure to defy the norms of the student culture. For this group of students, the problem became one of how to excel without offending their classmates. The *front* they chose to present was designed to soothe the anxieties of classmates and leave them with the impression that they had not been betrayed. The student culture did open a few avenues for excelling by occasionally providing the fleeting reference person who suggested something beyond the norm. However, the student culture on the whole, outwardly discouraged the education for excellence that the faculty desired for students, and it suggested rather an education for mediocrity. Yet, while competition was muffled in public, it flourished rather lustily in private and in less obvious ways in the subtle rivalry revealed in *fronting*. On the other hand, the authors observed that this student culture was a hindrance to socialization by its leveling influences and its perpetuation of the unsocialized self. On the other hand, the student culture also enhanced the socialization process by disseminating knowledge, by sustaining and assisting fellow students, and by promoting the competition that it overtly attempted to squelch.

The preceding two studies of student culture were based on a symbolic interaction approach to socialization. A contrasting perspective on student culture reported in the literature is that described by Merton et al. (1957). Their study *The Student-Physician* was based on a structural functional approach to socialization. The authors identified a student culture at Cornell which, compared with the Kansas case, was more integrated with the formal educational system. It functioned to maintain the communications network of the school, to clarify standards, and to control behavior based on norms that were mutually held by students and faculty. The Cornell students are portrayed as "physicians-in-training," while the Kansas students are viewed as "boys in white." The Cornell study reflects a context in which students were already accepted as colleagues, proceeding more or less smoothly to full membership in the profession. In contrast, the Kansas study illustrates a situation in which students and faculty were set apart, with distinctive and even conflicting interests, and with students in a position that was both isolated and subordinate, which made it clear that they were not yet professionals.

These two studies began with different conceptions of the socialization process and of the medical school and its relation to the profession. Also, the studies were conducted in different types of educational settings, Kansas being traditional, state supported, and Midwestern whereas Cornell was experimental in curriculum and philosophy, Ivy League, and private.

Development of A Professional Self-Image

By what interactional processes occurring throughout the socialization experience do neophytes develop a professional self-image and come to regard themselves as bona fide health professionals? Olesen and Whittaker (1968) propose two related processes, *legitimation* and *adjudication*, as a framework for analyzing and understanding the experiential transactions through which students develop their professional identities. Although Olesen and Whittaker studied the socialization of student nurses, their suggestions have potential utility in studying other health professional neophytes.

Legitimation as used by Olesen and Whittaker refers to the process by which others sanction the student's claim to the role of health professional. (Legitimation, then, consists of a series of *sanctions* applied to the student's claim on the general role of that health professional to which he aspires; the concept subsumes those sanctioning interactions encountered by the student as being generally accepted or rejected.) Adjudication as used by these same authors refers to the continual refereeing and negotiating of the minute, face-to-face transactions between students and faculty relative to the technical, refined aspects of role performance. During the adjudication process, the student's claim on his role is met with a variety of instructor styles that acknowledge it to be accurate or inaccurate. If the role is inaccurate, suggestions for corrections are made by instructors. The cycle comes full circle when the student has the opportunity to demonstrate awareness of appropriate altered behavior in the future. The adjudication process leads to legitimation for it is through the vivid presence and interaction of the other that students come to incorporate the role of the other in developing their own professional identities.

Olesen and Whittaker (1968) enumerated a variety of legitimation sources relevant to the role of nurse. They noted that students received legitimation in encounters with various persons in their role set. These legitimations included (1) nonofficial legitimation from parents, boyfriends, strangers, or former college friends; (2) legitimation from fellow students; (3) formal modes of legitimation derived from grades and evaluations given by the faculty; (4) legitimation from staff nurses, doctors, and supporting personnel such as aides, orderlies, and licensed practical nurses; and (5) legitimation from patients or clients.

The nonofficial legitmators included all those persons in the role set who gave only the most general acknowledgment of the student's claim on his role. Students derived great reassurance from these nonofficial legitimators, particularly in the early phases of their education. However, in the long run, faculty won out over these nonofficial legitimators as those who could most meaningfully legitimate and adjudicate sutdents' achievements and claims. Student legitimation resulted from an assessment of the manner and style in which students presented themselves to one another. Paradoxically, student judgment was influenced by the very same fronting that would earn the desired legitimation from faculty. The instructor's periodic evaluation of students and their grades served as reference points against which students could compare and legitimate themselves and, in passing, could assess their fellow classmates. In addition, Olesen and Whittaker noted that the student nurses' early contact with others practicing the profession to which they aspired resulted in legitimation from staff nurses. At times, legitimation from the staff was earned at the cost of that of the instructors, since the staff's ideas about techniques were frequently divergent from those of the instructors. Students frequently encountered radical differences in emphasis between the advanced notions of the faculty and the more conservative views of the hospital or agency practitioners. Where role conflict was high, students faced a problematic dilemma in obtaining legitimation from two divergent sources. Not surprisingly, physicians remained a significant legitimator throughout the socialization period. Legitimation from supporting persons such as aides, orderlies, and licensed practical nurses was paramount during the summers when many students found employment in hospitals. Finally, the patients constituted a particularly significant group of legitimators for students at the onset of their careers but diminished as the students became more able to evaluate and legitimate themselves.

Huntington's (1957) study of how medical students come to view themselves as doctors also draws upon an analysis of the student's self-images and role set. Huntington contends that students typically think of themselves primarily as students at the beginning of their medical training and come progressively to think of themselves as doctors as they advance through medical school. However, it is vis-à-vis patients more than with any other group in their role set that medical students tend to see themselves as physicians. Legitimation of a professional self-image can thus be seen as resulting from multidimensional transactions taking place with persons in their role set during the formal and informal encounters that occur throughout the professional socialization experience.

Ongoing Professional Socialization

Socialization that takes place during the formal years of education plays an important part in the development of a professional self-identity. However, students progress at different rates through the program and this has implications for role assimilation. Thus, while students in general assimilate a central core of values emphasized by the faculty and the profession, within a collection of graduating students there can be found wide divergence in types of professional role assimilation, varying degrees of self-awareness, and differences in professional behavior and knowledge. Furthermore, the process of socialization does not terminate with graduation from a program of study, but it continues as the neophyte commences his professional career. In reality, regardless of the outcome of the initial socialization, the process of professional socialization continues throughout life.

It has been noted that the greater the conguence of the norms, values, and behavioral expectations between the educational organization of the profession and the realities of the work setting, the smoother the transition will be from neophyte to full-fledged professional. Kramer (1974) proposes the concept of *reality shock* to highlight the discrepancies between the norms, values, and behavioral expectations existing in the educational setting of nursing and those of the work situation. She believes shock results from an inadequate socialization of the neophyte during formal schooling. Kramer contends that on account of these discrepancies the neophyte is unprepared to function effectively in the world of reality. Reality shock is a term Kramer used to describe the phenomenon of shocklike reactions of new workers when they find themselves in the work situation for which they have spent several years preparing and for which they thought they were ready, only to suddenly find that they are not. Kramer has suggested an anticipatory socialization program as a means for transmitting role-specific behaviors intended to meet the exigencies of the work world and to acquaint nursing students with the realities of the "Positive Now" (Kramer's term) without losing their vision and ability to function in the "Relative When."

The fact of the matter is that the initial work experience must be viewed as a continuation of professional socialization because it is in this situation, as the neophyte begins his professional career, that role-specific behaviors are learned. A major portion of professional socialization thus occurs after completion of the formal years of schooling. In the field of medicine, Olmstead and Paget (1969) and Bloom (1971) document the important contributions made by the internship and residency experiences. Initial work experiences in the other health professions likewise provide ongoing socialization in their respective disciplines. It is during this crucial period that the values, norms, and behaviors to which the individual has been exposed during his formal education are most likely to become internalized.

SOCIAL CONTROL WITHIN
AND BETWEEN PROFESSIONS

Society accords a monopoly to a profession with respect to its practice and standard setting on the premise that no lay person understands esoteric knowledge on which the profession rests, and therefore no lay person can judge what should be done. Society allows a profession to hold a monopoly because it is convinced that the profession is dedicated to an ethical or altruistic ideal in serving society. Society continues to allow this monopoly as long as it is convinced that a profession is exercising its privileges responsibly and aids and/or serves its clientele without exploitation.

Under its monopoly, a profession has the purpose of protecting not only the society it serves, but also its members, making it possible for them to practice effectively. Its protection, which occurs through methods passed on by socialization, takes different form as the profession confronts internal as well as external dangers.

Internally, a profession must protect society and its members against the incompetent or dishonest member whose actions may damage trust in the profession. A profession controls the number and kinds of persons who are allowed to enter and to study through the establishment of admission criteria and determining the length and types of programs allowed. These controls are imposed in order to prevent incompetent persons from entering the profession and to avoid an oversupply of practitioners as well. In addition, it controls the body of knowledge on which its practice rests and maintains the quality and standards of its education through a process of external accreditation. It further controls admission to the profession through licensing procedures as well as through various certification and credential procedures. It opposes efforts to establish conditions that would make its practice difficult or impossible. Each profession has an obligation to police its own ranks and to make certain that those who wear the name and display the license are in fact ethical and competent practitioners. From this obligation stem efforts to enforce the code of ethics of the profession even to the extent of expelling members who flagrantly violate provisions of its code. Thus, a physician can have his license revoked or a lawyer can be "disbarred." Professional associations aid practitioners in obtaining legal sanction for their monopoly. Once a profession is awarded legal status and is given the exclusive right to practice in the field of its competence, it can inhibit the practice of imposters by taking action in the courts to bring them to trial and punishment.

Each profession defines an area of practice in which it has a monopoly and it fights hard to preserve that unique area. A profession thus protects its members against nonlegitimate individuals and groups who may try to encroach on the area of practice reserved to the profession. In summary, a profession engages in a variety of activities that are designed to monitor and control itself while maintaining its claim as an autonomous body among other professional disciplines.

SUMMARY

Professional socialization is a process that continues throughout an individual's adult and occupational life. Concepts from role theory and reference group theory have been discussed and proposed as a framework for analyzing and understanding the mechanisms through which neophytes acquire norms, values, knowledge, and skills appropriate to a given occupation. Means of inducing compliance with normative expectations have been elaborated. Factors contributing to differential assimilation of a new professional self-image have been cited. Additionally, social control measures have been presented to illustrate the methods by which professions monitor themselves and legitimizes their claims as autonomous disciplines within society.

7

Stratification

BONNIE BULLOUGH

As indicated in earlier chapters, social roles are influenced by a variety of factors. Without minimizing the importance of other factors, it seems safe to say that stratification within the health care delivery system is a major variable in determining the roles or patterns of behavior of the occupants of the system. There are at least two major stratification systems within the health care profession. One of these is the stratification patterns of the health care workers themselves and the second is the system that links these providers with their patients. Each of these major systems, and their further subdivisions, will be discussed in this chapter.

STRATIFICATION

It is interesting to note that early American sociology texts tended to begin discussion of the stratification phenomenon with an elaborate rationale for its existence in view of the egalitarian ideology that held that ours was a classless society. Modern writers no longer feel that such an argument is necessary; stratification is now known as a pervasive phenomenon and its correlates are far reaching. Glenn (1969, p. 163) even suggests that stratification is the sociologist's favorite independent variable, if only because they are able to trace a correlation between stratification and almost any other social phenomenon. It is not surprising then that it has consequences for social roles.

The study of stratification is essentially a study of the levels of power, social class, and wealth within a given structure. The concept of *stratification* means the ranking of people using one or more of these variables. The structure that is the unit of concern can be as large as a society or as small as a dyadic relationship. Thus, the phenomenon spans all groups within a society as well as the levels of power within a single organization. *Power* is ordinarily operationalized as influence and it has been studied in the decision-making process. *Social class* is usually defined as prestige and it is measured using such indicators as reputation, lifestyle, and occupation. *Wealth* is usually measured in terms of income, property, or other possessions (Bendix and Lipset, 1966; Davis and Moore, 1945; Lenski, 1966; Light and Keller, 1975; Mills, 1956).

Differentiation is a term that subsumes stratification, since it covers a wide variety of distinctions that are made between people. Stratification involves a ranking system, but people are often differentiated by such factors as gender differences or ethnic characteristics which do not always include a ranking system (McGee et al., 1977). *Role differentiation* divides people by the set of expectations for performance that are associated with a social role. Roles can be differentiated into a stratified pattern when one role is superordinate and the other subordinate—as is the case between the registered and practical nurse—or they can be differentiated into separate specialty functions—as is the case in the differentiation between the roles of the coronary care nurse and the public health nurse. The concept of role differentiation that is used in this chapter refers to a process in which a single work role is divided or differentiated into two or more new work roles.

Stratification theory as it is discussed and studied by modern sociologists has its historical roots in the work of Max Weber, one of the founding fathers of sociology in the nineteenth century. He describes three different stratification systems: (1) the "class order," which is stratified by the production and acquisition of goods, and so it carries an essentially economic meaning; (2) the "social order," which is differentiated by the consumption of goods as represented by lifestyle and (3) the "party," which is the ideologic or political arena of power (Gerth and Mills, 1946; pp. 180-184; Weber, 1947; p. 152).

As social inquiry passed into its empirical phase (as opposed to the social philosophy of Weber and his contemporaries), a series of stratification studies was done in small American towns using a reputational approach. W. Lloyd Warner, a leader in this effort, worked through the third and fourth decades of the twentieth century. "Yankee City" and "Jonesville" were his major field research settings, although his students carried out similar projects in many other localities. These researchers could ordinarily identify five or six distinct social classes in the towns they studied (Warner and Lunt, 1941; Warner, et al., 1944). Using these data, Warner constructed an index of social class employing four factors to rank subjects: (1) occupation, (2) income, (3) source of income, and (4) dwelling area (Warner, et al., 1949). Similarly, August Hollingshead classified the families in "Elmtown" using four criteria: (1) lifestyle, (2) income and possessions, (3) participation in community affairs, and (4) prestige (Hollingshead, 1949). While these scales of social class are still appropriate for some types of research, their small-town roots and their emphasis on reputation limit their applicability to structures in which the distributive systems are more complex.

More recently, stratification researchers have tended to utilize discrete variables in order to rank subjects and study the stratification phenomenon (Glenn, 1969, pp. 171-172). Income, education, occupation, or some combination of these are most often used for this purpose, although almost any variable that differentially distributes people can be conceptualized as a stratifying variable. While researchers who use these discrete variables might well overlook the subtle power and prestige accorded the scion of an old family in a small town, these variables are more readily quantifiable and can be usefully employed in urban areas or nationwide studies where people do not have face-to-face contact as they did in Yankee City. Income as a discrete variable relates to the theoretical construction of stratification as measures of wealth; occupation and education are reasonably good indicators of social class. The aspect of stratification that is least emphasized by these indicators is power, although all three of them correlate with power to a certain degree.

The discrete variable that is probably most often used as a measure of stratification is occupation (Blau and Duncan, 1967). Occupational prestige seems to be a fairly stable phenomenon. In two separate studies done in 1947 and 1963, researchers connected with the National Opinion Research Center (NORC) asked a nation-wide sample of respondents to rank the occupational prestige of 100 major occupations. The ratings tended to be consistent over time; although a few scientific occupations gained prestige, most occupations remained virtually the same with street sweepers and shoe shiners at the bottom and supreme court justices and physicians at the top of the list. With few notable exceptions, such as nightclub singers and bartenders, the ratings tended also to correlate with both education and income (Hodge et al., 1964).

To facilitate the use of occupations as an index of social class, Bogue (1963) prepared a more detailed rating system of occupations and keyed it to the list of occupations used by the Department of Labor. These rating scores range from 184 for physicians to 44 for personal service laborers. Bootblacks, who were the baseline occupation in the 100 NORC occupations, score 47 on the Bogue scale. Nurses, who are not one of the NORC sample members, score 107, which is slightly above the midpoint on the scale.

THE STRATIFICATION
OF HEALTH CARE OCCUPATIONS

It is possible to look at the health care occupations using the Bogue scale. Table 1 lists them as they were included in the 1970 census, along with the median years of schooling achieved by their members. Although this list excludes occupations that are not related to health care, it is a broad list that spans almost the total health occupational power and prestige system. The spread of the system becomes more evident when the health occupations are compared with workers in the educational complex. Using the same ranking system as is shown in Table 1, college professors and administrators are rated 145; grade school teachers, 132; and the school office employees, 102. The power, prestige, and income of the physician is significantly higher than that of the college professor, and the nursing aide enjoys less power, prestige, and income than the person who works in the local grammar school office.

There are several reasons why the stratification system within the health care industry is so broad. Some of these factors seem legitimate, while others are more problematic and suggest that the system is in need of reform. First, the industry is large and rapidly growing; it now includes more than four million workers (National Center for Health Statistics, 1972). Although size and complexity do not always go together, they often do. Certainly the rapid growth in the number of health workers has paralleled the increased complexity of the system, and the simple doctor-nurse team of the early twentieth century has given way to the array of workers shown in Table 1.

A second factor in the development of the elaborate stratification system of the health occupations has been the emergence of the professionalization process as a significant factor in stratification. In earlier agrarian societies, wealth and property were more crucial variables in stratification. The scientific revolution has given primacy to knowledge as the basis of stratification and the learned professions have emerged as the most powerful occupations.

Although there are a variety of definitions of professionalization in use, it is basically a process whereby an occupation gains great power and

TABLE 1

SOCIOECONOMIC INDEX AND EDUCATIONAL LEVEL OF THE MAJOR HEALTH OCCUPATIONS

Occupation	Socio-economic Index	Median School Years Completed Men	Women
Physicians	184	17+	17+
Dentists	177	17+	15.8
Optometrists	144	17+	16.8
Veterinarians	142	17+	17+
Pharmacists	140	16.6	16.4
Chiropractors	132	16.8	16.1
Health Administrators	130	16.1	13.5
Therapists	120	16.0	16.3
Clinical Laboratory Technicians	117	14.7	14.6
Registered Nurses	107	13.5	13.3
Radiologic Technicians	106	13.0	12.7
Dental Hygienists	106	12.7	14.9
Health Records Technicians	112	14.5	14.0
Dieticians	96	12.7	12.9
Practical Nurses	80	12.4	12.4
Health Aides (non-nursing)	74	12.3	12.3
Dental Assistants	74	12.6	12.5
Nursing Aides and Orderlies	74	12.2	11.8

Sources: U.S. Census Bureau (1973); also Bogue (1963, pp. 516-521). 17+ is the highest classification level for education recoreded by the census bureau.

prestige because it holds a unique body of knowledge that is not shared by its clients. In part because of this protected knowledge, the public is forced to allow professions significant control over their own affairs (Daniels, 1971; Freidson, 1970). The learned occupations in turn have supported the professionalization process by lengthening training programs, organizing into collectivities, seeking support from the state through licensure or similar devices, and by taking pains to enhance the charismatic mystique that surrounds their expertise (Carr-Saunders and Wilson, 1933; Freidson, 1971; Greenwood, 1957; Jackson, 1970; Moore and Rosenblum, 1970; Vollmer and

Mills, 1966). Thus, professionalization has increasingly separated the high-status health occupations from the untrained or minimally trained health workers and has even increased the social distance between them and their patients. For example, the social distance between the modern specialty physician and his patients is greater than that between the old family doctor and his patients.

A third basis for the expansion of the stratification system is the fact that the health care industry is labor intensive. As the cost of labor has risen, health care costs have escalated. Moreover, the work is often of an emergency nature, and so staffing needs cannot be totally predictable; this in turn leads to overstaffing on the "quiet" days (Georgopoulos, 1972, p. 17). Although it is true that there have been significant technologic advances in health care in the last few decades, including the development of elaborate diagnostic and monitoring devices, automation has tended to broaden the spectrum of patients who can be effectively treated rather than cutting down the amount of labor needed to diagnose and treat patients. Some of the machines have in fact increased the requirements for personnel by necessitating a new class of technicians to monitor or utilize them. Consequently, the health care industry has not reaped the cost-saving benefits of the industrial revolution that have accrued to other industries.

In an effort to deal with the problem of escalating labor costs, hospital administrators, clinical managers, and physicians have sought to rationalize the system by breaking down work roles into component parts and assigning the simpler tasks to workers with little formal training. This had led to the development of a whole army of medical technicians. While a few of these roles—such as those of the physiotherapist and the inhalation therapist—have grown out of the nursing role, most of the laboratory and engineering specialties had their origins in the traditional job description of the physician.

The major thrust in the differentiation of the nursing role occurred in the decade following World War II and its full impact is only now being felt. During the war the office of civilian defense and the Red Cross had experimented with trained nurses' aides to augment the wartime shortage of nurses. At first these aides were allowed to perform only those tasks that were not directly related to patient care, but as the shortage of help worsened, they took on some of the less complicated patient care tasks. This precedent, which was begun as a temporary expedient, marked the beginning of "team nursing." It demonstrated that much of the work role of the nurse could be safely delegated to less-expensive workers. What previously had been one occupational role broke down into at least three levels: nursing aide, licensed practical nurse, and registered nurse (Bullough and Bullough, 1974, pp. 292-300).

Although contemporary nurses often decry this breakup of the nursing role as a source of fragmentation of patient care, there was little opposition from the profession when this division began. The American Nurses Association sponsored a series of studies and reports that recommended that the nursing role be differentiated. The most influential of these was done by Esther Lucile Brown, who surveyed the work nurses were doing in various settings and recommended the development of a "nonprofessional trained nurse" who could carry out the routine procedures and leave registered nurses more time to concentrate on complex procedures (Brown, 1948). Following this recommendation, schools for practical nurses proliferated rapidly and by 1952 thirty-nine states had established provisions for licensing practical nurses. The next year, Lambertson published a landmark book that described the stratified arrangement of nursing roles and called it "team nursing" (Lambertson, 1953). By 1960 all states had passed laws licensing practical nurses, or vocational nurses as they are called in two states (Roberts, 1961, p. 514). The hierarchical nursing team has remained the dominant staffing pattern, although the current experimental trend of providing primary nursing with a single nurse who has full responsibility for her patients over a 24-hour period may be the beginning of a new countertrend.

The role of the physician has been more resistant to differentiation than that of the nurse. While it is true that a myriad of technical specialties have developed from the basic discipline, this represents a slightly different process from that which took place when nursing split into the practical, registered, and aide levels. However, a similar differentiation of the medical role may actually be occurring at the present time with the development of nurse practitioners and physicians' assistants (Bullough and Bullough, 1974). Again, the basic driving force behind this differentiation is probably an economic one based on a historical trend.

Starting in 1910 with the Flexner report, medical education went through a period of upgrading. Many substandard schools were closed and others limited their enrollment. These reforms helped keep the physician-to-population ratio stable for the next half-century at the level of approximately 150 doctors per 100,000 persons (Fein, 1967). While the demands for physicians increased, medical science and technology were expanding the range of services that a physician could perform; and, concomitantly, consumer demand for services increased. These factors inflated the fees and salaries charged by physicians. While the number of physicians has now risen to a level of approximately 170 physicians and osteopaths per 100,000 persons, the specialty trend has complicated the situation. In 1910 most physicians were general practitioners; specialists now, however, outnumber general practitioners by three to one (National Center for Health Statistics, 1973).

This means that there are fewer physicians who are available for first level or primary care. Of course, general practitioners are not the only ones who give primary care; osteopaths, internists, and pediatricians are also engaged in this type of practice, at least part of the time. Osteopaths remain few in number, while both internists and pediatricians have gone through lengthy specialty training that is reflected in their fees. One approach to filling the primary care gap has been to try to replace the dwindling numbers of general practitioners with family practice physicians. Recently, private foundations, as well as state and federal agencies, have made grants to organizations to develop family practice residencies (MacBride, 1973, pp. 14-15). It is unlikely that this effort will completely solve the problem because the family practice training programs are as long as those of many other specialties; thus, another specialty is being created. Graduates of family practice residencies feel they are entitled to the same income as specialists in other fields, and while this argument is undoubtedly valid, it means that they do not fill the shoes of former general practitioners who were willing to accept lower incomes than specialists. It seems, therefore, that the problem is not so much one of a shortage of physicians, or even a shortage of physicians who can give primary care, but a shortage of people who can deliver safe, efficient primary care at a reasonable cost. Consequently, nurse practitioners, and to a lesser extent physicians' assistants, are moving in to fill this gap (Bullough, 1976).

Three major explanations for the broad stratification pattern of the health occupations have been offered: (1) the size and complexity of the industry, (2) the professionalization of the top occupations in the health field, and (3) the economic realities that stimulate role differentiation. Although these three factors appear to be legitimate causes of the many levels of power, income, and prestige within the industry, there are two additional factors that are more problematic: both gender and race seem to contribute to the allocation of power and perquisites within the system. Although these discriminatory elements of the system are currently under attack, it would be naive to think they are no longer operative.

GENDER AND RACE AS FACTORS IN THE STRATIFICATION OF HEALTH OCCUPATIONS

One of the most obvious characteristics of the health occupations is their marked sex segregation. Most jobs can be classified both statistically and in terms of their public image as being either male or female. Table 2 shows the percentage of male and female workers in each of the five major categories of

TABLE 2

SEX DISTRIBUTION FOR FIVE MAJOR CATEGORIES OF HEALTH WORKERS WITH OCCUPATIONS RANKED IN ORDER OF PRESTIGE

Occupational Group	Number	% Male	% Female
Physicians, dentists, and related occupations	541,453	91.7	8.3
Health administrators	85,252	55.3	44.7
Technologists and technicians	265,281	30.2	69.8
Nurses, dieticians, and therapists	966,585	5.6	94.4
Health service workers	1,230,454	12.0	88.0

health occupations. The group accorded both highest status and highest income is made up of physicians, dentists, pharmacists, veterinarians, optometrists, and chiropractors. This group is 91.7 percent male. The next group in terms of status and income is that of health administrators, 55.3 percent of whom are male. One of the reasons women fare so well here is that large numbers of nurses are included in the administrative category since they have day-to-day supervision over most institutional health workers. If the group were separated into a major decision-making category versus minor administrators, the breakdown would put the vast majority of men in the first category and most of the women in the second. The third group in the table is composed of health technicians and technologists: 30.2 percent male, 69.8 percent female. Within the technical group there are some occupations that are highly segregated, such as dental hygienists and record technologists who are almost all female. However, other technical occupations have a greater male representation, and so the total field looks more balanced. The next category in the table—nurses, dieticians, and therapists—are similar to the technicians in socioeconomic status but are separated in the census grouping, probably because of their overwhelmingly female representation. This group is 94.4 percent women, the most segregated of the major categories of health workers. The largest group shown in the table is composed of the more than 1,200,000 health service employees including licensed practical nurses, dental assistants, home health aides, nursing aides, and orderlies. This category is not quite so overwhelmingly female with only 88 percent of the group being women, although most of the male representation is clustered under the classification of orderly. There are more than 115,000 orderlies employed in hospitals and mental institutions (U.S. Census Bureau, 1973; Bullough and Bullough, 1975).

Table 3 shows a more detailed list with the sex distribution of each of the major health occupations. It can be noted that the high-status, predominantly male occupations tend to represent a much smaller population than the predominantly female ones. The distribution of women is a pyramidal one, with only a few women in the high-status health professions and heavy representation of women in the low-status occupations.

While the causal factors in this pattern are many and undoubtedly include all of the prejudices against women in the work force, these prejudices are mediated through the professional schools. In spite of the efforts of Elizabeth Blackwell (Blackwell, 1895) and the other nineteenth century pioneers, medicine and the other high-status professional schools

TABLE 3

SEX DISTRIBUTION IN THE HEALTH OCCUPATIONS RANKED IN ORDER OF PRESTIGE

Occupation	Number	% Male	% Female
Physicians	280,577	91.1	8.9
Dentists	92,776	97.0	3.0
Optometrists	17,550	99.6	.4
Veterinarians	19,176	94.4	5.6
Pharmacists	111,242	88.1	11.9
Chiropractors	13,459	84.3	15.7
Health administrators	85,252	55.3	44.7
Clinical laboratory technicians	119,955	28.3	71.7
Radiologic technicians	53,511	31.5	68.5
Dental hygienists	17,650	6.9	93.1
Health records technicians	11,084	6.2	93.8
Other technicians	60,174	43.9	56.1
Therapists	77,084	36.2	63.8
Registered nurses	848,182	2.7	97.3
Dieticians	41,319	7.9	92.1
Practical nurses	240,687	3.7	96.3
Health aides (nonnursing)	124,334	16.1	83.9
Dental assistants	93,242	2.2	97.8
Nursing aides	636,178	0.0	100.0
Orderlies	115,805	100.0	0.0

Source: U.S. Census Bureau (1973).

have until recently remained resistant to admitting women, or, as in the case of medicine, they have felt it sufficient to admit a few token women. In the early years, two women were admitted, rather than one, so that they could examine each other in their physical diagnosis course. That barrier is beginning to break down. The first-year enrollment of women in medical schools reached 24 percent in school year 1975-1976 (Dube, 1976), although, as indicated in the table, women remain underrepresented among practicing professionals.

Even schools of nursing are not without blame in the creation of the sex segregation pattern. According to the 1910 census figures, approximately seven percent of the student and trained nurses were men. Most of these came from schools connected with mental hospitals or from one of the few male schools, such as those run by the Alexian Brothers in Chicago and St. Louis. The twentieth century efforts of nursing to upgrade its educational programs forced the mental hospitals to close. This effectively cut out opportunities for men, except in the all-male schools, because the general hospital schools excluded men. This was done for an interesting reason. The hospital schools required student nurses to live on the hospital grounds in nurses homes in order to maintain surveillance over their behavior and keep them available for night work. The norms of that period would neither allow men to stay in these quarters nor in the higher status male interns' quarters. Consequently, men were simply excluded. By 1950, only one percent of the practicing nurses were men. (Bullough and Bullough, 1969, pp. 205-206). The current changeover to collegiate nursing is again opening up opportunities for men to enter nursing although there is still room for improvement. Approximately six percent of the registered and practical nurse students are now men (Educational Preparation for Nursing, 1976).

The educational system has also been a significant factor in excluding blacks and other minorities from the high-status health professions, although economic deprivation is certainly an added factor. Table 4 shows the percentage of nonwhite workers in each of the major occupational groups for 1970. The educational problem for minority students starts at the elementary school level with segregated educational patterns; and despite antibusing rhetoric, the fact remains that segregated education is inferior education (Bullough, 1972; Coleman, et al., 1966; Myrdal, 1944). Consequently, most minority members were unprepared for admission to professional schools. However, even those who managed to get a good basic education, faced overt and covert discriminatory patterns when they tried to enter high-status professional schools. Until the 1960s, when federal legislation outlawed discrimination in publicly supported educational programs, there were many American medical schools that had never accepted a single black applicant, and even those with reputations for open admissions had accepted

TABLE 4

REPRESENTATION OF NONWHITE MINORITY GROUP MEMBERS
IN EACH OF THE MAJOR CATEGORIES OF HEALTH WORKERS

Occupational Group	% Minority
Physicians, dentists, and related occupations	2.0
Health administrators	4.7
Technologists and technicians	8.9
Nurses, dieticians, and therapists	7.9
Health service workers	22.0

Source: U.S. Census Bureau (1973).

only a handful throughout their entire history. The only significant opportunity that was available for black students to enter medicine was through one of the segregated schools (Cogan, 1968; Morais, 1969; Norman, 1969, pp. 1-10). And the situation was similar in dentistry (Dummett, 1952).

The pattern in nursing was also segregated throughout most of the early part of the twentieth century. It changed somewhat during World War II because the Bolton Act, which created the Cadet Nurse Corps, included nondiscriminatory provisions. After the war some of the schools retained their nondiscriminatory practices, so the exclusion in nursing was less oppresive than in the higher status health professions (United States Public Health Service, 1950). In 1963 there were 22 segregated black schools operating; most of them were underfinanced and only 9 were accredited (Carnegie, 1964). A study of one segregated nursing school reported in 1971 documented the mental health and attitudinal consequences of this pattern and encouraged integrated nursing education (Gunter, Crecraft, and Kennedy, 1971). Since that time, the level of integration in nursing has improved, and nine percent of the nursing students are now black (Johnson, 1976). Nonetheless, the consequences of this discriminatory pattern remain evident in the present work force (Table 4): only 2 percent of the top-level professionals were classified as nonwhite, while 22 percent of the health service workers were members of nonwhite ethnic groups. Since approximately 12 percent of the total population is nonwhite, minorities are overrepresented in low-level jobs and underrepresented in high-status jobs (Bureau of Health Resources, 1974; Cogan, 1968).

THE STRATIFICATION PATTERNS
OF HEALTH CARE INSTITUTIONS

Up to this point in the discussion, the focus has been on the total health care industry. If the individual institution rather than the total health care delivery system is taken as the unit of analysis, it is again possible to note complex stratification systems and to see the impact of the stratification on the roles of its members. Since hospitals have been the subject of a significant body of sociologic inquiry, they will be the focus of this discussion; it should be noted, however, that many of the generalizations that have been made about hospitals could be applied to ambulatory care settings or nursing homes.

Evolution of the Hospital

Hospitals were an early medieval development. Although we can trace the rise of the Western hospital to the development of the concept of "Christian charity," there were parallel developments in the medieval Moslem world. Hospitals were originally generalized institutions, furnishing sanctuary for the poor, orphans, widows, and the aged as well as the sick. In the post-medieval period they gradually lost their more generalized functions and became lodging places for the sick poor and the victims of contagious illnesses or "pestilences," hence the name pest house is, somewhat paradoxically, a fairly recent term. (Clay, 1909; Rosen, 1963).

The bacteriologic revolution that occurred in the nineteenth century and the advent of the "trained nurse" revolutionized hospitals in the twentieth century. They were cleaned up to prevent cross infection and nursing care was markedly improved. The hospital became a place where one might well recover rather than die—in contrast to earlier history. Consequently, physicians moved their primary focus of practice from offices and patients' homes to the hospitals. Physicians had been almost unknown in the generalized medieval institutions, and even as hospitals became institutions for care of the sick, the physicians who entered them tended to be of lower status. Those university-trained physicians who were teachers with doctoral degrees treated their affluent patients in their homes. The physician's entry into the hospital in the twentieth century has been further stimulated by insurance company reimbursement policies that pay for hospital but not office procedures. While physician care is certainly a major factor in the improved recovery rates in hospitals, the presence of physicians has complicated the formal organization pattern of the institution. They are high-status, powerful professionals who essentially are outside the basic bureaucratic structure. That is, bureaucracies tend to be built upon clear lines of authority, written rules, and a hierarchical structure in which lower levels report to levels. Physicians complicate the structure because they are neither part of the hospital structure nor clearly clients of the hospital. In viewing the structural problem, one authority has described the hospital as "an organization at cross purposes with itself" (Smith, 1958). Nurses have tried to mediate this confusion but have never been completely successful (Croog and Ver-Steeg, 1972).

Economic Impact

In discussing the consequences of the steep stratification system of the health care industry, it may be well to start with the irrational elements in the system because they would seem to be the most ripe for reform. If we look at the economic implications of the steep status gradients—which seem to be further influenced by ethnic and sex discrimination—one finds marked salary differences. Current estimates of physicians' incomes place them well over $40,000 annually, although the 1970 census merely indicated that their incomes were in excess of $25,000. This figure is in sharp contrast with the salaries of male orderlies, approximately $4000 annually or less, and the salaries of female aides, $3000. Since there are more than 600,000 workers on the lowest rung of the ladder, their economic deprivation is not insignificant (U.S. Census Bureau, 1973). At the time the last census was taken, the Social Security Administration had pegged the poverty line for an urban family of four at $3700. Since the paycheck for the average nurses' aide fell below the poverty line, the aide might be better off quitting work and applying for welfare if there were children to support (U.S. Census Bureau, 1970). It is important to emphasize this marginal wage, since a few years ago during the war on poverty one of the strategies proposed for helping people escape from the debilitating consequences of the welfare "trap" was to train them for low-level jobs in health service fields (Reissman, 1969). Considering the salaries paid low-level health workers, particularly women, this strategy addresses only the cause of the problem rather than its solution. Reform is needed to bring the salaries of nurses' aides and other health service workers up to a reasonable level. Because the differentiation of the nursing role has given these workers crucial patient care responsibilities, their morale and performance are key elements in quality of care. In addition, it must be recognized that reasonable salaries are a prerequisite for attracting and retaining capable workers.

The disparity between levels and between men and women at the lowest level is only part of the economic picture. There are also significant differences between the male and female members of occupations at the higher levels. Female dentists earn only 29% of the amount earned by their male counterparts, while women physicians receive approximately 39% of the income earned by men in the field. In fact, women in the higher level professional fields seem to be closer in salary to middle-level technicians and nurses than they are to their male colleagues. By implication, it would appear that many of these women are used in the roles of assistant and technician rather than operating in their full professional capacity; so again, the discriminatory aspects of the system appear to have consequences for role performance.

However, a more important implication of sex segregation than income disparity in the system is the barrier to communication that is created between members of the health team. After studying one community hospital in depth, Duff and Hollingshead (1968) concluded that a lack of effective communication between the members of the health team, particularly between nurses and physicians, was a significant factor in explaining the poor patient care that they found. The communication gap that exists between nurses and physicians is not the normal one that occurs in complex organizations with multiple levels of workers; rather, it is an exaggerated one resulting from sex segregation with a peculiar stylized pattern that has been termed the doctor-nurse game. One of the best descriptions of the doctor-nurse game was written by a psychiatrist, Leonard Stein. He was fascinated by the strange way nurses made recommendations to physicians; as he observed, they pretended they had not done so. Physicians, in turn, pretended that nurses never made recommendations, yet Stein noted that the more highly regarded physicians were careful to follow nurses' recommendations. Stein called the pattern a *transactional neurosis* (Stein, 1967). It seems to be an exaggerated version of the traditional male-female game in which relatively powerless females gain power over men by manipulation. It is supported by reciprocal systems of reward and punishment, as well as by tradition. Most nurses are apparently unconscious of the game, yet they play it well and have been conditioned to do so throughout their professional lives. Unfortunately for patients, however, the tortured communication pattern of the game is not efficient. Crucial information is lost or its transmission slowed. Patient care suffers, and the dignity of both the nurse and physician roles is lessened. This seems to be another aspect of the system that needs reform.

Further Implications of Stratification

Even without its discriminatory aspects, the health care delivery system would still be highly stratified. Both the differentiation of the nursing role and the development of multiple medical technicians have fragmented and depersonalized hospital care. It is not unusual for a hospitalized patient to have contact with as many as 30 people in one day and yet feel lonely because the encounters are brief and impersonal. For example, consider the following hypothetical day of Mr. J.D., an ordinary postoperative patient with lung cancer:

> *Before breakfast, an aide checked his vital signs, a technician drew blood, and a registered nurse checked his chest tube and discontinued his intravenous fluid. An aide brought breakfast. The registered nurse returned with oral medication and a hypodermic for pain. The inhalation therapist helped him with Intermittent Positive Pressure Breathing (IPPB). A practical nurse helped him with his bath and allowed him to dangle his feet over the side of the bed. A messenger came to transport him to the x-ray department where a technician took chest x-rays.*

> *His surgeon stopped by (wearing his hospital "greens" with a mask around his neck); he checked the chest tube and said everything was fine. Another aide brought him water; a young woman from the diet kitchen asked him to select tomorrow's meals from a mimeographed menu; the inhalation therapist returned; a clerk from the business office brought insurance forms for him to sign and the television man came and replaced the set on the wall with another one that looked like the one he removed. Another aide brought him lunch.*

> *After lunch the head nurse came in carrying a clip board and asked Mr. J.D. how he felt, but she looked so busy he told her "fine." Another technician did an electrocardiogram. The practical nurse checked his vital signs and the janitor mopped the floor. He rang the bell once that afternoon to ask to have his urinal emptied. The ward clerk responded through the speaker using her "announcement" voice. She told him he would have to repeat the request, then she sent an aide. By three o'clock when the shift changed, Mr. J.D. had experienced 23 encounters with 18 different people. None of them stayed long*

enough for him to learn their names (he already knew the surgeon's name). He was unable to ask any of them the dreadful question that plagued him; he wanted to know if he was going to die.

Rationalizing the System

The process of breaking a role into its component parts and allocating the parts to individual workers in order to maximize efficiency is sometimes called rationalizing the system. Mr. J.D.'s experiences suggest that the nursing role has been rationalized to an *irrational* level. To a large extent nurses are aware of the negative consequences of role differentiation for patient care. In addition, many nurses feel personally deprived because the resultant fragmented roles are less satisfying to them (Kramer, 1974). Some of them also decry the fact that the role of the registered nurse has changed from that of direct patient care provider to that of coordinator, administrator, or technician. The nursing literature includes several papers addressing this role fragmentation, and nurses are urged to "come back to the bedside" to preserve the essense of nursing (Johnson, 1959; Norris, 1970; Reiter, 1966; Rogers, 1964).

To operationalize this suggestion, two related movements have emerged: in the mid-1960s the role of the clinical nurse specialist developed, while more recently there has been an experimental restructuring of hospital wards or units emphasizing primary nursing. Clinical specialists are nurses who have obtained educational preparation at the masters degree level—study designed to enable them to give expert care to seriously ill patients, act as role models, and spend time with patients who need emotional support (Riehl and McVay, 1973). Unfortunately, since the movement started in the educational system with nurse educators trying to reform the practice setting by preparing graduates to fill a new role, rather than in the service system itself, there have been problems institutionalizing the role. Since hospital and nurse administrators were the authors of the original differentiation of the nursing role, its reformation by educators—outsiders—has not been entirely successful. Some administrators have indicated that they are willing to accept clinical specialists if these nurses will also take on administrative roles, while others have suggested that clinical specialists should be willing to work for the same wages as basic registered nurses. Despite these obstacles to change, progress is being made in the acceptance of the specialists, at least in the more up-to-date centers.

A second, more recent effort to combat the fragmentation of care has been the development of primary nursing units. On these units the nursing team is replaced with registered or practical nurses who give total care on their shift to a group of patients, and plan for the patients' care on the other shifts. This gives the patient a person to whom he can relate (Brown, 1977; Marram, Schlegel, and Bevis, 1974).

Actually, these two movements are related. An early successful trial of clinical specialists used an administrative structure similar to the primary nursing model (Georgopoulos and Christman, 1973). Although the primary nursing approach sounds in many ways like a return to nursing care as it was delivered before the role was differentiated, it has some different elements. Probably the key element in its success is in the power that is given to the registered nurse when she is made accountable for a small group of patients, rather than simply using her in place of aides. In one California study, two models of primary care were compared: one in which primary nurses were held accountable for their patient load and one in which they were not. The nurses with the higher level of nursing responsibilities were found to produce the most favorable patient outcomes (Brault, 1976).

However, despite these countermovements aimed at reducing the fragmentation of patient care, it seems safe to assume that the overall picture will remain substantially unchanged relative to status differentials and that the health team will remain stratified. Once an occupational role has been created it is unlikely that anyone will consider eliminating that role or category. For example, there are nurses who believe that the role of oxygen therapist should never have developed because it is a narrow dead-end job that could have been handled by a nurse. This argument comes too late; oxygen therapists now exist and they want and need their jobs. Moreover, the teachers who prepare oxygen therapists want and need their jobs. Thus, the role has a momentum of its own. The same thing can be said for registered nurses or practical nurses, or any other category of health worker. As long as the occupation is cost effective and delivers a wanted service it will continue to exist.

IMPLICATIONS FOR THE PHYSICIAN'S ROLE

The differentiation of the physician's role that is occuring at the present time with the development of physicians' assistants and nurse practitioners has similar implications for the role of the physician. Using the differentiation of nursing as a model, it seems safe to say that medical care will become increasingly stratified. This will cause discontent among patients, who wish to have a warm personal relationship with their doctor rather than to be treated by the nurse practitioner. However, the new role may well improve patient care because physicians, preferring specialization, have already left the field of primary care underserved. Many physicians are being drawn away from the more emotionally satisfying role of primary care giver into teaching, supervisory, and coordinating roles. In the future, those who want to focus entirely on patient care will probably gravitate to the more complex specialties because at the primary care level they will have to compete with the lower salaried and lower status nurse practitioners. Thus, the trend towards specialization in medicine can be thought of as both a cause and a consequence of the differentiation of the physician's role. While recent figures suggest that family practice is growing in popularity, specialists still out number general practitioners by more than three to one.

STRATIFICATION AND THE CONSUMER ROLE

The professionalization of the high status health occupations and the increasing stratification of the health care delivery system is a significant factor in the current wave of consumer discontent. Consumers are expressing their discontent, not only in print, but more significantly in malpractice suits (Holder, 1975; Noble, 1976).

From the sociologic point of view, this growing social distance between the professions and their clients has some interesting implications. In this climate of consumer suspicion, the old concept of the "sick role" may well be out of date. The concept of the sick role as described by Talcott Parsons is a state in which patients are excused from their normal role responsibilities; but, in return, they are presumably obliged to comply with the medical regimen in order to get well. Physicians as described in this system were benevolent, knowledgeable authority figures who were not unlike fathers; patients were viewed as dependent, obedient, and childlike, although as they recovered they became less childlike (Parsons, 1951; Parsons and Fox, 1952). Conflict or even a legitimate difference of opinion is not a part of this conceptualization, although a failure to comply is possible and there is a growing body of sociologic literature that addresses the phenomenon of noncompliance with the medical regimen.

A more appropriate model of the patient role in light of the current state of affairs is the one proposed by Eliot Freidson (1960). He sees patients and providers as occupying different positions in the social system, and indicates that a clash in perspectives is not unexpected. According to Freidson, physicians are not just benevolent authority figures, they are members of a powerful monopoly who, by virtue of their position in the system, have the power not only to recognize illness but to define and even create it as a social role. In this respect, physicians are similar to judges and priests, who by their power to define can actually create crime and sin (Freidson, 1960, 1961, 1970). In *Professional Dominance*, Freidson extends his consideration of the medical monopoly to look at the power of physicians over other members of the health care team and the virtual inaccessibility of the health care industry to any effective consumer or quality control (Freidson, 1970). This approach necessarily modifies the "sick role" concept to include people who are ill but do not accept the childlike obedient stance, nor accept the physician and other health professionals as benevolent authority figures. These consumers want to be treated as adults and participate in decisions that are made about their health care.

SUMMARY

In this chapter the concept of stratification was reviewed. It was argued that the health care delivery system is highly stratified and several factors were advanced to explain this situation. Health care is a large and complex system marked by professionalization at the high-status levels and poverty at the lower levels. It is a labor-intensive system that has tried to cope with its economic problems by breaking up the medical role and differentiating the nursing role. The current differentiation of the medical role that seems to have started with the development of nurse practitioners and physicians' assistants was also discussed. Race and sex discrimination have entered into the system as irrational stratification variables.

Individual health care institutions are also stratified, and at this level the situation is made more complex by the emergence of physicians as high-status professionals who have complicated the functioning of the bureaucratic institutions.

The implications of this stratification system were traced. The steep gradient of the system is in many ways dysfunctional—blocking opportunities, making communication difficult, and fragmenting care. Although the system is obviously in need of reform, it is suggested that the broad picture will probably not be altered significantly in the near future.

8

Cultural Factors as a Source of Influence on the Health Professions

SANDRA MacKAY

INTRODUCTION

This chapter focuses on the training American physicians receive in the larger medical institutions. Because physicians are to a great extent "controllers" of the practice of other health-related professionals—a point explicated elsewhere in this volume—it is important to examine the basis of their beliefs and rationale for practice. These beliefs have consequences for the practice of those who occupy supportive or subordinate roles to physicians. To the extent that physicians take on or relinquish certain aspects of intervention in the treatment of the sick, there will be an accompanying realignment of the functions of other health professionals. That is, a number of role relationships will be altered. Nonphysician health care providers may be forced to negotiate newer roles for themselves in order to exercise fully their unique potential in the care and treatment of the sick. The perspective outlined here will, it is hoped, provide some insights into the nature of the socialization of physicians. The socialization process described here takes place within the context of an innovative physician-role-training program.

The training program at Inner City Hospital,[1] which was initiated in July 1974, represented an attempt on the part of one medical college to augment the number of physicians providing community-based primary care to consumers. As will be explained presently, the physician as primary care

177

practitioner represents what has generally been considered a less-valued medical role by the majority of physicians. Therefore, the transition from medical student to practitioner role for those in the Inner City program was attended by more than a usual amount of role strain. That is, the trainee was not only expected to take on a new role but one that was not highly regarded by his peers-to-be.

A brief overview of the cultural context within which American physicians are trained should be helpful in understanding both the traditional role of physicians and some of the cognitive dissonance surrounding emergent roles. As with other roles in the health care system, an explication of physician roles must consider the organization within which training takes place. Accordingly, attention is also directed here toward developing a deeper understanding of the kinds of organizations that are involved in the training of physicians in the two specialties most closely associated with primary care—internal medicine and pediatrics.

The majority of the data reported in this chapter are based on approximately one year of participant observation experience. In the course of this experience, I was privileged to observe first-hand some of the ways in which cultural factors influence physician training.

Despite the obvious need for more primary care physicians, there are fewer primary care training programs in existence than one might reasonably expect. Of the 114 medical schools in the country in 1975, 96 schools were teaching family medicine, but only 35 were involved in primary care programs. In other words, out of 131 programs available to medical students, no more than one-quarter were clearly identified with primary care (JAMA, 1975, p. 1344). At the graduate level, primary care training programs were even rarer. When the program described here became operational, only four primary care programs had been established within pediatric departments, and an equally small number of programs were available to medical house-officers who were interested in obtaining primary care experience during their internship and residency years. In spite of the scarcity of primary care educational programs and the fact that experts in the health field believe that the lack of a reliable system for primary or general medical care is the major problem in contemporary American medicine (McDermott, 1975, p. 34; Pellegrino, 1973, p. 47; Rogers, 1974, p. 224; White, 1971, p. 119), not enough is being done to alleviate the problem of inadequate primary care.

DEFINITIONS AND ASSUMPTIONS

Reduced to its barest essentials, the term *culture* is used by anthropologists to describe the way of life of a people:

The extreme generality, diffuseness and variability of man's innate (i.e., genetically programmed) response capacities means that without the assistance of cultural patterns, he would be functionally incomplete, not merely a talented ape who had, like some underprivileged child, unfortunately been prevented from realizing his full potentialities, but a kind of formless monster with neither sense of direction nor power of self-control, a chaos of spasmodic impulses and vague emotions (Geertz, 1972, p. 171).

However, because man is a symbol-using animal, ideas, attitudes, acts, and even material objects have meanings attached to them. These meanings are learned in relationship to other cultural traits as part of a particular world view; they are not imprinted in man as part of his genetic heritage. Because cultural patterns are models not only for perceiving reality, but for human constructions of that reality (Geertz, 1972; Harris, 1975; White, 1959), they have the power to "give objective conceptual form to social and psychological reality both by shaping themselves to it and by shaping it to themselves" (Geertz, 1972, p. 169). Since it is an underlying assumption of this book that role stress is a social structural condition, and that the subjective state of role strain is increasingly prevalent in modern health care settings, it makes sense to look at the institutions that train physicians, since the values and beliefs that these teaching hospitals impart contribute to the shortage of primary care physicians, as well as directly and indirectly affecting the roles of other health workers. For example, in the course of my own fieldwork, it was apparent that the shortage of primary care physicians created a situation in which clinical nurse specialists and nurse practitioners were hired to perform many clinical activities, such as taking a history, ordering tests, conducting a physical examination, and so forth—tasks that once were the sole prerogative of physicians—and that this practice, in turn, created gaps in administrative areas that had to be filled by others.

Primary care is health care oriented to the individual and family within the personal system of health care, rather than through the public health system. It is designed to provide "first-contact" medical care and longitudinal responsibility for care, whether disease is present or not. It is distinct, therefore, from treatment that is provided by physicians acting on a referral basis or by those who provide only secondary and tertiary medical services—highly sophisticated, technologically oriented medical care, such as the care of patients receiving vital-organ transplants—within the hospital. For whenever any other medical services are needed, the primary care physician is expected to function as the "patient's advocate" in the medical system, coordinating and integrating all of the other services for the patient. At the present time, general practitioners, internists, and pediatricians all have substantial primary care responsibilities. These, therefore, are the three groups that are usually mentioned as the "family doctors" of the future. However, the discussion in this chapter will be limited to a consideration of internists and pediatricians.

The reason for concentrating on internists and pediatricians will be clearer if the trend from general practitioners to specialists is taken into account. In the past, personal health care has always been provided by physicians in private practice. However, as Fahs and Peterson (1968) point out, we are currently witnessing the decline of general practice as an attractive career in this country (Fig. 1). This means that as older general practitioners either die or retire, they are not being replaced by younger physicians in the same field; hence, general practitioners will become extinct around the turn of the century.

More recent projections by the U.S. Department of Health, Education, and Welfare support these conclusions (Table 1). There were 66,870 general practitioners in 1963 and 56,266 in 1970; however, using 1972 first-year residency positions to predict future career patterns, there are expected to be only 36,510 general practitioners by 1990. Thus by 1980

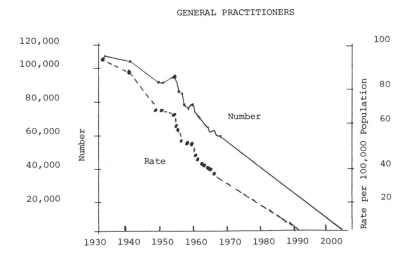

GENERAL PRACTITIONERS

FIGURE 1 Recent changes in the number and ratio of general practitioners in the United States, with furture projections. *Source: Fahs and Peterson: "Recent Changes in Numbers and Ratio of General Practitioners Per 100,000 Population, With Future Projections" in Public Health Reports 83:267, 1968.*

TABLE 1

NUMBER OF ACTIVE PHYSICIANS BY SPECIALTY:
ACTUAL 1963 and 1970; PROJECTED 1980 and 1990

Activity and Specialty	Number of Physicians				Percentage Distribution			
	1963	1970	1980	1990	1963	1970	1980	1990
General practice	66,870	56,260	47,140	36,510	25.6	18.1	10.9	6.4
Family practice	—	1,690	6,610	12,630	—	0.5	1.5	2.2
Internal medicine	30,430	41,870	71,650	106,880	11.6	13.5	16.7	18.7
Pediatrics	12,930	18,820	32,150	47,830	4.9	6.0	7.5	8.4
Surgical specialties	67,005	85,380	128,970	180,810	25.6	27.4	30.0	31.7
Other specialties	84,495	107,190	143,720	186,370	32.3	34.5	33.4	32.6
Total Active MDs	261,730	311,210	430,240	571,030	100.0	100.0	100.0	100.0

Source: U.S. Department of Health, Education, and Welfare, 1974, Table 40a, p. 75 (1963 figures, Table 34, p. 67 and Table 30, p. 60).

181

internal medicine can be expected to supply more primary care physicians than will general practice; and by 1990, internal medicine and pediatrics will be the two principal sources of primary care physicians in the United States (U.S. Department of Health, Education, and Welfare 1974, pp. 60, 67, 74-76).

To be sure, some of the decline in general practice will be offset by physicians entering the new specialty of family practice. However, before proceeding further, a few words of caution about interpreting family practice statistics may be in order. Most important, perhaps, is that there were no departments of family medicine in American medical schools until recently. Thus, when the first family practice boards were given on a pilot basis to 2,087 physicians in February of 1970, 99 percent of those taking the boards were members of The American Academy of General Practice and only 1 percent were graduates of approved, three-year residency programs in family medicine (Geyman 1971, p. 19). Furthermore, John P. Geyman, Chairman of the Division of Family Practice at The University of Utah College of Medicine, predicts that for at least the first decade following the establishment of a specialty board in Family Practice, the largest source of new physicians in this field will be drawn from the ranks of general practitioners. In line with this, manpower data from the U.S. Department of Health, Education, and Welfare (1974, p. 67) show that even though the number of family practioners increased from 1,690 in 1970 to 4,542 by 1972, most of this increase can be attributed to general practitioners who converted to family practice by taking their boards in that specialty.

Although no thoroughly satisfactory survey has been made of the entire primary care manpower situation in the United States, data provided by the Academy of Family Practice indicate that as of 1973 there were only 413 graduates of family practice programs in this country (Table 2). Family medicine appears to be gaining popularity, as there were 314 graduates in 1974, 565 in 1975, 872 in 1976, 1,190 in 1977, and, according to current enrollment figures, there will be 1,595 graduated in 1978; but since the total number of graduates from family practice programs will be only 4,952 physicians by July 1, 1978, it is still too early to predict whether family practice programs will continue to flourish in the coming decades.

What does this mean in terms of the availability of primary care physicians? Certainly, it is clear that large-scale demands for primary health care cannot be met as they have been in the past. Because the ratio of primary care physicians has *dropped* from 90 physicians per 100,000 people in 1931 to only 55 physicians per 100,000 people by 1973, even if one combines general and family practitioners with general internists and pediatricians as "family doctors," there are not enough physicians to meet the existing demands for primary care in this country (Table 3). This shortage cannot be attributed to any lack of physician manpower: at the same time that there

TABLE 2

ENROLLMENT AND GRADUATION TRENDS
IN FAMILY PRACTICE PROGRAMS:
1973-1978

	1973[a]	1974	1975	1976	1977	1978[b]
Number of residents	1,771	2,671	3,720	4,675	5,421	
Number of graduates	416	314	565	872	1,190	1,598

Source: American Academy of Family Practice (personal communication).
[a]*Graduates as of 1973.*
[b]*Expected graduates based on 1977 enrollment.*

has been a growing disparity between the availability of primary care physicians and the population size, the overall supply of physicians has been increasing. Whereas there were only 119 physicians per 100,000 people in 1931, there were 130 physicians per 100,000 people by 1973.

While it might be assumed that the presence of a medical school in a city would increase the number of physicians providing medical care to the sickest patients, this is not always the case. One of the many results of the declining standard of living within the inner cities of the United States has been the deterioration of community-based medical services available to this population. To illustrate this point, Boston has three medical schools, yet the number of general practioners practicing in this city declined by more than 50 percent from 1941 to 1961. Over this same twenty-year period, the distribution of internists and pediatricians became so markedly skewed that 90 percent of these primary care physicians were practicing in the most affluent neighborhoods, which comprised only 40 percent of the population (Dorsey 1969, p. 429-440). By 1971 the situation had deteriorated to the point where Dr. Andrew P. Sackett, Boston's commissioner of Health and Hospitals, declared, "There are areas of Boston that are deserts as far as medical care is concerned. . . . A whole system of medical care has collapsed" (Greenberg 1971, p. 118). In the worst ghettos, infant mortality was nine times higher than the national average and fifteen times higher than that of a nearby affluent suburban community. Nevertheless, most of the medical care that the poorest inner city residents received came from the emergency rooms and specialty clinics of Boston City Hospital (Greenberg 1971, p. 97, 100). Similarly, in 1940 physicians were fairly evenly distributed in Baltimore according to

TABLE 3

RATIO OF PRIMARY CARE AND ALL OTHER PHYSICIANS PER 100,000 POPULATION FOR THE UNITED STATES

Physician Category	1931	1940	1949	1958	1967	1973
Total physicians	150,385	156,970	173,129	179,485	247,256	270,412
Population (in 100,000s)	1240.4	1325.9	1497.7	1748.8	1986.3	2080.9
Physicians (per 100,000)	119.8	118.4	115.6	102.7	124.5	130.0
Primary care physicians						
general and family practice	82.4	90.6	73.7	39.2	36.2	27.9
general internal medicine	4.1	4.9	7.7	9.9	16.6	19.3
general pediatrics	3.1	1.8	2.9	5.3	7.2	8.0
Other physicians						
internal medicine subspecialty	NA	.5	1.3	2.1	2.0	4.3
pediatric subspecialty	NA	NA	NA	NA	.1	.3
dermatology	.8	.7	1.1	1.4	1.6	1.8

neurology and psychiatry	1.7	1.8	3.2	4.6	8.5	9.5
general surgery	10.7	5.0	8.1	13.0	13.9	14.3
neurosurgery	NA	NA	NA	.5	1.0	1.2
obstetrics and gynecology	5.2	1.9	3.4	7.3	8.0	8.8
orthopedic surgery	0.7	0.8	1.4	2.1	3.7	4.5
plastic surgery	NA	NA	NA	0.3	0.6	0.9
ophthalmology	NA	NA	NA	NA	4.1	4.6
otolaryngology	6.8	5.7	6.2	6.0	2.5	2.3
urology	1.9	1.3	1.5	1.9	2.4	2.7
anesthesiology	0.4	0.2	0.8	2.4	4.3	5.2
pathology	0.6	0.7	1.2	1.6	3.5	4.0
radiology	1.4	1.2	1.9	2.7	4.7	6.2
physical medicine and rehabilitation	NA	NA	0.2	0.2	0.4	0.5
other	NA	1.2	1.2	2.2	2.2	2.5

Source: Institute of Medicine, Social Security Studies Final Report Medicare-Medicaid Reimbursement Policies. National Academy of Sciences, March 1976, Table 2, p. 251.

185

Drs. M. Alpert Haynes and Michael Garvey and primary care services were readily available in most communities. However, by 1969, there were only 15 private physicians delivering primary medical services to 100,000 people in the vicinity of Johns Hopkins and no new primary care physician had opened an office in that area within the last twelve years. Ironically, this ratio was "lower than that of some so-called developing countries" (Norman 1969: 117-120), even though Maryland has long had more than its share of the nation's physicians. In 1963, Maryland had 163 physicians delivering patient care services per 100,000 population (Theodore and Haug 1968, p. 14); and in 1973, it had one of the highest physician-population ratios in the nation (Institute of Medicine 1976, p. 253). Boston and Baltimore are not unique: in many cities the outpatient department of a teaching hospital is replacing the personal physician as a source of primary medical care for the inner city poor.

In a society which is still dependent on physicians in private practice for most of its medical care, the consequences of this distribution pattern are obviously of grave concern. Indeed, one of the many results of the declining standard of living within the inner cities of the United States has been the deterioration of medical services available to this population. Already a substantial proportion of the medical care that the poorest inner-city residents receive comes from the emergency rooms and outpatient clinics of large teaching hospitals. The propensity for fragmenting services and dehumanizing care in these settings is so well known that it needs no further comment here. However, it is worth mentioning that the hopes for community-controlled neighborhood health centers—centers established during the 1960s to change this picture—have not been fully realized either; even the strongest neighborhood health centers find it extremely difficult to recruit and retain well-qualified physicians. Ironically, these are the same problems that have plagued outpatient departments of hospitals for years. Therefore, it is important to consider the possibility that the roots for such perennial difficulties may lie within the medical culture itself. For how else can one account for the low prestige accorded ambulatory medicine or the saying in medical circles that "the *outs* work in the outpatient department, while the *ins* take care of inpatients"? Indeed, largely because of the significance of such views, one of the most difficult places to start a new training program for physicians is the outpatient department of a major teaching hospital. As Mumford notes, because of the tendency to downgrade work in clinics, the best teachers are seldom found in the outpatient department, and faculty rank is likely to be at least a step lower if one's major allegiance is not to the inpatient service (Mumford 1970, pp. 195-196).

Nevertheless, the outpatient department is precisely where most of the training in primary care is likely to take place. Data presented by

Parker indicate that private physicians, outpatient departments, and emergency rooms were the three major sources of primary care in 1969, and that together they accounted for 86 percent of all visits falling into the primary care category (Parker, 1974, pp. 26-27). Furthermore, since it is known that almost one-half of all visits made to physicians for ambulatory care in 1975 were made to physicians in general or family practice (Koch, 1977, p. 18-19), and in light of the recent trends in this field, there is little doubt about the future significance of the outpatient department.

Thus, there are at least two reasons why it is important to pay close attention to patterns of practice in teaching hospitals. First, these hospitals provide most of the medical care that is available to low-income people, and can be expected to play an increasingly important role in the care of middle-income people as well. Second, a large number of physicians take a substantial part of their training in these hospitals. I have chosen to focus on these two reasons because I think that they are inextricably linked. However, there is an additional reason that is worthy of attention. The available evidence suggests that the medical profession has been attempting to retain its dominant position within the present high-technology field by strengthening its organizational base. The evidence for this statement is largely based on an analysis of the trends that are developing within teaching hospitals. Let us examine some of the changes that are taking place in these hospitals and the implications for primary care of their association with medical schools.

MEDICAL TRAINING AND THE
TREND TOWARD AFFILIATION

Until recently, most of the graduate medical training in this country was not under the control of medical schools. Even as late as 1965 only 27 percent of the hospitals with approved internship and residency programs were affiliated with medical schools (AMA, 1974-75). Yet over the next decade a remarkable change occurred (Table 4). Within five years, 55 percent of the hospitals with such programs had become formally affiliated with a medical school; and by 1975, the figure had risen to 67 percent. As Table 4 shows, of the 550 hospitals which became affiliated during the first five years, 329 hospitals (60 percent) developed major medical school affiliations extending to all levels of training. Since this mode of affiliation remained dominant throughout the decade ending in 1975, it is clearly the type of affiliation preferred over all others. One important reason for this is that major affiliations provide the kind of organizational structure in which it is possible to integrate all levels of medical training.

TABLE 4

TRAINING IN HOSPITALS AFFILIATED WITH MEDICAL SCHOOLS

Hospitals by Type of Affiliation

Directory Year	Hospital Affiliation			Affiliated Hospitals		Unaffiliated Hospitals		Total Hospitals With Programs*
	Major	Limited	Graduate	No.	(%)	No.	(%)	
1965-66	187	116	66	369	(27)	1017	(73)	1386
1966-67	275	141	101	517	(38)	850	(62)	1367
1967-68	339	137	121	607	(40)	905	(60)	1512
1968-69	327	174	120	631	(45)	781	(55)	1412
1969-70	376	182	141	699	(48)	750	(52)	1449
1970-71	516	243	160	919	(55)	766	(45)	1685
1971-72	567	288	141	996	(59)	696	(41)	1692
1972-73	473	276	134	888	(61)	573	(39)	1461
1973-74	694	364	107	1165	(68)	546	(32)	1711
1974-75	714	317	105	1136	(67)	547	(33)	1683

*Data included on non-inpatient institutions with residencies in preventive medicine.

Adapted from: American Medical Association, Directory of Approved Residencies 1974-75, p. 20. Copyright 1976, American Medical Association.

It is relevant to note that by the time the trend toward academic affiliation leveled off in the mid-1970s, the majority of hospitals with approved internship programs were already affiliated with a medical school (Table 5). In addition, as has been true for a number of years, internship programs generally took place in the largest hospitals. In 1972, 84 percent of all internship programs were in hospitals that had at least 300 beds. Of major significance, however, is the fact that 34 percent of the programs in the affiliated hospitals were in hospitals of 500 beds or more, while only 19 percent were in nonaffiliated hospitals of the same size. This emphasis upon large scale has enormous implications for primary care programs. When the primary care residency program began in 1974, the average hospital in this country had only 211 beds (Denton, 1976, p. 22). Yet by 1974, 44 percent of the affiliated programs (in contrast to only 27 percent of the nonaffiliated programs) were in hospitals with a minimum of 500 beds.

As might be expected, the group of affiliated hospitals also trained most of the physicians in the two fields most closely associated with primary care. As of 1973, more than 80 percent of the rotating internships in which either internal medicine or pediatrics was stressed were in affiliated institutions. And in the more prestigious specialty programs, such as those at Inner City Hospital, affiliation was even more common. By 1973, there were 311 internship programs in internal medicine, and 90 percent of these programs were in hospitals with medical schools. In pediatrics there were 89 comparable first-year programs, of which 91 percent were in affiliated hospitals (AMA, 1974-75, p. 2). Given the fact that it is virtually impossible to gain approval for single-specialty or "straight" internship programs in these specialties without also providing concurrent training for residents, affiliated hospitals actually monopolized the training of internists and pediatricians in the United States (AMA, 1973-74, pp. 2, 34-36).

There is some evidence that the trend toward affiliation slowed down, however, when medical schools were required to become involved in teaching in those hospitals that attracted a large number of foreign physicians. Inspection of the number of foreign-trained physicians in American hospitals—a fairly sensitive indicator of such hospitals' prestige—reveals a 3 to 1 ratio of American and Canadian graduates to graduates of foreign medical schools in affiliated hospitals, but a 1 to 2.5 ratio of these graduates in the nonaffiliated hospitals. Since it is known that affiliated hospitals are able to recruit at least 90 percent of the available house staff in this country, i.e., interns and residents, it appears that both medical schools and their graduates avoid less prestigious hospitals (AMA, 1974-75, p. 5), just as they avoid less prestigious programs. Given the strong trend toward affiliation earlier in this decade, this avoidance not only tends to isolate weaker hospitals and their staffs, but also helps to create a two-class system of medical

TABLE 5

INTERNSHIP PROGRAMS BY MEDICAL SCHOOL
AFFILIATION AND BED CAPACITY: 1972 and 1974

Classification	1972 Hospitals No.	(%)	1972 Programs No.	(%)	1974 Hospitals No.	(%)	1974 Programs No.	(%)
Affiliated hospitals								
Combined Hospitals	101	(14)	246	(7)	66	(15)	250	(16)
200 beds	50	(7)	87	(3)	18	(4)	65	(4)
200-299 beds	75	(11)	163	(5)	28	(7)	53	(4)
300-499 beds	236	(34)	1618	(51)	155	(36)	478	(32)
500 beds	241	(34)	1078	(34)	166	(38)	675	(44)
Totals	703	(100)	3190	(100)	433	(100)	1521	(100)

Nonaffiliated hospitals								
Combined Hospitals	4	(2)	12	(2)	4	(5)	15	(6)
200 beds	18	(10)	28	(3)	6	(7)	14	(5)
200-299 beds	48	(27)	101	(13)	20	(24)	56	(20)
300-499 beds	84	(47)	492	(63)	35	(42)	114	(42)
500 beds	27	(14)	145	(19)	18	(22)	75	(27)
Totals	180	(100)	778	(100)	83	(100)	274	(100)
Grand Totals	883	(100)	3968	(100)	516	(100)	1795	(100)

Sources: American Medical Association, Directory of Approved Internships and Residencies 1973-74; Department of Graduate Medical Evaluation, "Graduate Medical Education," JAMA 236, (1976), Table 5, p. 2974. Copyright 1976, American Medical Association.

training in this country. This situation may have short-term advantages for primary care, but it is likely to have long-term disadvantages.

The extent to which medical training is concentrated within a minority of exceptionally large and influential institutions is also worth noting, especially since these hospitals are not representative of the community hospitals in this country with respect to numbers of specialists, complexity of organization and physician training programs. As shown in Table 6, the majority of hospitals in the United States do not take part in training physicians. There were 7061 hospitals in this country in 1972; however, counting both the affiliated and the nonaffiliated institutions, only 25 percent of the existing hospitals participated in training physicians. Similarly, while the total number of hospitals increased to 7174 by 1974, the number of hospitals involved in training physicians decreased slightly. An examination of hospitals with medical schools indicates that the number of affiliated hospitals remained virtually constant during this brief period, but that the percentage of hospital beds which these institutions controlled increased from 29 to 42 percent. As a result, by 1974 affiliated hospitals controlled 80 percent of all the beds used for teaching purposes. Moreover, in both of these years, hospitals with major medical school affiliations accounted for only 10 percent of the country's hospitals, yet this small group controlled 39 percent of the beds used for teaching purposes in 1972 and 47 percent in 1974.

It appears, at least from a structural point of view, that American medical training is developing into a two-class system in which the dominant pattern is characterized by vertical integration of all levels of professional training and by the concentration of training efforts within a minority of exceptionally large and influential hospitals. And as has been demonstrated, these institutions have been reluctant to establish primary care training programs.

Thus, given the emphasis on and the prevalence of specialty training for medical school graduates, it is not surprising that the largest number of physicians entering practice choose roles as specialists rather than as generalists. In turn, this role patterning has implications for the role assignments of other professionals and paraprofessionals who participate in medical care delivery.

THE PREVAILING MEDICAL CULTURE IN THE UNITED STATES

A two-class pattern, not surprisingly, is what one could expect to find given the prevailing medical culture in the United States. In this culture, large,

TABLE 6

RELATIONSHIP OF HOSPITAL AFFILIATION TO U.S. HOSPITAL BEDS: 1972 and 1974

	1972					1974				
	No. of Hospitals	% of Hospitals	No. of Beds	% of Teaching Beds	% of Total Beds	No. of Hospitals	% of Hospitals	No. of Beds	% of Teaching Beds	% of Total Beds
Hospitals with approved programs										
Major medical school affiliation	697	10	255,023	39	16	752	10	375,927	47	25
Limited medical school affiliation	364	5	149,439	23	10	301	4	221,531	28	14
Graduate medical school affiliation	107	2	42,764	6	3	115	2	39,063	5	3
Total Affiliated	1,165	17	447,266	69	29	1,168	16	636,521	80	42
No medical school affiliation	546	8	200,471	31	13	503	7	156,744	—	10
Totals	1,711	25	647,697	100	42	1,671	23	793,265	100	52
Hospitals without approved programs	5,350	75	901,968		58	5,503	77	719,419		48
Grand Totals	7,061	100	1,549,665	100	100	7,174	100	1,512,684	100	100

Source: American Medical Association, Directory of Approved Internships and Residencies 1973-74, p. 19; Department of Graduate Medical Evaluation, "Graduate Medical Education," JAMA 236, (1976), Table 25, p. 2989. Copyright 1976, American Medical Association.

urban teaching hospitals with their approved graduate training programs and major medical school affiliations are often looked upon as "islands of excellence in a sea of mediocrity" by those associated with them (Knowles 1966, pp. 33-34). There are attempts both to impose inferior status on physicians who work elsewhere, and, to convince those physicians who want to strive for excellence that they should remain at a strong teaching hospital. Obviously, such ethnocentric views create an environment that is less than conducive to educating physicians for primary care. Indeed, the discrepancy between the demand for more primary health care and the production of physicians interested in this type of practice may be found in the attitudes and values which the teaching hospitals impart. For if structural considerations were all that mattered, it would be hard to find two medical subspecialties more suitably organized for integrating primary care training into every level of professional training than internal medicine and pediatrics.

Although medical academicians are not the only ones who display a high degree of ethnocentrism, such physicians are apt to be emulated by physicians-in-training. Research conducted more than 20 years ago on professional socialization during medical school (Becker et al., 1961) indicated that students are both coerced and guided into patterns of professional behavior that conform to the expectations and values of authority figures. Their conformity may be relatively superficial, as Becker and his colleagues (1961) discovered at the University of Kansas Medical School, or, in those cases where the students and their faculty are on somewhat better terms with one another, medical students may be socialized over a four-year period into roles that are more and more congruent with the faculty's own values and interests (Bloom, 1971; Merton et al., 1957). Clearly, there are numerous subcultural factors that affect relationships among physicians in different types of hospitals; however, until anthropologists conduct studies of such factors, we shall have to make use of the data that is now available.

Recent work carried out by Mumford (1970) indicates that most beginning physicians are initiated into the practice of medicine in such a way that older, more experienced physicians in the setting exert "direct, sometimes round-the-clock and near exclusive, influence or control" over them. All of this takes place in a "life-or-death" atmosphere that heightens the emotional intensity of the experience and establishes life-long patterns of behavior (Mumford, 1970, pp. 1-2). For as one physician told me, "internship is the crucible in which the identity of the physician is forged."

Studies of this type suggest that physicians-in-authority have a major influence on roles at all stages of training. Indeed, in 1975, when 3569 graduates of medical schools were asked to rank the importance of various factors influencing their choice of a speciality, 47 percent considered faculty members among the three most important factors in determining their future career choice (Institute of Medicine, 1976, pp. 295-296). Although the effect of graduate medical training on specialty choice has not been extensively examined, it is possible that physicians-in-authority have their greatest impact during internship. Despite subcultural variations in the norms that are established in these settings, it is clear from Mumford's (1970) work that physicians-in-training structure their professional behavior so that it conforms to the expectations of the particular setting where they train. This is not surprising when one considers that at teaching hospitals, including Inner City Hospital, access to each succeeding level of training requires the approval of a given department chairman. In addition, as Table 7 shows, there is a pyramiding of positions in both medicine and pediatrics. Under such conditions, it is considered essential to obtain a good recommendation whether one intends to remain at the training hospital or go elsewhere.

INNER CITY HOSPITAL

While it is true that standards for specialty programs are established at the national level, these standards are in fact flexible enough so that each teaching hospital can develop its own series of clinical experiences that will meet the formal criteria attached to the standards. This means, of course, that one of the best indicators of which clinical experiences are most highly valued in a department is the amount of scheduled time allotted to them throughout the year. At Inner City Hospital, the medical and pediatric departments were

TABLE 7

PYRAMIDAL STRUCTURE OF HOUSEOFFICER POSITIONS AT INNER CITY HOSPITAL: 1974-1975		
	Number of Positions	
Position	**Medicine**	**Pediatrics**
Chief resident	2	2
Senior resident	18	7
Assistant resident	33	11
Intern	36	13
Total	89	33

in separate buildings. As Table 8 shows, there were differences between
the kinds of clinical experiences considered important by the senior physicians in medicine and in pediatrics as measured by alloted time.

TABLE 8

NUMBER OF INTERNSHIP ROTATIONS OF 4 WEEKS TO 1 MONTH		
Service	Medicine	Pediatrics
Emergency outpatient	3	4
Ward	5	4
Ward (night float)	1	—
Intensive care*	1	3
Chronic disease, long-term hospital	1	1
Other†	1	1

*In medicine either on the intensive care unit or the coronary care unit; in pediatrics
experience in the intensive care nursery.

†In medicine at the affiliated medical school hospital; in pediatrics on the pediatric
surgical service.

In both specialties, rotations (time spent by an intern on each
service) were divided into blocks of time lasting several weeks. In medicine,
the rotations corresponded to the calendar months, whereas in pediatrics
they were based on blocks of four weeks. Taking these differences into consideration, medical and pediatric interns had roughly equivalent emergency
outpatient experience, similar exposure to another service within the medical
center, and comparable experience with the chronically ill, long-term patients
at an extramural medical facility. However, in both internal medicine and
pediatrics most of the rotations were devoted to acute care, "life-or-death
medicine," in which contact with the patient was strictly episodic (58 percent
of the time in internal medicine and 54 percent of the time in pediatrics). In
medicine, this episodic experience included six rotations on medical wards
(counting the "night float" rotation) and one rotation in either the intensive
care unit or the coronary care unit. In pediatrics, the seven rotations were
divided into four ward rotations and three rotations in the intensive care
nursery. Thus, despite some minor variations between these departments,
the overall pattern of clinical experiences was similar: very little time was
spent in primary care activities. Even in the primary care program itself,
only about 10 percent of the first year was devoted to primary care

experiences, and for the greater part of the time trainees were expected to function in either internal medicine or pediatrics.

Selection of Interns
at Inner City Hospital

At the time that the primary care program was initiated, Inner City Hospital was a 500-bed teaching hospital with major medical school affiliations and a long and distinguished tradition of training clinically oriented physicians. Consequently, it recruited students from some of the most prominent medical schools in the nation, (e.g., Harvard, Yale, Columbia, Pennsylvania, and the University of Washington, among other well-known schools). In addition, this hospital was affectionately spoken of in medical circles as "an interns' hospital," because of the unusually challenging clinical training that it provided and because interns were reputed to play a major role in this setting.

In 1973, when the decision was made to reorganize medical care under only one medical school rather than three as had been the case, the Department of Medicine had 500 applicants for 36 internship positions, and the Department of Pediatrics had 100 applicants for only 12 positions. In other words, there were 14 applicants for each internship position in medicine and 8 applicants for each internship position in pediatrics.

The following year, when prospective trainees were applying for internship positions, Inner City Hospital once again had a large pool of academically talented, highly recommended individuals competing for a small number of first-year positions. Only one new position had been added in pediatrics, however, so there were then 13 positions available in that specialty, as compared with 36 positions available in medicine. This is important to note since there was no separate matching program for primary care applicants. Those who were interested in primary care careers had to compete for a straight internship position in either medicine or pediatrics before they were eligible to be considered for acceptance into the innovative program. The rationale used to justify this double-screening procedure was that it would ensure "a higher quality program," and that a "separate track" for primary care would only create a group of "second class citizens" in the medical center. In other words, there was an implicit assumption that primary care applicants might somehow be inferior to applicants for the regular training programs. Nevertheless, the enthusiasm for primary care among young physicians was evident; when the selection committees met on June 10, 1974, there were twice as many applicants for the new program as there were available positions.

Admission to the primary care option for these new trainees

represented an important phase in their continuing socialization into the medical culture. Since, as I have documented above, specialty practice is the prevailing trend in medicine, it may be useful to examine some of the attitudes and expectations held by those individuals choosing a nontraditional training field with respect to the newer roles they would be expected to take on.

A Profile of Attitudes, Values, and Expectations of the Beginning Intern

A questionnaire was administered to all medical and pediatric interns during their orientation period. This questionnaire covered a wide range of topics about work, including future career plans, attitudes towards patients and staff, and the kinds of experiences that were most highly valued. The data provided a profile of some of the important similarities and differences between interns in the primary care program and interns in the specialty programs. Thus, it was possible to gain some insight into the self conceptions of these physicians at the beginning of the training year, before they had any actual experience working in either of the two programs.

The availability of the primary care training program "strongly encouraged" or "encouraged" 86 percent of the trainees to apply to Inner City Hospital, but according to the questionnaire responses it had little impact on those who chose the traditional internship. Only 32 percent of the traditional or regular interns reported being similarly influenced by this program. Nevertheless, interns who took their training at this hospital had several features in common. As a group, they can be characterized as clinically oriented physicians who were much more interested in developing new clinical skills and knowledge than in learning how to carry out research. All of the interns responded that it was "very important" or "moderately important" to gain new clinical skills in a training program, and all of the trainees and 87 percent of the regular interns felt the same way about gaining new medical knowledge. This is in sharp contrast to their attitudes about research skills. All of the trainees and 87 percent of the regular interns believed that it was "not important" or only "somewhat important" to prepare for a career in research. In keeping with their interests in patient care, all of the primary care interns and 98 percent of the regular interns considered it "very important" or "moderately important" to assume major responsibility for their patients' care during their training period. In addition, they indicated that they wished to assume responsibility not only for patients who were hospitalized, but also wanted the opportunity to follow their patients in the outpatient department. All of the primary care interns (trainees) and 80 percent of the regular interns considered this "highly important" or "moderately high" in importance at this stage in their careers. Given the fact that long-term patient care was so highly valued by the trainees, it is interesting that when they were asked how various other physicians would view a decision to spend "less time on the ward in order to spend more time in clinic," with few exceptions they perceived that their choice would not be widely supported by colleagues or superiors. In general, however, they expected to have such a decision supported by their own friends and social workers. However, they perceived that other professionals would "look down" on them if they made such a choice (Table 9).

TABLE 9

INTERNS' VIEWS OF HOW VARIOUS OTHERS WOULD REGARD DECISION TO SPEND MORE TIME IN CLINIC				
	"Dislike It or Look Down on It"		"Like It or Respect It"	
	% of Primary Care Trainees (*N* = 8)	% of Regular Interns (*N* = 41)	% of Primary Care Trainees (*N* = 8)	% of Regular Interns (*N* = 41)
Residents	63	56	—	10
Interns	50	51	—	7
MD faculty	50	46	38	19
MD friends	38	17	25	22
Nurses	38	25	12	14
Social workers	—	—	85	85
Other friends	—	2	100	46

At this point in their careers, these physicians were willing to work with a patient population that included large numbers of poor people from various ethnic minorities. The characteristics of the patient population either "had no effect" or "encouraged" all of the trainees and 83 percent of the regular interns to apply to this hospital. Indeed, 88 percent of the trainees and 73 percent of the regular interns "strongly agreed" with the statement that "health care is a right, not a privilege." Furthermore, all of the interns responded that it was important to develop the ability to deal with "problem patients" during their training. But while interns wanted a great deal of responsibility, they did not perceive themselves as entirely self-sufficient. They had strong views about the type of role models they believed they needed and of the extent to which they would need to collaborate with various other health care personnel in delivering medical care.

For example, when interns were asked to indicate the type of role models they valued most highly, all of the trainees and 91 percent of the regular interns gave "very high" to "high" importance to working with physicians who provided direct patient care. This is markedly different from their value rating of researchers, however, since only 26 percent of the trainees and 19 percent of the regular interns granted similar importance to "working with physicians who serve as role models in research."

Both groups showed considerable interest in working with a variety of health care staff (Fig. 2). While residents were clearly the preferred source of help for both trainees and regular interns, trainees expressed more willingness to consult nonphysicians when they needed help than did regular interns (Fig. 2). As might be expected, however, nonphysicians were more likely to be consulted in managing patient care than in making a diagnosis. For example, if a patient had a "broken appointment," all of the primary care trainees and 75 percent of the regular interns expected to turn

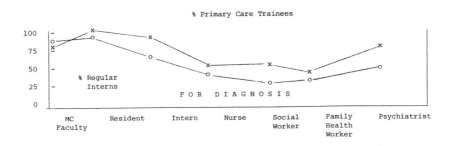

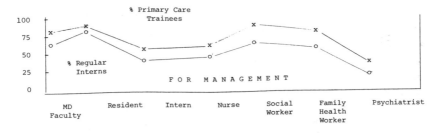

FIGURE 2 Expected patterns of consulting in clinic each week or every other clinic.

to a family health worker or social worker. Or, if the patient were found "making a medication error," 75 percent of the trainees and 80 percent of the regular interns expected to consult either a nurse or a resident.

Additional data suggest that there were certain differences between these two groups that had to do with their long-range career goals. For, even though trainees met the same standards for acceptance in post-graduate training as the regular interns, the directors of the program "left some room" for different interest patterns to develop. The trainees tended to be much more interested in working in the affiliated neighborhood health centers than did the regular interns (Table 10). And, unlike the regular interns, they indicated that they did not plan to remain in an academic teaching hospital. However, neither group planned on entering solo practice, or working in a governmental agency or an industrial/labor organization. On the contrary, both groups indicated a preference for organization settings in which they could practice medicine as part of a group.

TABLE 10

ORGANIZATIONAL SETTINGS PREFERRED
FOR FUTURE PRACTICE

Practice Setting	Primary Care Trainees (N = 8)		Regular Interns (N = 41)*	
	Number	(% Total)	Number	(% Total)
Academic teaching hospital	1	(13)	24	(59)
Neighborhood health center	7	(88)	8	(20)
Community hospital	3	(38)	9	(22)
Group practice	5	(63)	31	(77)
Solo practice	—		2	(5)
Government agency	1	(13)	—	
Industrial/labor organization	—		—	

Interns could choose more than one setting.

There were also differences in the patient population that each of these groups designated as "preferred" in their future practice. While both groups were oriented toward cities, primary care trainees generally expressed a preference for work with a lower income population than did regular interns (Table 11). The trainees also expressed more willingness than the regular interns to consider locating in rural areas. On the other hand, none

TABLE 11

DEMOGRAPHIC CHARACTERISTICS
PREFERRED IN FUTURE PRACTICE

Characteristic	Primary Care Trainees (N = 8)		Regular Interns (N = 41)	
	Number	(% Total)	Number	(% Total)*
Rural areas	2	(25)	5	(12)
Medium town (2,500-50,000)	2	(25)	13	(32)
Suburban area	—		11	(32)
Large city, low-income population	5	(63)	10	(24)
Large city, middle- to upper-income population	1	(13)	1 /	(42)

Interns could choose more than one location.

of the trainees wanted to practice in a suburban area, while 27 percent of the regular interns preferred such a location.

If one examines the kinds of experiences that were most highly valued, other consistent differences emerge between these two groups. However, there are sufficient overall similarities to suggest that these expressed preferences do not represent polar interest patterns. Rather, what *is* indicated is some variation around common themes. The data suggest that the preferences expressed by these interns may be a result of the selection process. That is, by carefully selecting a fairly homogeneous group of interns, Inner City Hospital educators assured themselves of recruiting physicians who would not challenge the dominant interest groups within this hospital.

THE MEDICAL PROFESSION AND THE HOSPITAL STRUCTURE

Since the modern teaching hospital symbolizes the power inherent in medical science and technology for alleviating life-threatening conditions (Stoeckle, 1976), it should not be too surprising that one of the reasons that the best

medical students often seek training in the largest teaching hospitals is to practice "a more scientific brand of medicine." Many students realize that only those hospitals that operate on a relatively large scale can afford the costly medical equipment and facilities associated with a scientific approach to medicine. But are physicians who work in large bureaucratic settings "free" to act solely on the basis of their scientific knowledge in caring for patients?

To the outside observer it may seem that professionals make no distinction among themselves between power based on professional expertise and power based on one's position in the organizational hierarchy. But careful observation reveals that such distinctions are made in a teaching hospital. Unfortunately, there is a misleading stereotype of the modern American hospital which assumes that such complex medical organizations are not bureaucratically structured. As a matter of fact, Freidson, one of the leading medical sociologists in the United States, recently suggested that so-called "professional organizations" should not even be classified as bureaucracies. Freidson's view is that

> while there is no comparative evidence to allow us to determine whether more or fewer workers are alienated from professional than from bureaucratic organizations, neither hierarchial nor authoritarian tendencies are missing in the professional organization of the division of labor, nor are alienation, absenteeism, low morale and high turnover insignificant problems. It is true for the worker as for the patient that the professionally organized division of labor has pathologies similar to those stemming from bureaucracy (Freidson, 1970, p. 145).

In my view the "pathology" is similar because the "anatomy" is similar. Professionals, like most others in this country, work in large-scale bureaucratic organizations, since this is where society's work is increasingly done. In fact, far from being mutually exclusive forms of social organization, professional and bureaucratic systems coexist in hospitals. The theoretical possibility that two or even three forms of social organization may be present simultaneously in complex organizations was recently suggested by Wallace (1971). From a cross-cultural perspective, Wallace sees the three major forms of social organization in human groups as kinship structures, community structures, and administrative structures. He defines administrative structures as the "crystalline form of the human group in which an accepted authority structure with recognized ranks and branches determines and coordinates those interpersonal relationships which are relevant to the group's task" and he defines community structures as those forms of social organization that define membership by "common residence in a territory (or, metaphorically, by common adherence to a profession)" (Wallace, 1971, pp. 1, 10).

Since the formal organization of Inner City Hospital includes professional groups, its social organization, by definition, also includes community structures. At the same time, however, all of the members of this organization work under administrative structures that have recognized ranks and offices similar to those found in any bureaucracy. Inner City Hospital, therefore, provides an ethnographic example of a bureaucratic organization that belongs to the most advanced type known—that is, a "permanent, continuous, full-time organization that has regular members and is constantly mobilized ... in the conduct of its business" (Wallace, 1971, pp. 1, 10). The business that is carried out at Inner City Hospital is delivering medical care seven days a week, 24 hours a day to area residents.

Of course, direct patient care is not the only business of a major teaching hospital. According to the 1974-75 Houseofficer's Manual at Inner City Hospital, teaching and research are needed to "strengthen" patient care. Manifestly, the greatest emphasis is put on patient care; however, there is presumably "no conflict" among these three important functions, because in an "effective" and "well-run service" everyone "works together" as a member of a "smoothly functioning team."

Paradoxically, although the interns' orientation to Inner City Hospital facilitated their smooth assimilation into the bureaucracy, it encouraged an adversary relationship with patients. If at orientation lectures each speaker painted a slightly different picture, all of them said that this was a difficult place to work. Typical of statements in orientation lectures are the following:

> *This is an exciting place to work but it is also dangerous. People do get stabbed in the corridors here and people have been shot while cleaning. Remember, this is a city hospital. There are no middle-class patients here. . . . As interns you will see everything. Among the snotty noses in the walk-in clinic are all the rare things you might expect to see on the floors. . . . And there are bugs here that aren't even in the literature yet. But there are also challenging social problems. Many children are battered by parents, boy friends, other children, etc. Others are left alone so you get the 3 P.M. to 7 P.M. syndrome of tired, neglected*

*children falling and having accidents. There is nothing
in the book about the feelings and reactions you
will have when you see your first battered child. But
I can tell you your first reaction will be anger. . . .
The type of violence you will see in regard to discipline, we consider battering. But that is normal
here. . . . By July 2nd you may be convinced that
no institution could possibly have all of the frustra-
tions of this hospital, but I can assure you this is
not so. There is no question that patients are sicker
here and that they have all of the social and behavioral characteristics of those who have been
excluded from the mainstream of society. But if you
look at the lead poisoning, the malnutrition, you
will conclude that this is a disenfranchized segment of
our society and that these are the people who most
need us. . . .*

*We don't want to scare you but there is a lot of
active TB in this hospital. Last year two house-
officers converted [i.e., tested "positive" for the
disease] and it can happen to you. Therefore, it is
important to wear your mask. . . .*

*You must get used to bearing the fact that some of
your patients are going to die. There is a 10 percent
mortality rate for patients who are admitted to the
hospital and some of your patients will die despite
everything you do to save them. That doesn't mean
you give up or accept this. On the other hand, this is
the real world and you must come to grips with these
things. (Author's notes)*

Besides being warned about the strain of caring for very sick
people, interns were taught to suppress their emotions and to regard their
patients as so culturally deprived that parents could not even be trusted to
take proper care of their own children. In other words, interns were encouraged to believe in the notion of a self-perpetuating culture of poverty—a
culture that would make their patients not only alien, but perhaps downright
dangerous.

What accounts for the fact that older, more experienced physicians reinforced the well-known culture of poverty concept, thereby dis-
couraging younger, less experienced physicians from learning how ghetto

residents organize and interpret their own experience? We have already seen that low-income families were stereotyped as broken, abusive, and patho-genic, and that the hospital was depicted as a dangerous place. In addition to these factors that were used to create distance from patients and to make interns acutely aware of their emotional and physical vulnerabilities, physi-cians in the system used the orientation lectures to promote dependence on the medical hierarchy.

During the orientation period many interns were apprehensive about receiving inadequate supervision. For example, in their discussions with one another, several of the interns mentioned that they had never seen any physicians do a complete history and physical examination, nor had the interns themselves been observed doing so. Subsequently, they were relieved to learn that many of their colleagues would be willing to help them if they needed them. It gave them immediate reassurance to hear statements like these:

> At the beginning you may get the idea that you will be lost in the halls with a patient and screaming for help. Ask for help, one of us is always available . . . call us any time of the day or night. We want to be called. We'll be doing those things too because it's part of the job; what we're really interested in is patient care.

> The fact that this is a resident's hospital implies that you can do what you want with relatively little supervision. . . . But the community considers it exploitation to be used as guinea pigs by physicians who come here for their clinical experience and then fly to the suburbs to practice. . . . At times you will be tired and there will be days when nothing goes right. But there are others to help you—junior resi-dents, senior residents, faculty—and no one will criticize you for asking for help.

> The key to survival in medicine is team responsibility. You can't do it alone. . . . If you have problems, let us know. The fact that this is a houseofficers' hospital means that there is a tendency to protect one an-other, which may not always be in the best interests of patients. If you have too many patients, it is not breaking a houseofficer's rule to call for help. If someone always calls for help to do his work we

will know that. But it has to be a cooperative effort.
If it is 36 interns versus the residents, it won't work.
(Author's notes)

Senior physicians gave the impression that the key to survival in medicine, both now and in the future, would depend on their relationships with colleagues rather than with patients. To reinforce the interns' sense of belonging to the medical profession, they were invited to informal luncheon discussions—held in the chairman's office—as well as to grand rounds, lectures by visiting medical scientists, and medical conferences. As further reinforcement they were told:

We know you have the capacity to be excellent.

All of you were our first choice. If this wasn't your first choice, it is now.

We want to make your year as atraumatic as possible. . . . This is a permissive service. We are not interested in upsetting your psyche, or putting you on the firing line, or that kind of thing.

We'll help you get a job. Once you are here you are one of our interns and we'll stand by you even if things are not going well. (Author's notes)

Belonging to a well-defined medical group would supply intellectual stimulation, emotional support, and assistance in obtaining future jobs, but it would also demand its pound of flesh in return. "No one is off duty when there are patients to be taken care of" was a recurrent theme throughout the orientation period. And interns were reminded that without help from colleagues no one would ever have any time off, since patient care was a full-time responsibility in the hospital. In this setting, unlike those settings in which physicians have been known to deal with very sick patients as if they were "professional equals" whose help and ideas were needed (Fox, 1959, pp. 89-95), patients were not viewed as potential collaborators. In describing orientation periods in hospitals, Mumford (1970) noted that the remarks made in lectures during this period often provided insight into a number of the problems in these settings. According to Mumford, senior physicians at the orientation meetings provided clues about the norms and values of their hospital, and as the interns moved through the various experiences, the directions implied during the first day were repeatedly confirmed (Mumford, 1970, pp. 50-68). Thus, it is important to recognize that the orientation speeches at Inner City Hospital encouraged an adversary relationship with patients while encouraging a collaborative relationship with other physicians in the system.

In light of the attempts to promote close relationships among physicians and to encourage more distant relationships with patients, it is interesting to note that before the new interns started work they were reminded that the community served by this hospital had identified the attitudes held by the hospital staff—including those of the physicians and nurses—as one of its major complaints. Largely in response to this, patients were now given a copy of a "bill of rights" upon admission to this institution. It is significant that such a document was developed in the first place. However, it is questionable whether such a pamphlet is an adequate means for protecting illiterate, non-English-speaking patients' rights when they are hospitalized. Obviously, a large number both of the professional staff and nonprofessional staff alike would agree with the rights detailed in the bill. How often such rights are violated, however, is unknown. It is not only at Inner City Hospital that there is explicitly stated concern for patients' rights. It is increasingly apparent that within the technology-intensive environment of the hospital the patient/consumer needs protection or assurance that medical therapy will not be applied against his will and that he will be given sufficient information within which to make informed choices about the treatment offered him.

In conclusion, we have seen that even those physicians who are committed to primary care careers when they begin their internship can be socialized into roles that discourage collaborative relationships with patients. They are expected to use their medical colleagues as a reference group and most of their career satisfactions are expected to come from these same colleagues. This role expectation does not facilitate the provision of primary care. With the rapid expansion of medical knowledge and the existence of scientific and technologic capacity to intervene in disease processes, the values and beliefs that are transmitted during medical training encourage physicians to practice in acute care settings where these technologies are available. Not only are there fewer rewards for those who practice in clinics or neighborhood health centers, but there is an implicit assumption that anyone who is interested in the delivery of such "ordinary" medical care must somehow be inferior.

SUMMARY

Attention has been given to the social context within which primary care training takes place. The discrepancy between the demand for more primary care, on the one hand, and the production of physicians interested in this type of practice, on the other, can be accounted for in part by the attitudes and values imparted to neophytes by their mentors in the teaching hospitals. Technology-intensive medical practice is clearly more valued by the profession than is primary care.

Advocates for the primary care model in medical education continue to make efforts to bridge the gap between physicians who are oriented toward providing general medical service in the community and those who have academic affiliation. One of these continuing efforts is the development of a primary care component that will be strong enough to perpetuate itself within an academic environment while retaining its community focus.

ACKNOWLEDGMENTS

Several people have been helpful in providing data that was not readily available at the time that this chapter was written. In particular, I would like to thank the following individuals: Dr. Joel Alpert, Boston University Medical School, and Dr. Thomas Almy, Dartmouth Medical School, for help in providing me with early statistics on the availability of primary care training programs for pediatricians and internists when such programs could not be listed separately on the National Intern and Residency Matching Program; Dr. Maurice Wood, Medical College of Virginia, for bringing me up to date on family practice trends; Dr. Graettinger, National Intern and Residency Matching Program, for help in understanding some of the discrepancies between statistics dealing with internship, first-year residency programs, and the like, during the 1970-75 transition to new terminology; and those staff members at the Academy of Family Practice, the U.S. Department of Health, Education, and Welfare, Division of Health Manpower, and the Institute of Medicine who have given generously of their time and advice.

NOTE

[1] Fictitious name for the hospital in which the author's study was conducted.

9

The Use of Knowledge

MARY-'VESTA MARSTON

During the past fifty years tremendous advances have been made in the knowledge basic to the prevention and treatment of illness. Implementation of this knowledge has resulted in the virtual disappearance of communicable diseases such as small pox, poliomyelitis, tetanus and diphtheria, and the development of sophisticated methods of treatment for patients with a wide variety of chronic diseases such as cardiovascular disorders and end-stage kidney disease. At present the major causes of morbidity and mortality in this country are chronic illnesses, especially cardiovascular diseases and carcinoma, and accidents. There is recognition on the part of professionals and the lay public of the need to clean up the environment and to do research concerning the potential etiologic role of the growing numbers of new substances being introduced in industry and in our everyday environment. Much needs to be done at the societal level as well as at the individual level if we are to improve the health of people. Increasing numbers of behavioral scientists are discovering health as a fertile field for applied research. Also, increasing numbers of nurses with advanced graduate preparation are developing their own theories and models for promoting health related behavior.

Several recent societal events have led to a developing interest in health by behavior scientists. Lower college enrollments with less demand for faculty have resulted in behavioral scientists entering applied fields. Health is a relative newcomer among applied fields. In recent years the federal government has shown preference for supporting applied rather than basic research. Also, enrollment in applied fields such as medicine, nursing and social work has increased relative to other college enrollments. Behavioral scientists have been invited by members of the medical and allied health professions to contribute their expertise to helping clients adopt more healthful life styles, participate in screening programs, and follow prescribed regimens in the case of patients with diagnosed illnesses (Cullen et al. 1976; Enelow and Henderson, 1975; Tillotson, 1975; Weiss, 1975). Interest in health care is evident in the professional organizations also. The American Psychological Association has a section on health behavior within Division 18 (Psychologists in Public Service), and the American Public Health Association has a Conference on Social Sciences in Health. Nurse sociologists have formed a special interest group within the medical sociology section of the American Sociological Association, focusing on health care and consumer concerns, and nurse anthropologists have organized themselves within the American Anthropological Association to address their concern for the relationship between cultural factors and the provision of health services.

Efforts are being focused on the application of theories and models of health and illness behavior to enhance patients' compliance with medical regimens as well as to promote more healthful life styles for essentially well people. For example, in 1973 the Fogarty International Center of the National Institutes of Health and the American College of Preventive Medicine set up task forces to develop recommendations concerning prevention of illness and improvement of the health status of people. The task force reports (*Preventive Medicine USA,* 1976) provided the basis for recommendations which later appeared in DHEW's *Forward Plan for Health* (1978-82). Both the United States' *Forward Plan for Health* and Canada's *A New Perspective on the Health of Canadians* (1974) have made an excellent case for the fact that the major causes of mortality and morbidity are influenced by life style and self care practices which are within the power of every individual to alter. We have reached the point where attitudes, values and customs are now recognized as major mediating factors which can limit the extent to which medical treatment can improve the health of people. Many behaviors suspected of being, or proven incompatible with health are valued by the general population, or by segments thereof. These include the use of alcohol, tobacco, and foods containing highly saturated fats, salt and other additives. There are limits to the amount of improvement in health status that can be accomplished by legislation, health education and social pressure. The alcohol, tobacco and food industries have available the same social science knowledge and techniques for promoting their respective interests as does the health industry. However, the health industry has much less capital for promoting health than do the commercial industries for promoting their products.

A number of models of health and illness behavior have appeared in the literature. Some, such as the Health Belief Model, focus on the perceptions of the individual concerning health and illness issues. Others, such as behavior modification, are concerned with enhancing health related behaviors; they may pay little direct attention to whether the individual's perceptions are in line with his behavior, although there may be the expectation that perceptions will move in line with behavior. The usefulness of models which focus on perceptions of individuals, to date, is limited by a lack of research, and by the fact that most research has utilized correlational designs. In these designs cause and effect are indistinguishable, and it is difficult to determine with any degree of certainty whether variables hypothesized to predict various health related behaviors were present *prior* to the time the particular health related behavior being studied was measured, or, whether the presumed predictor(s) co-existed with the behavior being studied. Furthermore, until recently, nurses—the largest number of health professionals—in particular, have been reluctant to take on an independent role beyond that of health educator in manipulating variables thought to influence health related behaviors.

The models developed, and the research thus far conducted, have been primarily by dentists, psychologists, physicians, and nurses who were concerned with the very specific problem of maximizing health behavior. For the most part concepts from role theory have not been used by these persons but the reader can readily make translations using such terms as cues for role behavior, role expectations, negative and positive sanctions associated with health related behavior, and sick role behavior. The author, purposefully, has not made these types of semantic alterations, and has chosen to discuss the models in their present state of development. At some future date these models of health related behavior may very well become part of the larger body of knowledge on roles.

The main focus of this chapter will be on those theories and models which have some empirical support, and which show the greatest promise for research and practice. Most attention will be given to models which use concepts that a health professional can alter or manipulate to bring about a change in health related behavior. Models which use concepts which are primarily descriptive and provide a sense of understanding about health behavior, but do not contain concepts that a health professional may selectively alter, will not be discussed.

HEALTH AS A PERSONAL RESPONSIBILITY

In the presence of illness there are well defined expectations concerning behavior appropriate to patients and health professionals. Sociologists have described these as the rights and obligations of the sick role. According to Parsons (1951): (1) the individual is not held responsible for becoming ill, and he is exempted from usual social role obligations of bread winner, home maker etc.; (2) the individual is expected to lay aside usual activities, and be taken care of, at least temporarily; (3) the individual is obligated to seek competent medical supervision; and (4) the individual is expected to co-operate with his physician in order to expedite recovery. Many illnesses are self limiting, and the individual is able to resume his usual activities within a relatively brief period of time. For patients with chronic illnesses, alterations in routine activities of daily living may become necessary because of long term treatment regimens and permanent disabilities. Although the sick role is assumed to be an undesirable state of affairs, most patients with chronic illnesses are never free of the obligations associated with it, but often they do not benefit from the advantages of being exempted from usual role obligations. Parsons' sick role does not explain why ill persons fail to take steps to promote improvement in health status. Also, his view of the sick role is not useful in explaining why essentially healthy individuals undertake health promotional activities.

During the past ten years there has been growing recognition of the necessity and obligation for people to assume responsibility for maintenance and improvement of their health, for treatment of episodic illness states, and for amelioration of chronic and irreversible medical conditions. Documentation of the fact that large numbers of patients fail to follow prescribed medical regimens came as a surprise to many professionals in the health care field (Caplan et al. 1976; Lasagna, 1976; Marston, 1970; Rosenberg and Raynes, 1976; Sackett and Haynes, 1976). Most of the literature on noncompliance with medical regimens has been concerned with failure to take enough of whatever therapeutic agent has been prescribed. Less well recognized is the problem of overmedicating which may occur by design or by accident. The prescribing of optimal therapeutic doses of drugs has been complicated by the finding that in drug trials participants failed to take medications as prescribed, sometimes leading to the prescribing in actual practice of larger than needed doses of medications to achieve desired therapeutic effects (Gordis, 1976). Noncompliance with aspects of the medical regimen other than drugs is an ever larger problem (Sackett, 1977). We have less sensitive measuring instruments and hence less good data on peoples' efforts to maintain healthy life styles or to adhere to aspects of therapeutic regimens which include dietary constraints, weight control, exercise regimens, and limitations on the use of alcohol and tobacco. People spend very little time in the classic sick role defined by Parsons; they are largely responsible for their self care in illness and in health. There are many gaps in desired self care practices which lead to unnecessary complications and disability. Health professionals are making a greater effort than ever before to apply health behavior models such as the Health Belief Model and to develop new models which can be used to enable people to improve their self care.

Kasl and Cobb (1966) have defined *health behavior* as "any activity undertaken by a person believing himself to be healthy, for the purpose of preventing disease or detecting it in an asymptomatic stage" (p. 246). *Illness behavior* is any activity undertaken by an individual who feels ill, for the purpose of ascertaining whether he is, indeed, ill, and if so, what steps should be taken to remedy this state of affairs. *Sick role behavior* is any activity undertaken for purposes of getting out of the undesirable illness condition (Kasl and Cobb, 1966). This definition is compatible with that of Parsons (1951).

The survival of people with chronic illnesses is to a great extent dependent upon their following certain self care regimens indefinitely. For the most part the task force reports referred to earlier (*Preventive Medicine USA*, 1976) were concerned with health behavior as defined by Kasl and Cobb. Distinctions between traditional health behavior, illness behavior, sick role behavior, and behaviors undertaken to control a chronic physical or emotional condition become somewhat artificial if our focus is directed toward improvement of the health of all people. It is not known whether distinctly different factors are operative in determining health behavior, illness behavior, sick role behavior, and behavior for care of chronic illnesses. Therefore, for purposes of this discussion, the term "health related behavior" will be used to cover all of these, unless otherwise specified.

Escalating costs and increasing consumer involvement in health care matters add urgency to the expectation that health professionals will be accountable for the quality of care given as well as for the outcome of this care. Practitioners concerned with health and illness issues are placing priority on the development of theories which are readily applicable in practice (Gortner, 1975). Nurses comprise the largest group of health practitioners.

During the past ten years nurses have been preparing themselves to take on expanded roles. Increasingly, emphasis has been placed on the independent functions of nursing. Independent, dependent and inter-dependent functions of nursing practice have come to be value laden, with the independent functions being the most prestigeous. The DHEW document, *Extending the Scope of Nursing* (1971), gave legitimacy to these distinctions. Nurses in expanded roles are in an excellent position to utilize theory and empirical knowledge of determinants of health related behavior to help their clients improve their health status.

National visibility for independent practice was highlighted by Kinlein (1972) who described her early experience with her own practice. More recently, Kinlein recommended that nursing's concern be with health rather than illness, and with helping clients to enhance their health (1977). She identified the self care concept as central to a definition of nursing, pointing out that individuals' life styles influence the way in which basic drives for food, sleep, work, love, play, etc., are satisfied. It is obvious that individual life styles and hence self care practices determine how people respond to their basic drives.

Self care practices are important in the development of healthful life styles to prevent the onset of chronic debilitating conditions such as cancer, stroke, coronary disease and arthritis. However, large numbers of persons now suffer from chronic conditions. An individual's comfort, independence of movement, and illness outcome for many chronic illnesses are dependent upon self care practices which are within the power of most individuals to influence. Levin, Katz and Holst (1976) have drawn attention to the groundswell of lay interest in assuming responsibility for self care wherever possible. To limit the self care concept to preventive health practices restricts the potential usefulness of the concept, and ignores the large numbers of individuals for whom self care means care for a chronic irreversible illness.

HEALTH EDUCATION

Usually, health professionals assume that clients are rational beings with respect to their health related behavior, and that they will adopt the professional's view of what steps should be taken to remain healthy or to regain health. Such a stance leaves little room for individual differences, or for differences in cultural perspectives on health and illness. The literature presents a dismal picture of the effectiveness of traditional health education techniques which emphasize provision of information (Green, 1970; Haynes et al. 1976; Marston, 1970; Richards, 1975; Sackett et al. 1975). One important exception is Maccoby and Farquhar's field investigation (1975) in three northern California towns which demonstrated that a multifaceted health education program made a significant impact on coronary risk behaviors. If we agree that people must assume responsibility for their own health and self care activities, then it is incumbent on health professionals to learn to use health education approaches along with a variety of other approaches to help them accomplish this. Health behavior models can be useful to the health professional in this task.

HEALTH BELIEF MODEL

The model which is the most fully developed, and the one which has received the most attention in the last five years is the Health Belief Model. The Health Belief Model was proposed by Hochbaum (1958), Rosenstock (1966) and their colleagues about twenty years ago, but did not receive the attention it deserved in terms of sparking research until Becker began his work (Becker, 1974). The Model focuses on social psychological variables, and is based on a phenomenological orientation. This orientation holds that "it is the world of the perceiver that determines what he will do and not the physical environment except as the physical environment comes to be represented in the mind of the behaving individual" (Rosenstock, 1974, p. 329). The Model has its roots in Lewin's Field Theory (1951). According to field theory, behavior is dependent upon the value an individual places on a given outcome, and his estimate of the likelihood that a particular action will result in that outcome. The Health Belief Model is sometimes described as a value expectancy theory. The way in which an individual perceives the world around him determines his behavior in any given situation. Two sets of perceptions are important: (1) psychological readiness to take a specific action; and (2) the extent to which an individual perceives that a particular course of action is effective in reducing or eliminating a particular threat (Rosenstock, 1975). Psychological readiness is composed of perceived susceptibility (or vulnerability) and perceived seriousness. Optimal conditions for taking action are thought to exist when, first of all, the individual perceives that he is susceptible to a health threat, that should the health threat materialize this would be a serious state of affairs, and that the course of action being recommended would be effective in reducing or eliminating the threat. Secondly, the individual must perceive that there is a relative absence of barriers to taking action such as expense, inconvenience, anticipated pain and negative attitudes of significant others. Thirdly, the individual must perceive cues or triggers to action, such as internal bodily states, physical symptoms, and new information bearing on the recommended health action.

The Health Belief Model has remained essentially unchanged since its formulation with the following exceptions.

1. In his 1957 monograph, Hochbaum included under "psychological readiness" the perception that an individual could have a particular diagnosis (in this case, tuberculosis) and not have recognizable symptoms. Hochbaum's findings indicated that this belief was related to the obtaining of voluntary chest x-rays, and interacted with perceived vulnerability and perceived benefits of early dianosis. For the most part, subsequent research has not taken account of subjective

perception that a particular health problem could exist without presenting symptoms. An exception is research by Kirscht et al. (1975) who included this variable in communications designed to encourage clinic patients to make and keep appointments for screening tests. In actual practice, perception that an individual could have a particular diagnosis and not have symptoms is currently used in recruiting people to have screening tests of various sorts.

2. Although the original Hochbaum monograph included some discussion of cues or triggers to action, recent papers have accorded more importance to this variable. Rosenstock (1975) has pointed out the difficulties of identifying and measuring cues which trigger specific health related behaviors for populations.

3. Becker, in two recent studies, has introduced the concept of "health motivation" (Becker et al. 1974: Becker et al. 1975). Components of health motivation reported in the 1974 research were: (a) perception of physical threat; (b) control over health matters; (c) attitude toward medical authority; and (d) general health concern. The subject population was composed of mothers or grandmothers caring for children with a diagnosis of otitis media for whom an oral antibiotic had been prescribed. Significant associations were found between all but the "control over health matters" variable and one or more criterion measures of compliance (medication taking, follow-up appointment, and appointment-keeping ratio).

In Becker's study of participation in a Tay-Sachs disease screening program (Becker et al., 1975), health motivation was operationalized as (a) desire to have children, and (b) typical health behavior (frequency with which the individual thinks about his own health, whether he goes to the physician as soon as he feels ill, assessment of present health status, and recency of latest physician visit. Desire to have children was significantly associated with participation in the screening program, but surprisingly, typical health behavior was not.

Some research has been done utilizing other motivators of health related behavior. For example, Leventhal (1970) and Janis (1967) have conducted and summarized a considerable amount of research on the use of fear communications in instigating health related behavior. Leventhal et al. (1965) investigated three levels of fear communication in motivating college students to obtain tetanus immunizations. Cue to action, as operationalized by specific information concerning hours and whereabouts of clinic facilities, were provided for half of the subjects. Subjects were exposed to high, medium and low fear communications concerning the prevalence and seriousness of tetanus. Fear communications were enhanced by the cues, with high fear and presence of cues proving the most effective. There is considerable hesitation among health professionals in the widespread use of fear communications as motivators, since: (a) too high a level of threat may cause a patient to deny the communication, and become more fixed in his noncompliance;

and (b) threat has a rapid decrement in effect, and therefore little usefulness for behaviors which need to be repeated over a period of time.

Becker and Green (1975) have suggested the use of appeals to a sense of responsibility to the family as a motivator of health related behaviors. This technique may have limitations also, since such communications could cause the person to whom they are directed to experience an overwhelming sense of guilt. No research utilizing appeals to family responsibility as a motivator has yet appeared in the literature, although short television commercials on hypertension are using this strategy.

4. Becker has proposed incorporation of modifying and enabling factors into the Health Belief Model. These include: (1) demographic variables; (2) structural variables such as complexity of regimen and side effects; (3) attitudinal variables such as satisfaction with clinic and physician: (4) interaction variables such as quality of patient-provider interaction and amount and type of feedback to patient; and (5) enabling variables such as prior experience with the illness or regimen and social pressure (Becker, 1974; Becker et al. 1977; Becker and Maimon, 1975). Becker proposes that the modifying and enabling factors serve as intervening variables and interact with the main variables of the Model.

The Health Belief Model was given a great deal of attention as a determinant of health related behavior at national conferences which have been held on cancer (Cullen et al., 1976), heart disease (Weiss, 1975), and nutrition (Tillotson, 1975). Since this Model has the soundest knowledge base of the health related behavior models now available it will probably continue to have high visibility because it can provide a reasonable theoretical framework for future research and practice. Also, as will be seen, the Model is compatible with other models of health related behavior to be reviewed later on in this paper.

There is a need for sounder research designs based on the Health Belief Model. Experimental, comparative and prospective studies are needed. Prospective studies give time ordering to the variables. Three prospective studies, those of Leventhal et al. (1960); Kegeles (1963); and Becker et al. (1972), are summarized.

Prospective Studies

Leventhal et al. (1960) conducted a field study designed to test the relationship between beliefs regarding Asian influenza and subsequent preventive actions taken. Because the outbreak of influenza materialized faster than anticipated, the sample size on which prior beliefs were measured and information concerning subsequent preventive action obtained was very small

(N = 86). Five of the 12 individuals who believed they were susceptible to the disease and were concerned about the seriousness of Asian influenza (42 percent), and 8 of 74 individuals (11 percent) who held either one of these beliefs or none took subsequent preventive actions. The difference between the two groups was statistically significant, thus lending support to the Model.

Kegeles (1963) studied the extent to which beliefs in susceptibility, seriousness and perceived effectiveness of treatment were related to preventive and symptomatic dental visits in a three-year period after the beliefs were measured. Subjects were factory workers who received free dental care as a fringe benefit. Those who believed that they were susceptible to dental problems were significantly more likely to make preventive visits than were those who did not hold this belief. However, no significant relationship was found between perceived seriousness or perceived effectiveness of treatment and preventive dental visits.

In the Becker et al. (1972) study, mothers of children attending a large city clinic were interviewed at the time of child's first visit for treatment of otitis media. Criterion measures of compliance with the prescribed medical regimen were: (1) medication administered, as determined by a urine test five days after the start of the regimen; and (2) knowledge concerning the regimen such as knowing the name of the medication, knowing the number of times the medication was to be administered, and knowing the follow-up date. Perceived susceptibility to reinfection was significantly associated with all compliance and knowledge measures except appointment keeping. Also, those mothers who perceived that previous treatment obtained at the same clinic was effective, and who agreed with the pediatrician's assessment of the child's illness showed more compliance.

Experimental Studies

Very little research has been conducted in which elements of the Health Belief Model have been manipulated systematically to influence health related behavior. Three such experimental studies were undertaken by Kegeles (1969); Haefner and Kirscht (1970); and Kirscht et al. (1975). These studies are summarized as follows.

In a field experiment with women in an urban ghetto, Kegeles (1969) administered standardized communications designed to influence beliefs concerning susceptibility to cervical cancer and effectiveness of cervical cytology for early detection, and to urge the women to visit a cytological clinic. Control subjects received a message on iron deficiency. Both groups received information concerning the cytology test, and the time and whereabouts of the clinic. Although experimental subjects did not change their attitude toward susceptibility to cervical cancer and the effectiveness of early detection significantly more than the control subjects, twice as many experimental as control subjects kept clinic appointments.

Kirscht et al. (1975) studied the effectiveness of positive messages and threat messages in persuading clinic patients to use the services of a new screening clinic. Positive messages emphasized the importance of maintaining good health, and suggested a thorough checkup as one way to ensure this. Threat messages suggested that people may have something wrong without their being aware of it, and that ignoring disease can have a serious result. Significantly more people who received the positive as contrasted with the threat message made and kept appointments.

Haefner and Kirscht (1970) presented films concerning the nature and prevalence of three diseases (cancer, heart disease and tuberculosis), consequences of the diseases, and preventive actions which could be taken. Subjects were paid volunteer subjects, recruited from among non-academic university employees. After viewing each film, experimental subjects were asked about their intention to carry out various preventive measures. Data were obtained concerning perceived susceptibility, seriousness, and effectiveness of measures being recommended to reduce the threat. Control subjects were not exposed to the films but answered essentially the same questions as experimental subjects. Eight months following exposure to the films both groups were asked to complete a questionnaire indicating which preventive behaviors they had undertaken. Haefner and Kirscht concluded that they were able to modify the participants' belief systems systematically, and that these changes were related to intended health behaviors. Intended and reported health related behaviors measured in this study provide less robust support for the Health Belief Model than do the Kegeles (1969) and Kirscht et al. (1975) studies.

In summary, the Health Belief Model proposes that perceived seriousness, susceptibility and effectiveness of treatment, and presence of cues to action along with a relative absence of barriers are important in determining specific health related behaviors. The studies which have been reviewed demonstrate that there is no clear cut evidence that the presence of all five variables, or any particular combination thereof, is necessary for any given health related behavior to be manifested.

ROTTER'S SOCIAL LEARNING THEORY

Whether an individual believes that illness outcome or the prevention of illness is under his control may influence what health related behaviors he will undertake. According to Rotter's Social Learning Theory (1966), people develop expectations concerning the amount of control they believe they have over their reinforcements in the course of everyday living. People with a belief in internal control think that for the most part what happens to them is due to their efforts, abilities and skills; people with a belief in external control think that what happens to them is primarily due to chance, fate, or the influence of powerful others. We would expect that belief in internal control would be associated with health related behaviors, and a number of studies have reported statistically significant associations between belief in internal control and health related behaviors such as successful loss of weight (Manno and Marston, 1972), cessation of smoking (James, Woodruff and Werner, 1965), use of contraceptives (MacDonald, 1970), and taking of influenza immunizations (Dabbs and Kirscht, 1971). However, the results of more recent studies have been disappointing. As noted earlier, Becker et al. (1972) found no association between belief in control and extent to which mothers adhered to a treatment regimen for children with otitis media. Lowery and DuCette (1976) failed to find an association between belief in personal control and control of diabetes, and Windwer (1977) failed to find an association between belief in internal control and choice of participation in a natural childbirth program.

There have been problems with measuring belief in internal and external control with patient populations. Items in the most widely used scale (Rotter, 1966) are either general, or associated with specific issues such as school grades, politics, and success at work. Wallston et al. (1976) have developed a health locus of control scale which may prove more useful in measuring belief in control of health and illness. As with the Health Belief Model, interpretations of findings of research on the relationship between belief in personal control and health related behavior have been hampered by the widespread use of correlational designs. However, some investigators have reported successful methods for changing clients' locus of control and behaviors thought to be associated with it (Dua, 1970; MacDonald, 1972). This makes locus of control an enticing variable for professionals working in applied areas. In all probability, belief in personal control will find its niche as one of several predictors of health related behavior. Conceptually, belief in personal control is related to perceived susceptibility and effectiveness of treatment, and the person with a belief in internal control would be expected to follow cues to action of a preventive or treatment regimen. Langlie (1977) reported that perceptions that the individual has some control over health and that preventive actions are effective were associated with self reported behaviors such as use of seat belts, exercise and nutrition behavior, medical checkups, dental care, immunizations, and participation in screening exams. With the exception of the Becker et al. (1972) study and the Langlie (1977) study no one has made a serious attempt to integrate aspects of Rotter's Social Learning Theory and the Health Belief Model although they are compatible.

JACCARD'S MODEL

Jaccard (1975) has proposed a social psychological model for predicting health related behavior based on a theoretical framework set forth by Fishbein (1967). This Model was developed because of the repeated finding of little relationship between attitude and behavior. The seriousness and magnitude of this problem for health education has been well documented by Green (1970) in his paper entitled, "Should we abandon health attitude change strategies?"

   Jaccard has listed those factors which he believes intervene between a behavioral intention and the actual carrying out of a behavior. These are as follows. (1) The time interval between the behavioral intention and the behavior is important because of events which may occur in this period to change the intention and/or prevent the behavior from occurring. For example, Finnerty et al. (1973) demonstrated that the number of no-show clinic appointments following blood pressure screening could be markedly reduced by arranging for clinic visits within 24 to 48 hours after screening. (2) Exposure to new information in the period between the behavioral intention and the behavior may cause an individual to change his behavioral intention. (3) The number of steps or sequences of behavior which must be completed before the target behavior is reached may be an impediment. (4) The desired behavior must be within the ability of the individual to perform. (5) Memory factors may interfere with completion of the desired behavior by way of forgetting. (6) An individual may intend to carry out a particular behavior but may exhibit another because of habit. (7) The relationship between behavioral intention and behavior may be influenced by: (a) the degree of correspondence between the measure of behavioral intention and the behavior; and (b) the extent to which an individual's stated intention is veridical to his real intention.

   According to Jaccard, a health related behavior is determined by an individual's beliefs about the consequences of performing a particular behavior and the value the consequences have for him, and by his beliefs about what he thinks relevant others think he should do.

   Jaccard (1975) reported results of a study of beliefs concerning the expectations of others and intentions to stop smoking. Belief systems were found to be consistent with intention to smoke or not smoke. Conclusions regarding the usefulness of this model are limited by the fact that behavioral measures were not obtained, and by the fact that belief system and intentions regarding smoking were obtained at the same point in time. No other studies designed to test this model have yet appeared in the literature although aspects of the Kegeles (1969) and Becker et al. (1972) studies bear on assumptions made by Jaccard.

Specifically, Kegeles (1969) noted that the acceptance of a clinic appointment card, or of a taxi card for a free trip to the clinic, might be regarded as an indicator of intentionality. Although the acceptance of clinic or taxi cards was not significantly related to clinic attendance, twice as many experimental as control subjects who had made appointments kept them.

Although not specifically designed to do so, Becker et al.'s study (1972) provides some support for Jaccard's model. These researchers reported that mothers and grandmothers who agreed with the statement, "I try to do exactly what the doctor tells me to do, without question," showed higher compliance with a medical regimen for care of children with otitis media. The same was true for those mothers who said they would not let anything interfere with keeping their child's clinic appointment. Both of these attitudes expressed by mothers seem to connote intentionality.

Jaccard's model shares with the Health Belief Model the assumption that behavior is determined in part by the value of the expected consequences. Jaccard notes that the concept of behavioral intention has not been incorporated as an intervening, or modifying or enabling variable, using Becker's terminology, between health beliefs and health related behavior in the Health Belief Model. There is no reason why this variable should *not* be added to Becker's list of modifying and enabling factors. Jaccard's model places considerable emphasis on the influence of social norms in determining behavioral intentions. Perhaps the influence of social norms could be subsumed under Becker's "social pressure" variable. Much research remains to be done to determine the influence of significant others on specific health related behaviors. Although both models have their origins in value expectancy theory, the Health Belief Model has measured beliefs in restricted domains, namely perceived susceptibility, seriousness and benefits, whereas the model Jaccard proposes accommodates *any* benefits the individual may believe to be relevant. Finally, Jaccard's model does not consider perceived susceptibility and seriousness to be integral parts of the model. The Health Belief Model and Jaccard's model emphasize somewhat different concepts, but the two are compatible. Research is needed to determine the relative usefulness of each model, and to determine whether some combination of the two is a better predictor of health related behavior than either model by itself.

SUCHMAN'S MODEL

In an early survey of more than 5,000 persons living in the Washington Heights section of New York City, Suchman (1965) studied the interrelationships between social organization factors such as ethnic exclusivity, friendship solidarity, and orientation to family tradition and authority on the one hand, and medical orientation, as measured by knowledge about disease, skepticism concerning medical care, and dependency in illness. Suchman concluded that demographic variables and social group factors were related to medical orientation, with individuals from tightly knit families and social groups, i.e., those with a parochial orientation, having an orientation toward more popular medical care, and those with a more cosmopolitan orientation being more oriented to scientific medicine. Demographic variables were independently related to source of medical care, with older upper class individuals seeking private medical care. Also, medical orientation was independently related to medical care, with a more scientific orientation being associated with private medical care. Ten years later Reeder and Berkanovic (1973) were unable to replicate Suchman's study in Los Angeles.

Suchman used knowledge concerning the influence of social groups gained in the 1965 study as a basis for a manipulation designed to increase use of a protective glove by sugar cane workers. Suchman's model (1967) for predicting health behavior is based on the traditional epidemiological model of host, agent, and environment. According to Suchman, this permits analysis of

> the individual factors present in the host which determine his "exposure" to the innovation and his "susceptibility" to its promises, the social factors present in the environment which influence his perception and interpretation of the innovation as "acceptable, appropriate, and desirable" from the point of view of his social group referrants, and the agent or attribute factors present in the innovation itself and the way it is introduced that affects his "image" of the innovation and his evaluation of its effectiveness or appeal (Suchman, 1967, p. 199).

Suchman points out that this formulation utilizes concepts of psychological readiness and social approval, both of which are contained in the Health Belief Model. In his 1967 study he attempted to introduce use of a protective glove in order to reduce the incidence of machete cuts. A community organization approach was applied to one group of workers and social pressure was applied to induce workers to accept use of the glove. A safety education approach was taken with a second group of workers who were supplied with information concerning the need, advantages and proper use of the protective glove. Host, or personal readiness factors were operationalized as recognition of seriousness of the problem, acceptance of personal vulnerability, predisposition to take action, motivation to act, ability to act, knowledge of desired action, and belief in desired action; environmental, or social control factors, were operationalized as social pressure to act, incorporation into role performance, and acceptibility of the action; agent, or situational factors, were operationalized as effectiveness of the action, previous experience, favorable environment, and attractiveness. Host, or personal readiness factors, were found to be highly predictive of adoption of the protective glove. This finding would be congruent with predictions of the Health Belief Model. Environmental or social control factors, and agent, or situational or action factors, exerted much less influence on the target behavior. Suchman concluded that direct health education measures were more successful than social pressure in gaining acceptance of the protective glove. This latter finding is at variance with most studies which have investigated educational manipulations to change health related behavior (Green, 1970; Marston, 1970; Sackett & Haynes, 1976). Much remains to be learned concerning factors which must be present in order for social pressure to be effective in promoting health related behaviors.

SOCIAL SUPPORT GROUPS

Haynes (1976) noted that patient compliance with therapeutic regimens has rather consistently been found to be associated with presence of support systems of family and/or friends. The literature on precisely what aspects of support systems are most important is in the embryonic stages. An early study by Gray et al. (1966) demonstrated that mothers who perceived that their neighbors thought they should have their children immunized against Polio were significantly more likely to have their children immunized than were those mothers who did not hold this perception. Pratt (1976) has shown that family structures which encourage individual autonomy and growth of members have members who are better able to manage their personal health behavior and to negotiate the health care system successfully. Langlie (1977) found that being part of a social network extending beyond the immediate family and characterized by relatively high socioeconomic status was related to self reported preventive health behavior. On the other hand, Caplan et al. (1976) failed to demonstrate that social supports were significantly associated with compliance behavior.

Becker and Green (1975) have suggested three reasons why the family may exert more influence on health related behaviors than has been recognized up to now: (1) Often healthy family members must assume responsibility for compliance behavior on the part of children, the aged and the disabled. The compliance literature to date has not distinguished between compliance behavior for which the patient was responsible and compliance behavior which was initiated by a responsible member. (2) Specific roles within the family may have important consequences for health related behaviors. The bread winner or mother with small children may, realistically, not be able to carry out some recommended health related behaviors. (3) Even when cost of medication—or cost in terms of time and energy—are not important issues, the attitude of others significant to the patient may be important. Although reference group theory has its own body of knowledge, it has not begun to receive the attention it deserves with respect to application in the health field. Becker's revision of the Health Belief Model incorporates presence of a support group as a modifying or enabling variable. Jaccard's is the only model which accords the influence of support systems a major role.

FABREGA'S MODEL

Taking an inductive approach, Fabrega has postulated a model of illness behavior which takes into consideration information an individual might be expected to process during an illness episode. Fabrega defines illness as a socially defined state on the basis of which a decision is made regarding medical treatment. He sees the need for a set of rules for organizing and explaining culturally appropriate behavior associated with illness in different contexts. Four open and interrelated systems, i.e., biological, social, phenomenological, and memory, interact within the individual and make possible the following stages:

1. Recognition and labelling of illness.
2. Evaluation of illness to determine "disvalues" (e.g., threat to life, degree of associated disability, etc.).

3. Formation of a treatment plan (e.g., home remedy, patent medicine, advice of significant other, etc.).
4. Assessment of treatment plan and assignment of probability that a plan will neutralize the disvalues noted above.
5. Assessment of treatment benefits.
6. Assessment of costs associated with treatment.
7. Assessment of net benefits (benefits minus costs).
8. Selection of a treatment plan to optimize benefits, to insure the lowest cost, and to attain the highest utility.
9. Repeat of above cycle if indicated, with new labelling.

Fabrega claims that one advantage of this model is that it can be applied in different cultural settings. This is the only model among those reviewed which takes into consideration individual differences of a cultural nature. The problem solving stages which Fabrega has set forth for treating an illness episode provide many appropriate points for intervention such as manipulation of the belief system, sharing up of social support systems, maximizing those variables known to influence the intentionality-behavior sequence, health education, etc. In addition to their use in illness intervention, similar problem solving stages could be utilized with health promotional activities. Testing of this model is needed.

BEHAVIOR MODIFICATION

The models and approaches which have been considered thus far assume that the individual strives to bring his behavior into line with his perceptions, attitudes, and beliefs. For example, health education presents a rational approach with explanations as to what behaviors are needed and why and how these should be carried out, and the Health Belief Model proposes that a set of perceptions or beliefs influence health related behaviors. Behavior modification makes no assumptions about the belief system, but sets about changing targeted behaviors. Sometimes, but not always, there is an assumption that change in attitude will follow change in behavior. According to behavior modification theory, all behavior is under the control of consequences in the external environment. In order for a behavior to be changed it must be observable and measureable, and its antecedents and consequences must be known. Change is brought about by systematically altering the behavior consequence contingency. Because of the lack of congruence between attitude and behavior, an assumption underlying the two major approaches to enhancing health related behaviors—health education and the Health Belief Model—increasing numbers of health professionals are embracing behavior modifaction, because empirically it is effective in bringing about desired change (Berni and Fordyce, 1977; Gentry, 1975; Katz and Zlutnick, 1975; LeBow, 1976).

SUMMARY

This paper has reviewed some of the more important models and findings concerning the extent to which individuals do or do not comply with medical regimens, or undertake health related behaviors which appear to be indicated at specific points in time. Attention has been focused, primarily, on those models whose components are capable of manipulation to enhance health related behavior rather than to those which, at this point in time, are restricted to description and explanation.

Based on an evaluation of available research on patient compliance up to 1974, Haynes (1976) concluded that health related behaviors were most consistently associated with three sets of variables: (1) elements of the Health Belief Model; (2) presence of meaningful social support systems within and/or without the family; and (3) the quality of the patient provider relationship, including satisfaction with care received. For the most part demographic variables and health education efforts were found to be ineffective in predicting health related behaviors. Haynes did not review the growing body of research on the use of behavior modification to change peoples' health related behaviors.

Attention has been drawn to the fact that some of the models and approaches which have been reviewed share concepts in common. Becker has suggested incorporation of modifying and enabling variables such as demographic factors, quality of the patient provider relationship and support systems into the Health Belief Model. The Health Belief Model is the most comprehensive model of health behavior available at this time. It is in need of further testing since we have insufficient data concerning results of systematic manipulation of the elements under controlled experimental conditions. With the exception of approaches derived from behavior modification, we have even less good data concerning the other models on which to base practice.

This chapter has provided a commentary on these models and theories which can be used in the practice of health professionals. There are many gaps in the models, and the research based on them. The models presented have elements in common; however, until more work has been done on the individual models, it would be premature to attempt to interrelate those which have been outlined thus far. Eventually, a workable model of health related behavior which would serve as an alternative to behavior modification is needed for use by health professionals, regardless of their discipline.

10

The Queen Bee Syndrome: One Solution to Role Conflict for Nurse Managers

SUZANNE HALSEY

With the growing awareness of human rights in the 1960s, women became politically active in seeking new ways to effectively influence their place in society. Nursing, a predominantly female profession, presents a microcosm of this movement. Just as the women's movement has its leaders, nursing too has advocates who are working to gain power for nurses in the health care system. The nursing literature of the 1970s frequently implores nurses to become politically astute, claiming that, given their numbers in comparison to other health professionals, nurses wield little power (Kalish and Kalish, 1976, p. 29; Stanton, 1974, p. 580). The future for women and nursing will be significantly influenced if nurse leaders can gain support of their constituency and if nurses can look to these leaders for direction.

In *Hospitals, Paternalism, and the Role of the Nurse*, Ashley emphasizes the importance of this recent thrust for the nursing leadership. Ashley contends that nurses have long been subjugated and abused by physicians and hospital administrators. She notes that, as a women's profession, nursing reflects many of the problems and attitudes faced by women in general. Furthermore, she sees the role of nursing as "the epitome of the women's role" (Ashley, 1976, p. 125). For example, nurses are not given full status professionally or equal educational opportunity, nor are they expected to make a lifelong commitment to a career. Ashley points out that socialization into the profession has "stifled initiative by rewarding subservience. Caught in circumstances they could not easily alter, nursing leaders have done

231

their profession and the public harm by acquiescence to male-dominated groups in the health field" (Ashley, 1976, pp. 126-127).

As advice to nurses who are working collectively for a better future, Ashley emphasizes the need for quality leadership. She urges that "professional nursing must begin exerting open and public leadership in meeting consumer health needs" (Ashley, 1976, p. 133).

In nursing the leadership role is not viewed positively. As Ashley indicates, few women enter nursing seeking the power, prestige, and status often associated with leadership. This may be because of the relatively low status accorded the nursing profession. A key factor in this lack in nursing leadership is the "prevailing negative socio-cultural attitude toward authority, management, and leadership" (Leininger, 1974, p. 30). This may be because women and nurses have traditionally been socialized to be caring, helpful, and obedient. Leininger goes on to say with respect to the negative attitude toward authority that "it militates against the recruitment and retention of nurses in top leadership and administrative positions; [this is] clearly manifested by the many unfilled deanship and nursing service positions in the country" (Leininger, 1974, pp. 30-31). Nursing is a profession with reluctant leaders and noncommitted followers as indicated by these long-unfilled administrative posts and that well-prepared nurses consistently opt for research and teaching posts.

Unlike the case for men, the leadership role for women has not been studied in depth. And, "Research has generally reinforced the popular mythology that women are essentially nurturant, expressive, and passive" (Freeman, 1970, pp. 36, 39). This may be particularly true in nursing. In fact, the idea that a woman might be successful in any enterprise outside the realm of her household is contrary to the traditional American way of thinking. Perhaps the paradoxical relationship between the traditional role of women and the contemporary model of a successful professional woman or leader makes it difficult for women and nurses to accept other women as leaders or to take a leadership role themselves (Putnam and Heinen, 1976, p. 48). This attitude may lead to polarization among women; and in nursing, where leadership is not highly valued, the goals and behaviors of the leaders may be viewed with suspicion by the rank-and-file nurse.

THE QUEEN BEE SYNDROME

Staines recently coined the term "Queen Bee syndrome" (Staines, Tavris, and Jayaratne, 1974). It was used to describe antifeminist behaviors in women who had successfully secured positions of leadership in the traditionally male career world. Staines' idea was an adaptation of his countermovement concept. However, from a role theory perspective, the Queen Bee syndrome may be viewed as a role-resolution pattern for the woman who must contend with the conflicting demands of traditional and professional roles. In his work, Staines identified the women's movement as the initial social movement, the proponents as feminist women, and the opponents as antifeminist women. According to Staines et al., the most common feminist opponent is the woman who is content in her traditional role and reluctant to take on the new roles advocated by feminists.

The Queen Bee, however, is an unusual antifeminist because she carries out both the role of the traditional woman and that of the contemporary professional woman. While succeeding as a contemporary role model, the Queen Bee supports the traditional female model for other women and opposes the aims of other career-motivated women within her role system.

Staines et al. sum up the Queen Bee syndrome this way:

> There is a group of anti-feminist women who exemplify the Queen Bee syndrome. Their countermilitancy has its roots in their personal success within the system: both professional success (a high-status job with good pay) and social success (popularity with men, attractiveness, a good marriage). The true Queen Bee has made it in the "man's world" of work, "and if I can do it without a whole movement to help me," runs her attitude, "so can all these other women." . . . Successful people in general, and Queen Bees in particular, tend to be countermilitant for several reasons, each of which has to do with self-interest (Staines et al., 1974, p. 45).

Spengler, using diverse nursing literature to support her belief, concludes that the Queen Bee syndrome exists in nursing (Spengler, 1976, p. 102). Spengler explicitly describes the nurse Queen Bee. She states:

> The Queen Bee syndrome, developed by some nurses, is diagnosed by characteristic symptoms. To begin with, they (Queen Bees) are different from many other nurses. They are not ordinary in the area of motivation and achievement. They are talented individuals who have excelled in their chosen area of interest. . . . They view themselves as successful. They think of themselves as different from other nurses and do not want to associate closely with their own

> *group. Like other Queen Bees, they want to identify up, not down, and therefore, they identify with others out- side of nursing. Very often, these others are men. . . . They then maintain an allegiance to these men and to the system. Queen Bees in nursing are usually found to hold higher paying, more prestigious positions (in nursing, that is). They do not necessarily hold posi- tions that are as well-paying and prestigious as men in the same system. . . . Since the Queen Bees enjoy a privileged position (especially for a nurse) they are not necessarily concerned about making changes in the system they are in (Spengler, 1976, pp. 124-125).*

Many of these characteristics are similar to those outlined by Staines et al.

Spengler goes on to describe what it is like to work with a Queen Bee:

> *It is very frustrating to work with a Queen Bee. To begin with, if she is in a position of authority, she de- mands allegiance from others to her rather than an idea, a program or the profession. If she has special skills, she will not teach other nurses those skills; she keeps them to herself. If she is in a practice setting working with a patient who has special needs that she cannot meet, she will not refer the patient to a nursing colleague; she will find someone else after she finally decides that she herself cannot do it. Some Queen Bees will work with groups of nurses but only on cer- tain levels. They will either have to be the star attrac- tion "who receives special treatment or recognition," or they will have to "run the show." The decision to get involved with other nurses is made on the basis of how it will benefit the Queen Bee—not how others might benefit (Spengler, 1976, p. 126).*

If this exposition of the behavior of the nurse Queen Bee is accurate, then it raises many questions about the role of the nurse leader and her effectiveness in the nursing profession.

Relevance to Nursing

Nursing, like other professions, offers a career ladder for the aspiring. For career development, each upward step features different professional responsi- bilities, opportunities, and associations. The prospects for success for aspiring nurses may well depend on the attitudes of those nurses already in control. When nurse leaders thwart the career mobility for other nurses, they are, in the terms of Staines et al., Queen Bees. Such behavior in nurse superiors engenders frustration and dissatisfaction on the part of the rank-and-file nurses. On the other hand, some nurse leaders may help their subordinates develop new skills and gain career mobility. This behavior is not Queen Bee-like and fosters cohesiveness and colleagueship among nurses on all levels.

A Theoretical Framework

The nurse who takes a leadership position as a head nurse, supervisor, or director in a hospital or health care institution assumes what theorists call a role, which may be determined by others in a particular role setting; role may also refer to expectations or actual behaviors. For instance, Secord and Backman (1974) refer to roles as the expectations that persons hold in common toward any person who falls in a particular category by virtue of his position in the social system" (p. 457). In contrast, other theorists see roles arising from the role incumbent himself. Sargent says, "A person's role is a pattern or type of social behavior which seems situationally appropriate to him in terms of the demands and expectations of those in his group" (Shaw and Costanzo, 1970, p. 335). Whatever the vantage point, the nurse leader must develop a behavior pattern that helps her to cope with the demands and expectations of those around her.

In her professional position, the nurse leader must, however, deal with role prescriptions from a variety of sources. Often, she discovers that the demands and expectations of one group of people are inconsistent with those of other groups. For instance, the medical staff may expect the nurse to spend her time obtaining equipment and assisting with medical procedures, while patients expect her to spend her time instituting comfort measures and teaching good health practices. To compound these ambiguities, the nurse leader must also deal with traditional expectations and behavioral norms related to her other roles of wife, mother, sister, daughter, community member, and so on. As a leader in her work setting, she may be expected to be outspoken, decisive, and assertive. Away from work, as wife or mother, she may be expected to be compliant, obedient, and passive. Because these expectations conflict, the nurse leader may have difficulty assimilating them. This incongruency between traditional expectations and the contemporary professional model for women creates a stumbling block for the professional woman who wishes to be successful in all of her endeavors.

Role theorists call such incongruencies a variety of names. As applied to the hospital setting, Knutson would say the nurse leader has a "role dilemma":

> *Role dilemmas may arise when an individual experiences conflicting pressures regarding the demands of his position. The administrator (nurse leader) must often face choices between the needs and desires of an individual and those of the group. . . . Role dilemmas . . . may arise from either pressures within the organizations or pressures within the individual himself, but, however they arise, they lead to difficult problems for the person who must make decisions (Knutson, 1965, p. 122).*

Knutson would also acknowledge that because the nurse leader is a member of other social groups—such as her family, community, and church—other role conflicts arise. Knutson says that "when a person finds himself filling more than one position and therefore performing more than one role at the same time . . . the demands of the two roles or the conception of how they should be performed may be in conflict" (p. 128). While the term role conflict is popular among theorists, other terms such as role stress, role imbalance, role incongruity, and role ambiguity have been introduced to describe similar phenomena (Lindesmith and Strauss, 1968, pp. 374-376). The subjective experience associated with these role problems has been described as role strain (Goode, 1960).

Merton, while using the term role set to describe "the complement of role relationships which persons have by virtue of occupying a particular social status," acknowledges that the expectations and demands of various others within a social setting do not always complement each other (Biddle and Thomas, 1966, p. 282). According to Merton's terminology, the nurse leader experiences role disarticulation. An example of this might be that the hospital administrator asks the nurse leader to make a budget cut in her department to facilitate financing equipment for another department. The nursing staff might object because a budget cut would severely compromise patient safety and the quality of nursing care. The nurse leader must make a decision for or against the budget cut based on either her personal or professional values, each of which may be in conflict with the other.

In a theory of role-conflict resolution, Gross et al. (1957) identify a process intended to overcome both intra- and interrole conflict. In the case above, the nurse leader experiences intrarole conflict. Gross et al. identify three factors that are considered before resolving a conflict. These are "(1) the relative legitimacy of the expectations, (2) the sanctions incumbent upon the non-fulfillment of each of the expectations, and (3) the moral orientation of the actor" (Shaw and Costanzo, 1970, p. 340). Thus, the nurse leader must formulate her position on the basis of the legitimacy of the administrator's request, the reasonableness of the nursing staff's objections, the potential rewards and punishments including loss of personal job security, and the possibility of professional ostracism. Her professional values and standards will be the key determinants in her decision making. This active process is called role-conflict resolution. A more general process called role bargaining has been identified as a means for managing role problems and the associated role strain (Goode, 1960).

Because the nurse leader is frequently caught in such conflicts requiring decision making based on both expediency and morals, she is forced to take on those attitudes and behavior patterns that will minimize such conflicts and maintain her position. Knutson calls this step "role definition." Knutson says:

> How an individual defines his role and carries it out within a group is likely to differ greatly from the way it is defined by other members of his group. Each person coming into a new group may be told what his rights and responsibilities are, together with how he is expected to perform them. In reality, however, these definitions cannot be complete and precise, with the result that each person must go through a period of adjustment or adaptation to his new role. In the process of this adaptation, the definition of the role and the manner of its performance is likely to change somewhat from the initial definition. (Knutson, 1965, p. 122)

In explaining the dynamics of the role-definition process, Knutson emphasizes the importance of the individual's previous socialization:

> How an individual adapts . . . depends not only on how the position is defined by significant others but also how he himself defines the situation together with his own unique capacities, abilities, experiences, and style or manner of coping with problems in performing his duties and carrying out his responsibilities. Understanding the personal role definition therefore involves understanding both how the role is conceived and how the role is performed (p. 123).

The socialization of the nurse leader may come not only from her home and culture but also from her nursing education where she undergoes the process of professional socialization.

Closely related to role definition is a process called role making. This is a strategy consciously undertaken by the role incumbent or nurse leader. She actively works to modify her role. Turner describes role making as a process in which "the individual confidently frames his behavior as if [it] had unequivocal existence and clarity" (Lindesmith and Strauss, 1969, p. 216). In the instance of the nurse leader, behaviors identifiable as Queen Bee-like can be construed as an example of role making, an attempt to make certain aspects of the role explicit.

The nurse leader who recognizes that role expectations and role demands conflict may actively seek a behavior pattern that is consistent and productive, at least from her point of view. One strategy the nurse leader may choose for managing role conflict is to keep the roles separate and to give priority to the role at hand. However, the nurse leader may want to be successful in the traditional woman's role and simultaneously to succeed in the career of her choice. To do this, she adopts the characteristics that have come to be labeled the Queen Bee syndrome.

This Queen Bee syndrome enables her to prescribe the traditional family role model exclusively for other women. She uses various strategies to keep other women down. By projecting this point of view, i.e., approval of the traditional role, she wins the favor of men in her work setting and minimizes the competition from other talented women who wish to succeed as she has. In so doing, she is able to carry out her leadership role of outspokeness and assertiveness. While this antifeminist posture on the part of the professionally successful woman is paradoxical, it minimizes role strain for the Queen Bee by serving to reduce professional competition. For the nursing profession, nurse Queen Bees can limit nursing's potential and can hinder its development in the health care system because the Queen Bee's values remain static.

THE QUEEN BEE SYNDROME
IN NURSING MANAGEMENT

Recently, I conducted a study to determine whether the Queen Bee syndrome actually exists in nursing and, if so, whether it becomes progressively more manifest in the higher the level of nursing (Halsey, 1977). The sample included persons in the management positions of head nurse, nurse supervisor, and director of nursing in selected hospital settings. The director of nursing sample was taken from a random sample of directors from the Massachusetts Hospital Association list for the Commonwealth of Massachusetts. The supervisor and head nurse responses were elicited from 14 metropolitan Boston hospitals. This was not a random sample.

The nature of the sample and that of the concept to be tested determined the type of investigation. Because the sample was composed of persons who had demanding time commitments and because a relatively large sample was needed, a tool that was quick and easy to complete and that would reach many people was needed. For these reasons a questionnaire was selected.

The questionnaire contained 44 items, including personal data questions, statements believed to be descriptive of Queen Bee characteristics, and distractor statements. These statements were measured on a seven-point Likert scale. The questionnaire was pretested on nurse educators, nurse assistant directors, and nursing coordinators. Queen Bee ness was measured in terms of several discrete characteristics. The scores on these characteristics were combined into a composite score of all Queen Bee characteristics. Distractors were designed to make the questionnaire interesting and to disarm the sophisticated respondent.

The statements designed to elicit Queen Bee-ness were based on seven distinct conceptual categories. The first category related to the Queen Bee's reference group. For example, it is known that she likes to identify with those in positions above her. The second category deals with the Queen Bee's alignment with the establishment and resistance to change. Closely related to this is the third category: the Queen Bee holds antifeminist beliefs that she projects onto other women. The fourth category deals with the Queen Bee's desire to run the show at the expense of other competent women. Fifth, the Queen Bee, as a decision maker, works independently of others and avoids group work or group solutions. Sixth, because she feels that she is appropriately rewarded for her expertise and "specialness," she views the system in which she works positively. The final conceptual category, which is specific to nurse Queen Bees, is that of perceived nurse-doctor conflicts (Spengler, 1976, p. 125). Low Queen Bee characteristic statements were developed to parallel Queen Bee-ness in a contrasting dimension.

The questionnaire return rate was 51 percent, which is unusually high for such a mail survey. The data base was thus compiled from 140 questionnaires. The questionnaire returns comprised the responses of 50 head nurses, 43 supervisors, and 47 directors of nursing.

Characteristics of the Sample

The hospital representation from which the questionnaires were returned varied. Hospital size ranged from 30 to 1200 beds. For the hospitals from which the directors came, the modal size was 225 beds; whereas for head nurses and supervisors, the modal hospital size was 420 beds. This difference reflects the fact that the director sample was drawn from all over Massachusetts, including rural areas, whereas the head nurse and supervisor group was drawn from 14 metropolitan Boston hospitals.

The respondents themselves, while all women, varied considerably in age, experience, and educational preparation. The average age was 40 years, and the range was from 24 to 67. It is interesting to note an increase in the mean age the higher the level of the managerial group (significant at the 0.001 level): the mean age of head nurses was 33; of supervisors, 39; and of directors of nursing, 50 years.

The average number of years of experience of respondents also showed an increase for the higher levels of nursing management: the head nurse average was 12 years experience; supervisors, 18; and directors of nursing, 26. The mean number of years of experience for the group as a whole was 18½.

The educational preparation of the nurse respondents also varied: 2 percent of the respondents were graduates of associate degree programs, 40 percent were graduates from diploma schools of nursing, 27 percent were baccalaureate-prepared, and 31 percent of the respondents possessed Master's degrees in nursing. This is a surprisingly large percentage. The director's group had by far the most Master's degrees. Most head nurses and supervisors had less than a baccalaureate education.

Since the purpose of this study was to look at Queen Bee-ness with respect to job categories, it was important to examine the demographic trends with respect to the categories of head nurse, supervisor, and director. This was done by an analysis of variance. Clearly, and not unexpectedly, the means for age, years of work experience, and education increased with each progressively higher level of management. As indicated, the composition of each managerial level was unique with respect to age, experience, and education (see Table 1). It is important to note that not only did the means increase with each higher level but also that the differences were statistically significant. This may indicate that these were critical variables in influencing the Queen Bee-ness of nurse respondents.

The Findings

Before testing to see if the Queen Bee syndrome was more prevalent at progressively higher levels of nursing management, it was necessary to see if any Queen Bees existed in the total sample. In fact among the 140 respondents, 40 (28 percent) were judged as Queen Bees (Table 2). A respondent was considered a Queen Bee if her Queen Bee score was greater than four, i.e., above the median value on the seven-point Likert scale used to measure Queen

Bee-ness. This score was developed by reversing the numerical value of low Queen Bee statements, then summing high and low Queen Bee responses and dividing by 21, the total number of statements.

TABLE 1

DEMOGRAPHIC CHARACTERISTICS FOR DIRECTORS, SUPERVISORS, AND HEAD NURSES

	Head Nurses	Super-visors	Directors of Nurses	All Re-spondents
Age (mean)	33	39	50	40
Nursing education (mode)	diploma	diploma	Master's	diploma
Experience (mean in years)	12	18	26	18

TABLE 2

QUEEN BEE STATISTICS FOR THE TOTAL SAMPLE AND FOR QUEEN BEE RESPONDENTS

	Mean Queen Bee Score	Standard Deviation	Respondents
Total sample (including Queen Bees)	3.61	0.93	140
Queen Bee respondents	4.75	0.51	40

The hypothesis of the study was that the Queen Bee syndrome is more prevalent in increasingly higher levels of nursing management. To confirm this the findings had to be significant at least at the 5 percent level. The relational hypothesis was accepted by using three different analyses, all yielding significant findings.

For the first analysis, the number of Queen Bee nurses in each managerial group was determined. This was done by selecting only those nurses with Queen Bee scores greater than four. In the sample, there were

33 director Queen Bees, 6 supervisor Queen Bees, and 1 head nurse Queen Bee. This means that the Queen Bee syndrome existed in 2 percent of the head nurse group, 16 percent of the supervisor group, and in 70 percent of the director group. Clearly, this indicates that Queen Bees were more prevalent in increasingly higher levels of nursing management.

The second analysis revealed the statistical significance of the Queen Bee scores with respect to each management group. Here, the mean Queen Bee scores increased with each higher level of nursing management. The proportionate variance explained, r^2, was 0.60. This explained the proportion of variance of the influence that job category had on Queen Beeness. Finally, the F value of 102.77 was significant at the 0.001 level (Tables 3 and 4). This was considerably better than the 5 percent level of significance believed necessary to accept the finding as significant.

TABLE 3

STATISTICAL SIGNIFICANCE OF THE QUEEN BEE SCORES FOR ALL RESPONDENTS ACCORDING TO MANAGEMENT LEVEL			
	Proportionate Variance Explained (r^2)	r (Pearson's Correlation)	F
Queen Bee score	0.60	0.77*	102.77*

*p = 0.001.

TABLE 4

QUEEN BEE SCORES FOR TOTAL SAMPLE ACCORDING TO MANAGEMENT LEVEL				
Management Level	Mean Queen Bee Score	Standard Deviation	No. Queen Bees With Score > 4	No. in Group
Head Nurses	2.75	0.55	1	50
Supervisors	3.69	0.42	6	43
Directors	4.47	0.75	33	47
Total	3.61	0.93	40	140

Finally, a third analysis, a Pearson's correlation, between the Queen Bee score and job level was computed. This gave an *r* value, or coefficient, of 0.77, significant at the 0.001 level. Because age and education seemed to show similar trends with respect to management level, a partial correlation was done between Queen Bee scores and management levels, controlling for the effects of age and education. The correlation between Queen Bee and management level was relatively strong and changed little when controlling statistically for education. The partial correlation yielded an *r* of 0.67, which is significant at the 0.001 level (Table 5).

TABLE 5

		PEARSON CORRELATION COEFFICIENTS FOR AGE, EDUCATION, AND MANAGEMENT LEVEL WITH THE QUEEN BEE SCORE		
	Job Level	Age	Education	Job Level Controlling for Age & Education
Queen Bee score	0.77*	0.53*	0.27*	0.67*

*$p = 0.001$.

To consider the implications of Queen Bee-ness, it is necessary to look not only at the Queen Bee score, but also at the individual components and their theoretical formulation. The first conceptual Queen Bee category related to the Queen Bee's reference group. The findings indicated that the reference groups for nurse leaders change as they move up the career ladder. And the results show that nursing directors and supervisors tend to identify with people outside of nursing, placing little value on input from lower level nurses. This makes one wonder about the priorities of nurse leaders and the extent to which staff nurses' suggestions and ideas have an impact on the administrative nursing care decisions. The second Queen Bee category addressed the question of her alignment with the status quo. She prefers to keep things running smoothly and avoids situations in which the staff may become agitated. However, the differences between each managerial level were significant. Head nurses indicated that they were most willing to try something that might change the status quo, while the director group was least willing. The third category dealt with the Queen Bee's desire to exclude competition for her position. In this area, nursing directors showed greater interest in "running the show" or controlling a work situation than did supervisors or head nurses. Similarly, directors indicated the most uneasiness when expertise and knowledgeability equal to her own were demonstrated by subordinates. The next category dealt with the crux of the Queen Bee syndrome. The Queen Bee, although liberated herself, projects antifeminist beliefs on other women. Here, while the goals of feminism are acknowledged, there are distinct differences in the responses of the groups. It was clear that directors are more apt to project traditional values on other women. The fifth category dealt with the Queen Bee's leadership style. This characteristic was also identified by Spengler (1976, p. 125). Here, the Queen Bee prefers using individual strategies for problem solving rather than tapping the resources of a peer group. Generally, the findings indicated that this sample of nurse leaders used some degree of participative management. However, it was clear that the director's group used this style less frequently than did supervisors and head nurses. The next category dealt with the Queen Bee's perception of the system in which she works. Characteristically, the Queen Bee believes she is being properly rewarded for her talents, and she reasons, therefore, that the system is right and just for all. It is interesting to note that, in general, respondents indicated that promotions and hirings were carried out fairly, but that reimbursement for services was inadequate. Despite this discrepancy, it was clear that the differences between groups were significant and that directors were the most inclined to say that hospital promotions were fair but salaries were not, reflecting a Queen Bee-like attitude. The last Queen Bee category is the one that deals specifically with the nursing setting. Here, Queen Bees see "the many problems of nursing as a problem of individual nurses," and they deny conflicts between nurses and other health care professions (Spengler, 1976, p. 125). The findings related to this category indicated that lower level nurse leaders perceive tension and conflict when dealing with the medical profession. On the other hand, the director's group seemed to negate or deny this belief. This is consistent with the first category, which indicated that the director's group tended to identify with persons outside of nursing, and, in a hospital setting, this may well be with doctors.

In conclusion, it was clear that, for these seven categories, there were significant differences in the responses between head nurse, supervisor, and director levels of management. These findings were consistent with the finding that the composite Queen Bee score showed significant differences among the job levels of nurse administrators.

Results of Factor Analysis

In order to empirically verify the Queen Bee scale, a factor analysis was computed to identify underlying concepts around which Queen Bee statements clustered. This analysis identified four factors around which all Queen Bee statements were correlated. Because the magnitude of the correlation was small with respect to two of the four factors, only the two factors where correlations are high are considered. The factors are illustrated in terms of the continuum shown in Table 6.

TABLE 6

THE QUEEN BEE CONTINUUM IDENTIFIED BY FACTOR ANALYSIS
FACTOR ONE: Orientation with Society

Feminist	Antifeminist Authoritarian Establishment Status quo

FACTOR TWO: Orientation with Nurses and Organization

Pro nurses Group participation Salaries unfair	Cooperative nurses, a priority

QUEEN BEE CONTINUUM

Low Queen Bee	High Queen Bee

The concepts encompassed in these two factors were related to Queen Bee-ness. The primary factor identified statements relating to the Queen Bee's orientation to society or adherence to the status quo and to traditional and conservative beliefs. The statements that positively correlated with this factor were those that were antifeminist, those that indicated maintenance of the status quo, and those that acknowledged a need for endorsement from hospital administrators and medical staff. In contrast, the statements that were negatively correlated acknowledged rejection of traditional authoritarian management styles with a preference for participative styles. Also included in this category were feminist statements.

The secondary factor identified the respondents' relationship with their nurse constituency and with the organization. This is best conceptualized in terms of the classic role conflict of the professional working within an organization (Etzioni, 1964, pp. 81-87). Statements that related to this concept concerned nurse reference groups, perceptions of the organizations, and individual methods of making changes. Thus, the factor analysis empirically verified the seven conceptual categories of Queen Bee-ness developed by the investigator; the seven conceptual categories, however, were reduced to two more general conceptual areas.

DISCUSSION

The findings of this exploratory study indicate that the Queen Bee syndrome exists in nursing, a female-dominated profession. This finding is important because, in the original article on the Queen Bee syndrome, Queen Bees were identified only in male-dominated professions (Staines et al., 1974, p. 55). Of greater importance, however, is the fact that this study shows that the Queen Bee syndrome becomes more prominent in progressively higher levels of nursing management. This finding has many implications for nurse leaders and for the nursing profession.

To date, the constellation of behavior that earns the label "Queen Bee" is generally thought to be negative and counterproductive. Berry and Kushner condemn the "hard-headed, two-fisted woman executive" image that is labeled as Queen Bee (1975, p. 173). They are concerned about the reaction of aspiring young women to the stereotype of the Queen Bee, about which they say:

> To young women considering future careers, the "Queen Bee" can become a sociological icon highly charged with negative connotations and the power to drive away female seekers of prestigious positions for fear of their being labeled Queen Bees (Berry and Kushner, 1977, p. 173).

The authors categorically refute each negative aspect of the Queen Bee. First, they assume that the Queen Bee is the victim of other women. They think it is right that the Queen Bee is engaged in an ongoing struggle to prove herself in a competitive system. Furthermore, the Queen Bee is seen as "a high achiever who needs few rewards from others in order to gain satisfaction from what she does" (p. 174). They argue that it is logical that the Queen Bee identify with the "male reward system" because, having been a victim of "psychological sabotage from other women, [she] is apparently quite aware of their motives." They conclude that it is necessary for the Queen Bee to identify with male colleagues in order to gain a support system against opposition from outside groups, including women. However, in nursing there are few male nurse colleagues. Therefore, the female nurse adminsitrator seeking a male support system may identify with the medical chief of staff or hospital administrator. By identifying outside of nursing, the nurse adminsitrator may create a "credibility gap" between herself and the nursing staff. Her nursing staff may well view her motivations with suspicion and may carry out her goals and plans with limited cooperation. Berry and Kushner do concede that the Queen Bee prefers individual strategies over group strategies. They maintain that this is appropriate because she is an efficient decision maker. They seem to disregard current management theories that emphasize the need for delegation and participative decision making. They conclude that the Queen Bee label is too narrow in focus to describe successful women.

I believe that the Queen Bee syndrome may not represent a set of role behaviors consciously selected by the nurse leader but one arrived at by trial and error, through professional socialization and experience. The nurse leader develops the Queen Bee syndrome by role making and role taking, a process of trying and discarding different sets of behavior until one is found that fits.

A Queen Bee nurse leader has probably had to contend with conflicting role expectations and obligations. For her, the Queen Bee behavior offers a way of coping with the conflicting demands of the contemporary professional role model and the traditional family role model. It permits her to operate on a double standard; what is right for her is not always right for other women. Due to this double standard, the nurse Queen Bee may frequently be haunted by decisions that she has made from these two conflicting frames of reference. Chesler seems to understand the plight of the Queen Bee who must contend with two different sets of role obligations when she says, "Paradoxically, while women must not 'succeed,' when they succeed at anything, they have still failed if they are not successful at everything" (Chesler, 1972, p. 88).

In her work role, the Queen Bee may function in one of two ways. She may be very hard-working and productive in her career. In this case, the organization will benefit from the short-term gain of her personal endeavors. However, in the long run, the organization will suffer because her subordinates are not trained or developed, and her expertise is hoarded rather than shared. On the other hand, she may be ineffective because of her reluctance to initiate changes and because of her strong orientation toward maintaining the status quo—her organization remains static and immobilized. Because the Queen Bee is unwilling to take risks, few if any changes are initiated. This results in poor staff morale, low interest in work, poor motivation, and poor performance. Regardless of her personal level of productivity, Queen Bee behaviors in nurse leaders have a negative effect on the institution, other nurses, the nursing profession, and on the quality of nursing care.

At a time when nursing has a critical need for quality leaders to help shape the future of the health care system, decisions by nurse Queen Bees may be detrimental to the role of nurses in health care planning. Colton maintains that it is the reluctance of nurses in leadership positions to make decisions and to take risks that keeps nursing behind the scenes in health care planning (Colton, 1976, pp. 29-31). It is also clear that nurse leaders who tend to identify with other health professions may forsake the goals of nursing. Similarly, nurse Queen Bees, by maintaining their double standard of values, are postponing the development of role competence both for nurses and woman in general. By avoiding such role development, the Queen Bee forfeits opportunities to be a positive role model to other nurses. Also, by hindering the development of their subordinates' skills, the Queen Bee may squelch potential leaders. By maintaining the status quo, these Queen Bee leaders may prevent nurses from learning the skills necessary for advancement. And finally, the Queen Bee's projection of the traditional family role onto other women prevents nursing from fully utilizing its resources.

The author believes that the solution to the current leadership dilemma in nursing rests in training nurse leaders to combine the role-making process with the role-taking process. In role taking, the role incumbent takes the roles of significant others in a setting. In so doing she develops an attitude of empathy so that she can predict how her role, communications, and behavior will affect not only herself but others and society. Mead describes this conscious and active process in this way:

> It is through taking the role of the other that [one] is able to come back on [oneself] and so the role of the other . . . is not something that just happens as an incidental result of the gesture, but it is of importance in the development of cooperative activity. The immediate effect of such role-taking lies in the control which the individual is able to exercise over his own response (Mead, 1962, p. 254).

This process enables the person or actor to assume a role that is dynamic and that maximizes the needs or goals not only of the actor but of the significant others in the situation. By combining role taking with role making, nurse leaders will learn to recognize the long-term consequences of Queen Bee behavior. It would require the careful analysis of their personal and professional values and the development of one single, harmonious, and operational code of behavior.

Thus, it is clear that the Queen Bee syndrome is one solution to role conflict frequently used by nurse managers. It offers the nurse leader comfort and safety in her role by helping to control and limit the power of her subordinates. Simultaneously, the syndrome, with its orientation to the status quo and traditional values, helps her to maintain a nonthreatening image for her superiors, who are often men. Clearly, these characteristics of Queen Bee-ness benefit only the role incumbent. However, other nurses, the profession, and patient care delivery may well suffer from the Queen Bee style of leadership. Staff development, colleagueship, and creativity are compromised when the nurse leader adopts this method for resolving her own role conflict. Nurses and nursing must learn to look beyond the role of the Queen Bee for leadership styles that will complement not only the needs of the role incumbent but those of the profession and its clients as well.

11

Professional, Political, and Ethnocentric Role Behaviors and their Influence in Multidisciplinary Health Education

MADELEINE LEININGER

INTRODUCTION

Bringing together individuals having diverse backgrounds of interests, needs and goals to discuss common matters of social concern is a noteworthy achievement. But to bring together a core group of scientists and professional people to work on critical multidisciplinary issues and tasks in a harmonious and productive manner is truly a major challenge, a challenge seldom met to the fullest extent of human potential available.

Within the last decade there has been a clear movement in the United States toward the development and implementation of multidisciplinary professional health education programs within university settings (Hogness, 1976; Leininger, 1971; Pellegrino, 1975, p. 224). This movement reflects a rapidly growing effort to achieve collegial multidisciplinary types of education with the ultimate intent of improving health care services to people. In general, this trend is viewed as an encouraging one that should help bring about more optimal utilization of health professionals—utilization consonant

251

with their educational preparation or experience backgrounds. Furthermore health professionals are becoming aware of the need to share ideas and to work together as a partnership of equals in order to maximize educational talents and resources. Thus, the movement toward multidisciplinary efforts seems promising, but there still remains a variety of unresolved problems to be addressed.

In this chapter I shall identify some of those factors that encourage or facilitate movement toward the establishment of interdisciplinary health education programs. Some of the barriers to effective interdisciplinary collaboration will also be identified. Both a nursing and an anthropologic perspective are employed in examining interprofessional behavior. Ethnocentrism is singled out as an anthropologic construct particularly useful in examining such behavior.

Within the current multidisciplinary process of "discovering" and studying the aspirations, accomplishments, and interests of those in the health disciplines, one can find that there are contributions more or less unique to a specific discipline, areas of overlap, and, of course, areas of common interest among the disciplines. At the same time, one can identify interpersonal tensions, uneasiness, problems, and concerns among those health professionals (Leininger, 1975) participating in multidisciplinary activities. The past efforts undertaken by disciplines to become autonomous and independent of each other are being challenged today by those committed to multidisciplinary philosophy and goals. Furthermore, shifting from highly independent behavior to more interdependent role behavior necessitates changes in attitudes, goals, and actions. From an anthropologic perspective, present multidisciplinary efforts of the health professions resemble a loose tribal organization in which many separate clans and subclans are trying to find the common identity, interests, and goals by which they can live and work together. Whether this tribal group and its organizational structure will survive is to a great extent dependent upon knowledgeable and skilled leaders committed to multidisciplinary efforts.

Presently, the five traditional health disciplines—nursing, medicine, dentistry, pharmacy, and social work—remain the principal groups that are exploring ways to make multidisciplinary efforts effective, satisfying, and helpful to consumers and themselves. As the members of these disciplines struggle and work together, a variety of questions have surfaced together with ambivalent feelings about multidisciplinary participation. There is, however, little question that the movement toward establishing multidisciplinary programs in both health education and service delivery will continue unabated. There are a number of reasons why this trend can be expected to continue and some of these will be identified presently.

In general, multidisciplinary health work means bringing different disciplines together to plan, implement, and evaluate their educational and practice services, and to discover how each can work together in effective and satisfying ways. Establishing a climate of trust in multidisciplinary work in order to share experiences and plans is essential; it helps to promote a climate in which partners can listen to and learn from each other.

THE ESTABLISHMENT OF MULTIDISCIPLINARY HEALTH EDUCATIONAL PROGRAMS

There have been a number of important factors contributing to the development of interprofessional health educational programs during the past decade. Seven of these will be discussed here. First, there has been *societal concern about access to and availability of health care services for all social, economic, and cultural groups* in the United States. Ideally, all Americans want health care services to be accessible at a reasonable cost. Increasingly, people are demanding such services as a human right, and, understandably, there have been a number of questions raised publicly about ways of making health care fully accessible and available to all persons irrespective of socioeconomic status and cultural or ethnic differences.

For a number of reasons—including economic, cultural and political considerations—equal access to care and the right to health care are ideals that have not as yet become a reality. Consequently, several minority cultural groups and lower income groups have not received adequate health care through those professional services now available (Oseasohn, 1975; Paul, 1963; Sanchez, 1973). Moreover, the general shortage of well-prepared health personnel together with their maldistribution have limited the availability of health care services to many groups in this country. But even if there were adequate numbers and proper distribution of health personnel to provide care, some people would not use the services either because of prohibitive costs or cultural value differences between health care providers and recipients (Leininger, 1974; LeVine, 1974; Paul, 1963; Saunders, 1954). Acquisition of knowledge about differences in beliefs and values of professionals and of cultural groups they serve is an essential aspect of multidisciplinary health education. In turn, such critical social value factors serve as major incentives to developing multidisciplinary health education and to encourage efforts to improve the availability and accessibility of health services to people.

Second, multidisciplinary health education has been initiated largely because of the continuing concerns expressed by legislators, health consumers, faculty, and students about the *high costs of educational programs in college and university settings* (Carnegie Commission on Higher

Education, 1973, pp. 2-3). Concomitantly, there has assuredly been a growing national concern about the educational costs of medical and dental schools, and to some extent about the costs for schools of nursing, pharmacy, and social work. Attempts to reduce costs of education during periods of high inflation have been given increasing attention by health professionals and by some legislative groups. Attempts made to control costs in an across-the-board manner have adversely influenced the quality of educational programs in several health disciplines. For example, in some public colleges and universities, faculty salaries have been cut from budgets, instructional supplies have been severely cut, and research linked with teaching appears to be regarded by state budget technicians as more of a luxury than an essential enterprise. Health education costs, therefore, continue to be a critical issue, forcing health leaders to try to contain costs while at the same time maintaining quality programs. Multidisciplinary education appears to be one promising way of reducing costs insofar as it can reduce some of the duplication now present in health professional education programs. For example, educators in nursing and medicine often present identical cognate content in separate courses; this content could easily be offered in a single course for students in both of these disciplines.

Closely related to the cost factor is a third factor—that of *encouraging the development of common multidisciplinary basic and advanced health science courses in order to reduce duplication of offerings and enrich student learning.* Where similar courses and larning goals exist, common courses could be initiated to enhance learning and reduce costs. For example, physicians, nurses, social workers, pharmacists, and dentists could well share some graduate core courses together and additionally gain insight about one another through the learning process. In the baccalaureate health science programs, health students could be enrolled together in courses dealing with basic physiologic and psychologic aspects of health care, prevention modalities, health education interviewing, disease processes, diagnostic assessments, and other common content domains relevant to nearly all health professionals. The establishment of both basic and advanced common cores of "service" courses for all health science disciplines would appear to be essential to future health education programs if costly duplication of courses and programs is to be avoided. Such common core courses would provide the added benefits of stimulating interprofessional learning opportunities, wiser allocation of faculty time, and more cost-effective utilization of available financial resources (Leininger, 1971).

A fourth factor influencing the development of multidisciplinary health programs is the explicit intent of some educators to *increase interprofessional humanistic sensitivities and to reduce unnecessary interprofessional competition and tensions.* Helping each profession to learn about both the traditional and current dominant interests, goals, and unique health care contributions of the other professions has been a salient goal of multidisciplinary leaders in recent years—enhanced by the trend toward humanistic nursing, medicine, and social services (Bulger, 1974; Leininger, 1974). In the historical development of the five major health disciplines, each had gone its separate way until approximately 1965. Consequently, shared knowledge was meager and humanistic understandings about each other was minimal and superficial. Clearly, action was indicated to facilitate humanistically oriented interprofessional education in order to help professional students become comfortable with and sensitive to one another as they pursued their shared goal of providing health services to people. Students have often served as the impetus to encourage faculty and other students to share clinical learning experiences and plan interprofessional curricula. Clinical conferences and clinical projects both inside and outside the hospital setting have been important attempts at some universities to bring together faculty and students from the different health disciplines. As these interprofessional conferences and projects were encouraged and increased in number, the learning opportunities for each profession likewise increased. In addition, interprofessional sensitivities, awareness of the goals of other disciplines, and mutual expectations were heightened. Some projects were expressly established to facilitate faculty-student exchanges across interdisciplinary lines and to discover attitudes, feelings, and professional life interests among these groups. An implicit assumption behind such efforts was the belief that if students from different disciplines were socialized together in multidisciplinary program experiences, they would then become more sensitive to each other and would be likely to work more effectively together upon completion of their programs of study.

A fifth factor and an assumption supporting multidisciplinary health education is the belief that *positive and effective interprofessional education can change the quality of health care services to people.* At the onset of the movement toward interprofessional education and services, many health personnel were aware that they offered uniprofessional services to consumers and that many of their services were coordinated only to a very limited extent with those services offered by other health professionals. As a consequence, health care delivery problems arose. Gaps in services to clients, role confusion, poor communication, and many other problems arose in attempting to provide comprehensive health care. In turn, these problems became concerns for health educators developing multidisciplinary courses for students in the health field. Within the framework of these early multidisciplinary efforts, educators in each discipline assumed the charge of becoming aware of one another's service contributions, of watching for fragmentation and duplication of services among the disciplines, and of remaining alert to interprofessional service-related problems. The planning and implementation of collaborative health services, with a focus on continuity and cooperation, have continued to be extremely important objectives for interprofessional education.

Still another factor facilitating collaboration in education—the sixth in this discussion—is the *occurrence of a number of major role changes within the health disciplines over the last several years* (Bullough, 1976; Ford, 1968). As the roles of health professionals changed, it became apparent that there existed a need to examine and discuss such role changes among the health science disciplines. Role changes, role negotiations, and new role images needed to be explicated for students while they were in their basic educational programs, rather than after they left these programs to take on their professional roles. In addition, it was believed that students needed to have interprofessional clinical experience in the home, hospital, clinics, and other settings where health professionals worked.

As many new health worker groups entered the health care field over recent years, it became important that health professional students be given opportunities to interact with these different groups—many of them auxiliary personnel. One not unexpected outcome of such increased interaction has been the incidence of interprofessional and intergroup competition, jealousy, and role claims related to "expanding" or "extended" roles between and among health disciplines (Bullough, 1976). A recognizable need to bring health groups together to examine these tensions and to debate new or emergent roles manifested itself. At the same time, it was evident that there was a need to project which types of health roles would be required to meet consumer needs in the future. Thus, establishing multidisciplinary health educational programs appeared to be both a logical and promising means of discussing interprofessional roles, conflict areas, and relationships. It was anticipated that as diverse health groups came together with their vested interests, norms, and cultural values, they could address role changes and negotiate modifications in their respective goal-related role functions. New role encroachments upon traditional role behaviors led to the "turf syndrome," in which each health discipline claimed rights to certain role activities, physical space, and areas of practice that they felt belonged to them. Thus, the need to examine such behaviors and role claims, together with the need to reinforce, relinquish, or modify role expectations, were important guiding factors in interprofessional studies. The *health science councils* that had been formed in a number of universities for the purpose of coordinating multidisciplinary education took on the additional task of attempting resolution of these role-related tensions and conflicts.

An interesting phenomenon subsequently developed. With heightened interprofessional interests and its consequent political maneuvering, some powerful disciplines—chiefly, medicine—tended to cast other disciplines into roles those disciplines were unwilling to accept. For example, during the late 1960s the discipline of medicine tried to place nurses into the roles of "physicians' assistant" or "nurse practitioner" in order to meet medicine's economic needs for increased numbers of less costly assistants. With their political power, physicians were able to generate strong federal funding aimed at achieving their goal of increasing the supply of nurse practitioners or physician assistants; in addition, many physicians were willing to employ these "extenders" at salaries much above the prevailing rate for professional nurses in general. Until recently, the nursing profession has had to accept these imposed medical-model role patterns, despite their incompatibility with nursing's own identity strivings toward professional autonomy.

A seventh factor leading to the development of multidisciplinary health education programs is the *marked increase in the numbers of students who sought admission to the health professions following World War II.* In addition to students from the five traditional health schools, a large number of different professional, semiprofessional, and nonprofessional students have entered the health field. While the health field has become an increasingly attractive career field for students, in part because of increased consumer needs for health care and in part because of the growth of scientific knowledge, there were no explicit advance plans to accommodate this sharp increase in the number of students. Thus, the sheer increase in the number of students in the health professions gave an impetus to attempts to maximize available human and financial resources. Educators, who were faced with tight budgets, viewed multidisciplinary programs as a possible means of coordinating educational resources and avoiding the spawning of a great variety of similar programs. The combined force, therefore, of a number of factors encouraged the initiation of multidisciplinary sharing in core course offerings for health professions students. A certain amount of experimentation occurred as attempts were made to find the best possible model and to organize groups and programs into some innovative patterns.

EMERGENCE OF NEW ORGANIZATIONAL STRUCTURES

As a consequence of the above factors, a need to develop and establish new kinds of organizational structures to facilitate cross-disciplinary education and their related research programs became evident. This need, in turn, led to the establishment of multidisciplinary health science councils or health science boards within university settings. Within such organizational structures, multidisciplinary curricular councils, research units, and special projects were established—all intended to facilitate cross-disciplinary learning. Another aim of this reorganization was that of sharing expensive teaching equipment, classroom space, and a variety of other physical resources—an all-important objective in light of the diminishing financial resources available to universities in the late 1960s. These objectives were realized in the emergence of newer types of relationships among professional schools and departments where cross-disciplinary learning could and did take place.

In sum, the factors cited above gave impetus to the rise and establishment of multidisciplinary administrative units and interprofessional educational programs; these have been recent evolutionary developments on most university campuses. In a related development some measurable progress has been made to facilitate the interests and goals of the professions involved. Unquestionably, various health manpower groups organized under the aegis of the United States Federal Government have played a key role in helping to support interprofessional curricular, clinical, and research projects, particularly since 1968. These groups, composed of national health leaders, were quick to recognize the economic, political, and professional implications inherent in multidisciplinary education. The economic implications were that health care costs might be contained; the political implications were that consumers would have tangible evidence of efforts by the professions to be responsive to consumer needs; and the professional implications were that better health care could be provided through coordinated group efforts.

ETHNOCENTRISM: A THEORETICAL EXPLANATION OF INTERPROFESSIONAL BEHAVIOR

In any human enterprise in which old practices give way to new developments affecting its function and meaning, the application of a theory, conceptual framework, or hypothetical formulation can aid the study and explanation of such phenomena, insofar as these affect behavior. As noted earlier, I have chosen the construct of ethnocentrism and some theoretical formulations derived from it to help explain interprofessional group behaviors. These formulations include the professional, political, economic, cultural, and social manifestations that together help to explain certain behaviors which might otherwise be inexplicable to the ordinary observer.

The construct of *ethnocentrism* is a familiar term to anthropologists, but only recently has it become of interest to members of the health professions. Ethnocentrism refers to *the attitude or outlook by which an individual or group holds that its own cultural values are the desired, preferred, or best ones* (Leininger, 1969; LeVine and Campbell, 1972). Individuals almost unknowingly take their own cultural values as objective reality and use them automatically as criteria against which to judge situations, perform acts, and anticipate the actions of others. Generally, ethnocentric individuals seldom realize that their outlook or values may be quite different from those of others. In fact, such individuals may quickly decide that behavior that deviates from their expectation is inferior, immoral, or incorrect. LeVine (1972) helps to illustrate these points in his cross-cultural investigations based upon the theoretical construct of ethnocentrism. He makes the point that "ethonocentrism is not simply a matter of intellectual functioning but involves emotions that are positive and negative." Symbolic referents related to ethnocentrism can also be identified through verbal and nonverbal ethnocentric behaviors. Unquestionably, ethnocentrism is a pervasive phenomenon influencing human behavior—aspects of which can be observed and predicted in a variety of interactional contexts and common life situations.

While social scientists have been intrigued with ethnocentric behaviors since Sumner's work of 1906, the concept itself was never fully explicated, defined, or even studied extensively until anthropologists became involved in cross-culture endeavors and personality studies around 1950. The work of psychologic anthropologists such as Campbell (1972), Frake (1969), and LeVine (1972) inspired social and health scientists to explore further the phenomenon of ethnocentric behavior.

In the early 1960s, I was involved in an anthropologic study examining the ethnocentric behavior of two villages in the Eastern Highlands of Papua, New Guinea, and at that time I came to realize that similar kinds of ethnocentric behaviors tended to occur in multidisciplinary health groups in America (Leininger, 1966). Hence, an ethnocentric model suggested itself as a framework for studying interprofessional group interactions. The use of ethnocentric principles and related research can assist not only in understanding interprofessional role conflicts, stresses, and behaviors, but appears useful in attempts of social scientists and health professionals to bring about more functional interprofessional relationships.

Ethnocentrism and Multidisciplinary Behavior

The following theoretical formulations are presented here to stimulate the reader to examine multidisciplinary health behaviors and to discover the value of using ethnocentric formulations in explaining such behaviors:

1. The greater the manifestation of strong ethnocentric role behaviors among health professional groups, the greater the likelihood of interprofessional role conflicts, stresses, and barriers to achieving desired norms for effective multidisciplinary endeavors.

2. The more pervasive and arbitrary the political or power behavior manifestations of a professional group, the greater the social distance, intergroup stresses, and heightening of ethnocentric behaviors.

3. The greater the behavioral differences related to ethnocentric cultural norms and values between health professional groups, the less the evidence of effective intergroup collaboration among the disciplines involved.

4. The more marked the signs of ethnocentric behaviors manifested by each professional discipline, the more difficult will be the achievement of harmonious and cooperative multidisciplinary educational goals.

5. The greater the signs of marked ethnocentrism and social status differences among health professional groups, the more frequent will be the occurrence of interprofessional conflicts, stresses, and covert hostilities.

6. The more ambiguous the role expectations of cultural or subcultural groups, the greater will be the need to resolve such role ambiguities through role negotiation, role clarification, and role performance activities.

These hypotheses, then, provide some theoretical statements for examining multidisciplinary health behaviors, both past and present, and might well help to identify areas for further study. Some examples of ethnocentric multidisciplinary behaviors will be provided.

Professional Ethnocentrism and Political Role Behaviors

PRE-1965 ERA[1]

In the cultural evolution of multidisciplinary health education in university settings prior to and following 1965, there can be found themes and manifestations of heightened ethnocentric behaviors among the several health disciplines. Prior to 1965, formal multidisciplinary health educational programs in universities were given limited recognition with virtually none of them offering interprofessional health courses or projects. Where the few health science centers existed, they were very loosely organized. Some of the existing centers were used primarily for communication and for conceptual orientation purposes. That is, although administrators, faculty, and students from the five traditional professional schools (nursing, pharmacy, social work, medicine, and dentistry) were cognizant of each other and administrators may have met periodically, formal organizations or programs meant to bring them together were very limited. Informal modes of interaction and inter-professional sharing among faculty and students tended to occur in college cafeterias, hallways, clinical areas, libraries, or at public health lectures. Each health discipline was aware to some extent of the physical space the other professional groups occupied, and there was at least implied interest in the spirit of interprofessional work. In those early days, each professional disci-pline appeared highly ethnocentric—promoting its own cultural norms, curricula, clinical experiences, research interests, and general professional styles of thinking and acting. Furthermore, most health disciplines seemed deeply involved in developing their own physical and psychologic territories and the types of professional identities in which ethnocentric attitudes, thinking, and action patterns prevailed. For example, many nursing colleges had their own buildings. They attempted to protect their building from a "take over" by physicians when medicine saw fit to deem it politically expedient.

In considering further the historically strong ethnocentric tend-encies of the health professions, it is apparent that there existed an implicit expectation that each profession would contribute directly or indirectly to medical care education and research. Medicine was by far the most influential, dominant, and powerful health discipline, compelling the allegiance and dependency of other health groups (Freidson, 1970; Kane and Kane, 1969). Indeed some health disciplines drew vicariously upon medicine to more fully achieve their own goals. That is, dentistry and nursing faculty often relied upon medicine for its acknowledged political and financial power (as backup support) and medical course content, which could be used in courses to be taught to students in the nursing and dentistry programs. Despite this reliance upon medicine, both disciplines were simultaneously making efforts to explicate their own body of knowledge and establish a distinct identity. Such ethnocentric behaviors were prevalent until multi-disciplinary education became more widespread in the late 1960s. In part because of their dependence on medicine, nonmedical health personnel were vaguely aware of experiencing role conflicts, tensions, and ambivalent atti-tudes vis-a-vis medicine. There were both overt and covert beliefs and feelings that medicine was trying to control the identities and the development of the nonmedical professions. These ambivalent attitudes and covert hostilities undoubtedly greatly influenced the development of multidisciplinary health education. That is, there was no consensus among the concerned groups that multidisciplinary education was the preferred objective. In fact, there was considerable reluctance on the part of the professional groups involved to support such multidisciplinary educational programs and projects they did begin to get started.

Prior to 1965, the idiosyncratic cultural values and norms of each discipline could be readily identified by social scientists. However, many of the disciplines were not fully aware of their own norms and behaviors (Leininger, 1968, 1976). Ethnocentric behaviors were clearly evident in the attempts of each discipline to maintain its own territory, roles, and functions and in its posture of noninterference with the major educational or service goals of the other disciplines. Indeed, most health disciplines felt they had considerable freedom to develop and advance their professional interests. Perhaps the single exception was nursing, in that many nurse administrators, educators, and clinicians seemed unduly dependent upon medicine and willing to function according to its rules of behavior. Although most nursing schools controlled their own curricula, faculty, and students prior to 1965, the prevailing norms in teaching, research, and practice content tended to reflect the discipline of medicine. Furthermore, some physicians in university settings actually tried to control nursing programs by controlling their resources—especially their fiscal resources—in the pre-1965 years. For example, the budgets of some nursing schools were subject to review and final approval by deans of schools of medicine rather than by the administrative officer responsible for coordinating all professional schools on a given campus. Those schools of nursing located within a department of medicine were under especially tight control. Thus, medical ethnocentrism and norms engulfed nursing, often without substantial opposition on the part of nurse educators and administrators.

With respect to nursing curricula prior to 1965, there were only a few programs that were clearly nursing centered; most curricula were based on the medical model of disease, diagnostic processes, and curative therapy. Some nurse administrators and faculty felt they were under mandatory constraints to teach substantive medical content. Physician disapproval, and even sanctions, could be imposed in some instances if a physician took issue with nursing course content. For example, I recall the case of a nursing instructor who was made to feel guilty when her lesson plan—which focused on nursing care—was criticized by a physician. The physician's comment was, "There is nothing substantive to your instruction as there are virtually no medical diseases included in your outline."

During the 1960s, a number of nurse educators began to shift their teaching content and clinical experience away from the medical model to a nursing model. This shift in emphasis generated distrust and doubt on the part of some medical faculty toward nurse educators. However, the trend continued as nursing achieved more autonomy and self-directedness—most noticeably in institutions of higher education. At the same time, as more nurses were prepared in college and university settings, a healthy degree of autonomy and ethnocentrism began to emerge. This autonomy was especially evident in the development of nursing (as opposed to medical) curriculum content by nurse faculty. Theoretical and conceptual frameworks began to appear in the nursing literature to explain nursing practices, processes, and phenomena (Orem, 1971; Rogers, 1970; Roy, 1974). Such changes led to signs of cultural shock among physicians and gave rise to further attempts by them to control nursing through their power and authority roles in universities. So as nurses became more ethnocentric and autonomous, they simultaneously encountered more power struggles in protecting their budgets and defending their physical space, research laboratories, and instructional media. Direct confrontations took place in some instances between nursing and medical faculty as these value shifts occurred. Unfortunately, some nursing leaders were not competent to deal with the political role behaviors of physicians, and some were afraid to risk a separation from medical norms and lifestyles (Leininger, 1974).

In contrast to the situation in nursing education, and prior to 1965, the professions of dentistry and pharmacy enjoyed a relatively high degree of autonomy and their ethnocentric tendencies were strongly evident as they developed their own professional goals, largely without interference from medicine. It is of interest that these disciplines remained loyal to medicine and, in fact, looked to it for professional, financial, and moral support. An attitude of "collective ethnocentric brotherhood" appeared as the predominantly male disciplines of medicine, dentistry, and pharmacy supported each other both in formal and informal collectivities within university settings. The author found this behavior noticeably in contrast to the predominantly female disciplines of nursing and social work in which no similar "collective ethnocentric sisterhood" alliance was manifest. Such data support the author's cross-culturally derived observation that women tend to have more difficulty than men in uniting themselves in crisis situations or in times of societal value shifts. The reasons for this failure to unite include lack of value consensus, intergroup jealousies, and inappropriate use of women's talents and roles.

Prior to 1965, the disciplines of nursing and social work were slow to manifest strong political role behaviors or to use their potential for decision making in their universities. Both of these largely female disciplines were greatly influenced by medicine. Psychiatric social workers and psychiatric nurses did, however, seem to exhibit more efforts to deal with political role and power behaviors vis-a-vis the male-dominated disciplines than did other social workers and nurses and, additionally, they participated in interprofessional team work.

In sum, pre-1965 multidisciplinary health education efforts were very limited in the majority of university settings. Interprofessional conflicts, restlessness, role strains, and problems were pervasive throughout higher education. The major health disciplines, except for nursing and social work, manifested generally autonomous and marked ethnocentric behaviors but showed signs of medical influence. There is no question that the political and authoritative role of medicine had a pervasive influence on other health professions with respect to personnel selection, curricula, physical resources, and financial allocations. Covert concerns and uneasiness about medical influence were particularly evident within the professions of nursing and social work. These largely female disciplines were substantially less ethnocentric than the male-dominated professions of medicine, pharmacy, and dentistry.

POST-1965 ERA

Since 1965 and continuing to the present, there has been a steady increase in the numbers of health science centers within the large universities in the United States. As of July 1977, there were approximately 85 health science centers, and others were being developed (Dixon, 1977). One of the major organizational groups promoting the development and support of these health science centers in universities was the Association of Academic Health Centers (AAHC). Initially, the Association was organized primarily as a self-help group for physicians who were serving as the vice-presidents, chancellors, or directors of health science centers.

When first established, most of the health science centers in universities were called medical centers—a label that accurately reflected the medical orientation of these units and their administrative control by physicians. Concurrent with the establishment of these units, nursing leaders evidenced anxiety about these potentially large organizations concerned primarily with medical affairs. They knew that the centers would be controlled by physicians, who would tend to focus on problems of medical education rather than on the broader problems of health or the interests of other health disciplines. These centers seemed to reinforce medicine's traditional control at a time when nursing was trying to move away this dominance and its related influences. Some nursing deans held to the position that the centers should be called *health* centers in order to provide for the inputs from nursing and other disciplines; indeed, several Deans were successful in having this title designated for their centers. To some extent, the use of the term *health center* made it explicit to the public that a number of health disciplines, rather than medicine alone, contributed to the delivery of care to people.

Essentially, curricula, research, and related projects of the health science centers developed in accord with the collective philosophies, health practices, and political behaviors of the deans or their designates. Today, most of these centers now focus upon the broad dimensions of health, including maintenance of wellness, the prevention of disease, and the restoration of persons to health. Research related to these aspects, as well as to the study of *health-seeking and behavior that promotes healthy lifestyles*, is gradually becoming one of the major program goals of health science centers (Leininger, 1974). The health science center concept is coming to be more widely endorsed by the health professions, although some disciplines continue to remain ambivalent about its value. This ambivalence, where it exists, appears to be related to concerns for professional autonomy, the adequacy of financial support for each discipline, and the effectiveness of the leadership provided in the various centers.

Since the inception of the health science centers—and despite the persistent efforts of the other health professions—the authority, leadership roles, and power continue to reside largely with physicians. Physicians, almost as a matter of course, have been appointed by university presidents as vice-presidents or directors of these centers. Some of these physician appointees were primarily prepared as epidemiologists, surgeons, endocrinologists, internal medicine, or community medicine practitioners. Few of these heads of the health science centers have had educational preparation in the theory of formal organization, group process, or in the management of complex social systems. While there were and are other health professional leaders prepared in such areas, virtually none occupies a vice-presidency or similar position. It is interesting to note that most of the physicians appointed as vice-presidents of health science centers had been deans of schools of medicine; thus, their authority, power, and role behavior have tended to span two large, distinct, and powerful divisions in the universities. A few deans within the health science centers were aware of both the specialized medical preparation of physicians and their lack of formal preparation in administration. Role conflicts, role strain, and role ambivalence were predictable outcomes in those centers in which physicians served as presidents or vice-presidents.

Some discernible patterns of control become evident within the various health science centers. For example, firm "line" relationships were generally established between the vice-president of health affairs and the deans of various colleges or schools in the university. The new vice-president of a health science center generally was the only health professions representative having direct access to the president or chancellor of the university. Thus, deans of other health programs generally did not have direct access to the president but reported instead to the vice-president of the given center. This state of affairs, again, posed concerns among nursing deans, in particular, who had only recently achieved some gains in their professional autonomy and full control of their school or college resources. In sum, within the health science centers, medicine regained some of its former authority and control of other disciplines. Nonetheless, the rational arguments for establishing multidisciplinary centers in universities continued strong and the pattern of establishing the centers continued.

Medical Influence
in the Health Science Center

As the health science centers have endeavored to promote multidisciplinary education and research, many substantive issues have arisen. For example: (1) What are the major functions and role responsibilities of a health science center? (2) What is the role of the vice-president or director of the health science center? (3) What autonomy do the individual health professions have under this type of organizational structure? (4) Shall (or can) these centers become truly multidisciplinary places for collaborative work? (5) Will (or should) the health science center remain a part of the university? Might it become an independent entity? (6) Shall the traditional health colleges remain separate, as they were at the time of the center's inception? (7) Shall these centers continue to be managed only by deans of medical schools? If so, why? (8) What organizational structure or model is likely to be the most effective in ensuring that multidisciplinary collaboration will occur among all health science disciplines? These questions and many others have been debated within and outside health science board meetings, and to some extent continue to be debated as unresolved questions. To date, no universally accepted health science center model has been developed. Instead, a variety of organizational models representing a variety of philosophies exists (Leininger 1976).

While some health educators continue to be unenthusiastic about the health center concept, other health science deans and faculty have welcomed the establishment of the centers, believing that they are long over-due. Deans of nursing schools, particularly those deans with social science backgrounds, seemed to comprise the majority of those with doubts about or objections to the centers. They questioned the new structures largely because they believed that such centers would enable physicians to wield more influence and control, when what was required was the freedom and incentive for the several disciplines to engage in interprofessional collaboration.

It is of interest that while the health science centers were being developed, three medical subgroups in the health science centers could be identified. The first subgroup consisted largely of surgeons, obstetricians, internists, and the chairpersons of the academically based medical-surgical units in hospitals. The physician members of this group questioned support of health science centers. By implication their view was that there is nothing to gain by aligning themselves with other disciplines. They appeared satisfied with their role position. Figuratively speaking, they held the broad medical world in their hands and, practically speaking, they controlled the resources essential to their needs (Leininger, 1974). The second subgroup consisted of the upwardly mobile and politically astute academic physicians who had a broader orientation toward medical-health affairs than the first group. Most of these men were actively seeking top positions in health science centers, either as presidents or vice-presidents of universities, or some other strategic position. It was from this group that presidents of universities tended to appoint physicians as the vice-presidents of health science centers—obviously viewing them as the most logical persons to lead the centers because of their knowledge, high status, power, and their potential as fundraisers. Thus, from approximately 1968 to 1975, the majority of vice-presidency roles within health science centers were given to highly politically oriented male physicians. There were no women appointed as vice-presidents of health science centers of the older, major universities in the United States from 1968 to 1971 (Leininger, 1974).

Finally, there was a third subgroup in medicine composed of the very young and a few older physicians who had worked effectively and cooperatively with other health disciplines in the past. These physicians supported the ideal of students of the various health professions studying and working together and, consequently, supported the center concept. The younger physicians, who in recent years had been socialized somewhat differently from the previous generation, showed marked interest in collaborative group work and seemed more amenable to distributive authority and responsibilities within the academic milieu. For the most part, these physicians occupied positions in departments of community medicine, pediatrics, and psychiatry.

In general, some health professional disciplines—especially those of pharmacy, dentistry, nursing, and social work—have continued to have reservations about the ultimate possibility of truly multidisciplinary health centers in universities. (I can recall, for example, that the deans of dentistry and pharmacy on one campus more than once said, "I will wait and see what happens, and if the center does not work, then I do not know what we can do.") In recent years, there seems to be more acceptance of the centers among all the health professions involved than was the case in the early 1970s. There is reason to believe that some of this change in attitude is related to physician leaders having learned to function in their new roles, having altered their behavior as the result of feedback from other deans, and having adopted the norms of distributive power as opposed to centralized control.

A Retrospective and Prospective View

During the past decade, institutionalization of multidisciplinary health education programs has both progressed and encountered problems. One positive outcome is that several health science centers have been fairly successful in facilitating the development of interprofessional health educational programs (Dixon, 1977; Leininger, 1976). A core of professional faculty and nonprofessional staff are now employed in the majority of centers to help promote multidisciplinary health education. There seems to be a heightened awareness that interdisciplinary education can be accomplished given sufficient commitment, cooperative planning, and interprofessional efforts. A focus upon wellness and health maintenance as dominant themes is gradually pervading interdisciplinary health education programs. Presently, one can find university catalog listing more multidisciplinary health courses than were found in the mid-1960s. One other positive feature of the health science centers has been the increase in shared knowledge among faculty and students about common multidisciplinary problems, issues and achievements in the health field. More recently, one finds a waning of strong ethnocentrism on the part of physicians and more willingness on the part of these once highly ethnocentric professionals to participate in interdisciplinary projects. Other health professionals participating in teaching, research, and policy setting are becoming more assertive in their respective roles. In addition, there is recent evidence that health professionals are giving more attention to the relation of their roles with client care and, to a lesser extent, with interprofessional status concerns (Ford and Silver, 1968).

PROBLEMS IN MULTIDISCIPLINARY
HEALTH EDUCATION

There are problems about role definition, role practice, education and professional norms that will need to be addressed as health science centers become institutionalized. Only a brief enumeration of these problems or issues will be attempted here. First, there are urgent problems related to the need to clarify the role expectations of the various health professions practitioners so that their potential contributions can be recognized and used appropriately. Role socialization, negotiation, and refinement of roles all are major problem areas needing study. In addition, if better client care is to occur, role conflicts in the health professions will need to be identified and ways found to lessen or redirect those conflicts toward more effective interprofessional relations.

Second, the concepts, definitions, and practices related to the meaning of *multidisciplinary teams* and *health education teams* need to be examined for their practical consequences related to practice, research, and education. The concept of *team*, for example, continues to be vague and open to conflicting definitions.

Third, there are real problems faced by professional schools in their attempts to find time both to develop and to teach interdisciplinary courses. Presently, the curricula of each health science school seem to be "packed" and have only limited time or space for any new courses and experiences. Much curricular work remains to be done before true interprofessional courses can become established.

Fourth, there are several problems inherent in the hypothetical statements posed in this chapter regarding ethnocentrism, political role behaviors, social status, and interprofessional stresses. Each of these hypotheses lends itself to systematic exploration and possible reformulation based on further evidence. There is a continued need to increase interprofessional group sensitivity so that ethnocentric behaviors preventing listening, learning, and working with others can be reduced. Reducing interprofessional tensions and conflicts related to ethnocentric behaviors should help facilitate work. Based on the descriptive data presented here, it is apparent that the greater the authority and political power held by particular health professionals, the greater will be the role conflicts, tensions, and social distance between and among the health professions. In addition, it appears that the more frequent the occurrence of social distance, the more problems there will be in achieving collaborative relationships in multidisciplinary work. These hypotheses and others warrant further study.

Fifth, there are problems related to conflicts about interprofessional norms. Undoubtedly, there are some idiosyncratic cultural values that tend to complement each health profession's values, but there are also some values that can be sources of friction and interprofessional tensions. For example, the subculture of medicine values control of people with acute, dramatic, and unusual illnesses. Nursing also seeks control of these same clients since it provides care for them. The value of control for nursing and medicine is a conflict area insofar as it involves perceived "rights" to the client. Examining such cultural values—and others—should help to determine how disciplines fit in their orientation, values, and action patterns, thus providing a key to developing more functional relationships than heretofore.

Sixth, there remain the problems of motivating faculty of the different health professions to participate in interdisciplinary education, and research, and of providing time for them to work on multidisciplinary projects. As yet there is no universally accepted or best type of faculty appointment, where faculty can become participants in multidisciplinary education activities. Tenure considerations in universities have not generally taken such activities into account. Furthermore, where non-job-related salary differentials exist among the health schools, together with inequities in academic rank for similar preparation and role responsibilities, there will continue to be problems of morale and organizational instability.

Seventh, there are issues that relate to the kinds of organizational structures more likely to facilitate interprofessional work. To date, there are too few organizational models that have been mounted and tested. The traditional university model consisting of semiautonomous departmental subunits seems to be the prevailing model. Whether departmental structures are appropriate or functional over the long run for interdisciplinary college training remains to be seen.

Last, but not least, there is a need to look at problems inherent in the use of power, control, and authority. Political power behaviors can be functional or dysfunctional for the achievement of shared goals. The relationship of ethnocentric behavior to political processes is an intriguing area for further study and such study, if undertaken, could develop additional insight into how interprofessional collaboration can be achieved without violating strongly held professional values.

SUMMARY

In this chapter I have identified several factors leading to the establishment of so-called health science centers within the university. Evidence has been offered to support the prediction that this trend is likely to continue within the framework of higher education. It has been suggested that multidisciplinary health education is one of the more intriguing yet complex phenomena for study because of the number of people involved, the diverse organizational structures, and the differing values intrinsic to interprofessional work. Seven factors that have contributed to the development of multidisciplinary education were identified in this chapter. Ethnocentrism was identified as a construct potentially useful in understanding interdisciplinary behavior. Finally, it was recommended that ethnocentrism and its behavioral implications should be studied in a systematic manner, to enlarge our understanding of how such behavior on the part of health professionals can be reduced. It is assumed that the next decade will provide a much clearer notion of the directions multidisciplinary education will take. Indeed, the health professions and their public are only beginning to become aware of the nature, scope, function, and future impact of multidisciplinary education.

NOTE

[1] The 1965 date was selected as the dividing line of the pre- and post-multidisciplinary era since there was a notable increase in the numbers of multidisciplinary health science centers after 1965.

12

Role Attitudes: A Measurement Problem

ADA SUE HINSHAW

Attitudes toward the performance of roles are subjective phenomena learned from cultural and social experience. Role attitudes include both preset opinions of what to expect from the performance or enactment of roles as well as evaluative opinions of completed role performance. In both cases, the role attitudes represent subjective phenomena that are difficult to operationalize or tap in the "real world." Two questions are important: Why are social attitudes as related to health care roles and role performance important to study? What are the problems in operationalizing social attitudes toward health care roles?

The delivery of health care depends on the enactment of a number of roles. Individuals occupying these roles hold expectations for their own role performance and also have opinions concerning the performance of roles held by others in the health care setting. Nurses hold certain opinions of how patients should act. When patients comply with these expectations they may be labeled as a "good" patient." Physicians have specific expectations of nursing staff that create intense conflict when not met. In turn, patients hold definite expectations of both nurses and physicians, resulting in considerable dissatisfaction if violated. Thus, incongruency in role expectations can create conflict among individuals occupying major health care roles and retard their ability to function together effectively. In situations of role conflict, the quality of health care delivered can be drastically curtailed and consumer satisfaction with health care may be negatively influenced.

In order to counteract the negative consequences arising from incongruency in role attitudes, understanding and prediction of the various sets of expectations from different role perspectives is necessary. Understanding and prediction can be gained from studying the attitudes of individuals who occupy the various health care roles. However, a crucial problem is the ability to operationalize or tap various attitudes concerning the performance of different health care roles in the "real world." A major operational problem is one of measurement error. The traditional techniques for measuring subjective phenomena, such as social attitudes toward roles and role performance, result in a sizeable degree of measurement error. The error problem results from several conditions of the basic scaling techniques; i.e., the production of primarily ordinal level scales and the use of the scales in designs that do not control for inter- or intrasubject variation on many extraneous variables or factors.

Magnitude estimation, a measurement technique adapted to the social sciences from psychophysics, shows promise for handling the problem of measurement error with subjective phenomena such as attitudes toward role performance. Innovaters of the technique suggest that measurement error is reduced by producing ratio level scales of the attitudes, and by operationalizing the techniques within mathematical designs. Correlational and experimental mathematical designs reduce error by holding conditions statistically constant, averaging out random measurement error arising from nonsystematic intersubject variation, and specifically testing for the function best fitting the data rather than assuming a linear function.

This chapter will review the concept of role, summarize the traditional measurement procedures for subjective phenomena such as role attitudes, delineate the theoretical paradigm and general measurement technique for magnitude estimation, and discuss the use of magnitude estimation for measuring subjective role phenomena in several nursing studies.

ROLE: DEFINITIONS AND ORIGINS

Role, as a construct, has consistently been difficult to define and systematically analyze due to its multidimensional nature. As Neiman and Hughes (1951) noted in their classic survey of the use of the term *role*, it may be defined in terms of the personal dimension that deals with the dynamics of personality development or in terms of a structural dimension that speaks of social roles that are the functional units of systems such as formal and informal groups or society in general. The first orientation to a personality dimension suggests that individuals are socialized into specific life roles; e.g., being a male, being a father, being white, being black. The second orientation to roles as a structural dimension defines sets of expected values and behaviors that are specific to given functional positions in social structures; e.g.; teachers in school systems, secretaries in business offices.

Several commonalities in the two orientations to role are evident: role always involves either an individual's definition of a specific situation *or* an individual's acceptance of a group's definition of a specific situation. In addition, the concept involves the assumption of a process of interaction and communication as a prerequisite preparing the individual for enacting a specific role.

Scott (1970, p. 58) defines role as a "set of shared expectations focused upon a particular position; these expectations include beliefs about what goals or values the position incumbent is to pursue and the norms that will govern his behavior." The set of shared expectations evolve from the incumbent's socialization experiences and the values internalized while preparing for the position as well as the incumbent's adapting to the expectations socially defined for the position itself. For every social role, there is a complementary set of roles in the social structure among which interaction constantly occurs. The term *shared expectations* includes the idea that the values, attitudes, and behaviors of the position are shared or held by occupants of complementary roles in the social structure as well as by the position holder (Hunt, 1965).

A role consists of three components: values, attitudes, and behaviors (Linton, 1945). Values are defined as ideas held in common by members of a social structure, such as a group, that guide the identification and prioritizing of goals or objectives (Scott, 1970). Attitude is considered a tendency, set, or readiness to respond to social objects or events in the real world in terms of a favorable or unfavorable evaluation, while an opinion is defined as expressed attitude (Katz, 1960). According to Anderson et al. (1975), values generally refer to stable aspects of an individual's overall belief system, while attitudes are more specific and usually are indicative of the values held. Attitudes are assumed to guide role behaviors. (The assumption of a relationship between role attitude and behavior is controversial. Expressed attitudes may be a poor predictor for subsequent behavior.) The readiness or set perspective implicitly suggests that an individual will be preset or predisposed to enact certain behaviors because of certain attitudes.

The process of child and adult socialization provides a body of information and values or attitudes from which roles are either defined by their occupants or by which occupants are able to learn and accept society's definitions of the role. In learning roles, the socialization is a two-pronged process. It involves (1) the internalization of specific values and attitudes and

(2) the acquisition of skills for the enactment of appropriate behaviors. Operationally, the concept of socialization refers to individuals learning the necessary knowledge and skills, as well as internalizing the values and attitudes of a particular social system, in preparation for fulfilling a specific role in that system.

Thus, life roles that are to be enacted in society are learned. Early informal socialization prepares individuals to function in personal roles such as woman and mother. In addition, formal educational processes and experience provide the basic knowledge and skills that individuals require as prerequisite to adult socialization. Adult socialization is a continuing process of internalizing new values, attitudes, and behaviors appropriate to adult positions (Rosow, 1965). One of the most important adult socialization processes is that of preparation for occupational roles. This process involves internalizing the values and attitudes specific to a particular occupational or professional group and learning the knowledge and skills required to enact the behaviors of the occupational or professional role.

Individuals enact multiple roles in society in a variety of social systems. For example, a woman may be a daughter to her parents, a mother to her immediate family, and a professor to her students. These roles are interactive and individuals move between them. Internalized values, attitudes, and learned behaviors accompany each of the roles. The interaction of such roles brings the values, attitudes, and behaviors into juxtaposition; continually forcing integration or generating conflict.

MEASUREMENT OF ROLE ATTITUDES

Understanding and predicting the role behavior of individuals in roles of patients, nurses, or other health professionals requires isolating certain identifiable aspects of the internalized role values and attitudes for investigation and developing methodologies that will allow valid and reliable measurement of those role dimensions. In attempting to study human behavior as exemplified in life roles, it is necessary to deal with how individuals define and subjectively judge their roles. Measurement of role values and attitudes is a complex process requiring a knowledge of scaling theories, scaling techniques, and the issues of validity and reliability. This chapter will focus on measurement of role attitudes, since they theoretically reflect the values basic to internalization of a role.

Role attitudes, which are subjective social phenomena, have been extensively studied. The study of role attitudes requires clear conceptual and operational statements of definition. The conceptual definition of a construct, such as role attitude, refers to the meaning the term or phrase has within an abstract theoretical system. In role theory, the term attitude generally refers to a readiness, tendency, or set to act or react to some social object or event in a particular way (Himmelfarb and Eagly, 1974). Thus, an attitude about a role may predispose an individual to expect certain behaviors from an occupant of the role. Furthermore, role attitudes are formed through prior socialization; both from informal life experiences and formal educational processes. For example, depending on a patient's attitude toward nurses, the patient may be predisposed to favor certain behaviors as expected or valued. The patient's attitudes toward nurses and expectations regarding how nurses ought to function or behave stem from a set of values gained from prior individual and family experiences with nursing care, hospitalization, and health care in general. Role attitudes function in several ways: (1) they predispose individuals to hold certain expectations of role performance and (2) they guide an individual's evaluation of actual role performance.

An operational definition is specified for a concept by defining it in terms of a set or sets of measurement techniques. For the construct of attitude, many studies describe role attitudes or attitude formation and change through the use of some form of self-report questionnaire or measurement scale. The purpose of the scale is to identify and quantify an individual's present attitudes and their formation or possible change regarding a specific social object or event. Several methods or techniques have been developed for empirically quantifying role attitudes and expectations (Likert, 1932; Thurstone and Chave, 1929; Guttman, 1956). These methods will be discussed after general principles of attitude measurement are examined. An additional measurement technique, magnitude estimation, will be explored as a potentially useful scaling method for studying subjective phenomena such as role attitudes.

General Principles of Attitude Measurement

The purpose of attitude measurement is to construct a scale that allows numbers to be assigned to individual opinions. Such quantification leads to the objective standardization of attitude variables for the purpose of identifying the central patterns evidenced by many individual respondents. It is the central pattern from which researchers are able to explain and predict. For example, patients' attitudes toward the technical care they receive can be assessed by requesting a number of them to judge the nursing care they receive. The judgments could be obtained by choosing a strongly satisfied to strongly dissatisfied response on a set of items portraying technical nursing care functions. The strongly satisfied to strongly dissatisfied categories can be converted to numbers. Then, by averaging or summarizing across the quantitative scale for the respondents, the general attitude toward technical nursing care could be estimated.

Both the concept of attitude and the process of measurement require further consideration. In measurement theory, attitude is defined as an "implicit cue-drive-producing response" to socially relevant characteristics that is basically evaluative in nature (Anderson et al, 1975, p. 32). The word *implicit* suggests an attitude or opinion inherent within an individual, while the phrase *drive producing* means that the attitude will tend to predispose an individual to form or hold certain expectations and act in a selective manner. The term *response* suggests that a behavior reflecting an attitude or opinion can be elicited by providing appropriate stimuli. Appropriate stimuli refer to socially relevant characteristics with which individuals have had experience. Lastly, the word *evaluation* in the definition of *attitude* suggests that such opinions are based on values held by individuals and will vary from positive to negative (Anderson et al., 1975).

The measurement definition of *attitudes* is not in conflict with the definition generally used in the role theory literature. Both definitions speak of attitudes as predisposing individuals to certain expectations and behaviors, which in role theory can be discussed in terms of expectations and behavior involved with role performance. In addition, both definitions emphasize the evaluative nature of attitudes. For example, Himmelfarb and Eagly (1974) suggest that operational definitions of role attitudes scale opinions toward items of social objects or events on a favorable to unfavorable dimension.

"In its broadest sense, measurement is the assignment of numerals to objects and events according to rules" (Stevens, 1951). The term *numerals* refers to the use of numbers (1,2,3...) to describe a variable response. *Assignment* involves mapping the numerical response from one set of objects onto the response of another set. In attitudinal measurement, numerals representing levels of response to socially relevant stimuli are assigned to individuals according to their attitudinal responses on a measurement scale. The rules are the set of guidelines, that is, explicit instructions for assigning the level of attitudinal response to the social stimuli presented (Kerlinger, 1973). For example a rule might say:

> *Assign the numerals 1 through 5 to nurses who have worked with you according to how satisfied you are with their care. If a nurse gives very, very good care, assign the number 5. If the nurse gives very bad care, give the number 1.*

The measurement definition of the concept attitude dictates two key properties that are necessary in constructing a measurement scale. First, a measurement tool or scale must present the subject with a series of socially relevant stimuli in order to provoke an attitudinal response. Second, in order to assess the evaluation component, the scale must allow the individual to give his response on a positive to negative dimension according to specific rules.

Accuracy of Measurement Scales

Several major conditions must be considered in constructing and using attitudinal measurement scales. These are validity, reliability, and precision. The accuracy of the information obtained and the sensitivity of the data depend on these measurement characteristics.

Validity. Validity is defined as the extent to which the scale measures the theoretical dimension it is constructed to measure. In other words, does the scale measure what it is intended to measure? For example, while a scale may be constructed to measure a client's perception or satisfaction with the amount of teaching a nurse included in her care, *does* the scale measure that perception or satisfaction level? Among the kinds of validity generally considered with measurement scales are: face validity, content validity, criterion validity, predictive validity, and construct validity (APA, 1966). Face validity, the weakest form of validity, consists of "eyeballing" or reviewing the scale in relation to the theoretical dimension it is constructed to measure, and deciding from such a cursory exam that validity seems to exist. Content validity is defined as the extent to which the scale represents the generally held consensus about the concept under measurement. This type of validity primarily reflects the degree to which the measurement tool contains the elements of the attitude that are agreed upon in the literature and by known experts in the field. This type of validity can also be referred to as consensus validity, since the process involved with estimating content validity is to determine the consensus of the literature or of a set of expert judges on the validity of the scale content. Criterion validity refers to the degree to which the scale under consideration correlates with other scales constructed and tested to measure the same attitude dimension.

Predictive and construct validities are more powerful types of validity testing that are quite similar. As Kerlinger (1973) notes, the power of these forms of validity comes from their unification of "psychometric notions with theoretical notions." Predictive validity is estimated by studying the degree to which defined theoretical concepts and predicted relationships are empirically substantiated (Cronbach & Meehl, 1955). It first requires a clear definition of the concepts or variables under study and a prediction of their relationships. Second, it is necessary to identify clearly the scales that will measure each concept. If the study data substantiate the predicted relationship, then the scale can be estimated to yield a valid measure of the concept. Construct validity requires judging the validity of a scale in relation to its underlying theoretical dimension by estimating its meaning or relationship to other constructs. The issue is similar to predictive validity, except the "meanings" or relationships specified are not predictive. With construct validity, two types of relationships are specified: (1) relationships to constructs that should converge or be correlated positively to the construct scale under test and (2) relationships to constructs that would be different or divergent from the construct scale under test. In the latter, the construct scale measurements would correlate negatively or have no correlation. Initially, the constructs are defined and the convergent and discriminant relationships are specified. Then, measurement scales are selected or constructed for each construct. Construct validity can be estimated to the degree that the study data substantiate the specified like and unlike relationships between the theoretical variables. Corroboration of predictive and construct validity can be obtained only through replication.

Reliability.   Reliability refers to the consistency with which individuals are ordered, or scored, on a measurement scale. "If no true change occurs in a given attitude an individual holds, does the attitude scale consistently yield the same ordering (or score) for him relative to others?" (Bohrnstedt, 1970). Since reliability is a matter of degree, it can generally be defined and tested since "the greater the correlation between two parallel forms the greater the equivalence is presumed to be" (Bohrnstedt, 1970). Essentially, three types of reliability are estimated: stability, equivalence, and internal consistency (Mehrens, 1973). Stability refers to the degree to which an individual's score on an attitude scale varies from one measurement to another. The technique generally used to estimate stability is that of test-retest; that is, testing is repeated. Equivalence refers to the degree to which several items in an attitude scale appear to measure the same theoretical underlying attitude. Equivalency is generally measured by using a two-form technique. Two forms of a test with equal content are given to individuals on the same day and the results are correlated (Mehrens and Lehmanon, 1973). The focus of internal consistency tests is to estimate the degree of homogeneity of the items within the scale as well as the degree to which the item responses correlate with the total test score. (See Bohrnstedt, 1970; Kerlinger, 1973; and Mehrens, 1973 for detailed discussion of the conditions of validity and reliability and for the techniques used in their estimation.) A variety of techniques are used to estimate internal consistency (e.g., Kuder-Richardson estimates.)

Precision (sensitivity).   Precision is defined as the level of measurement that can be assumed about the scale. Four levels of measurement are described by Stevens (1951): nominal, ordinal, interval, and ratio. For nominal scale measurement, attitudes can only be determined to be in one of several exhaustive, mutually exclusive categories. With ordinal data, in addition to being categorized, an individual's attitudinal response can be ranked or ordered in contrast to other possible responses. That is, the response can be judged as greater than or less than a contrasting response. The internal level of measurement encompasses the categorical and ordering properties of the responses and also suggests there are equal intervals between the categories, which have an arbitrary beginning or zero point. The fourth level of measurement is a ratio scale. The ratio scale includes all the properties of the nominal, ordinal, and interval levels in addition to possessing an absolute zero point. Attitude measurement scales generally attain an ordinal level of measurement, although several techniques—the Thurstone scale, for example (Thurstone and Chave, 1929)—profess to characteristics of interval scales as well.

If quantification of data is desired, then the highest possible level of measurement is preferable. The higher the level of measurement, the more information is available about the attitude under study. For example, an interval scale gives information about the type or category of attitude response, where it ranks in contrast to other possible responses, and asserts that there are equal intervals between the categories of possible responses. With greater amounts of information available about the attitudinal response, more precise and powerful statistical procedures can be utilized, e.g., correlation and regression statistics rather than lambda or gamma techniques.

The accuracy of information gained from attitude measurement depends on the assurance of validity, reliability, and precision. With respect to validity and reliability, evidence of the degree to which these conditions are fulfilled in the scale needs to be reported. In terms of precision, the goal is to use the highest level of measurement possible.

Traditional Methodologies for Role Attitude Measurement

Three major methods have traditionally been used to measure role attitudes and opinions: those of Thurstone and Chave (1929), Likert (1932), and Guttman (1956). All three of these measures are self-report methods for the scaling of verbalized attitudes.

Thurstone. Thurstone's method of equal-appearing intervals (Thurstone and Chave, 1929) is a technique for achieving interval level scales. The scale items are constructed to measure an attitude on a positive-to-negative dimension, which assumes the underlying theoretical attitude is continuous (Nunnally, 1967).

Thurstone's technique involves scaling predetermined attitudinal statements. Initially, a set of judges ranks a series of attitudinal statements (e.g., 1 to 5) from strongly negative to strongly positive. The mean or median of the set of judgments is assigned to each attitudinal statement. These judgments locate each item on the positive-to-negative attitude continuum. Individuals whose attitudes are to be measured are asked to agree or disagree with the prejudged statements. Scores for each individual are obtained by adding the scale values preassigned to the statements from the judgment procedure (Anderson et al. 1975).

Likert.   Likert's method of summated ratings (1932) directly scales individual attitudinal responses to social objects. This summative technique constitutes a linear model for scaling; i.e., the sum of the attitude statement scores has a linear relationship to the attitude under study and the model leads to a linear combination of items. These characteristics and their underlying assumptions are basic to the argument that scales based on this model can be assumed to produce an interval level of measurement. However, there is a lack of consensus as to whether the scaling technique produces ordinal or interval level data.

Initially, a set of positive and negative attitudinal statements is formulated. The group of individuals whose attitudes are to be measured respond to each statement by using a multiple-point scale such as: 5 = strongly agree, 4 = agree, 3 = not certain, 2 = disagree, and 1 = strongly disagree. Each statement is assigned a score of 1 to 5 depending on the response selected and the scores are then summed. The total scale score for an individual on the attitude is the sum of the statement scores (Anderson et al., 1975; Shaw, 1966). Research suggests the Likert technique can provide equally as valid and reliable data on attitudes as the Thurstone technique and with greater economy in terms of the time required for instruction and grouping of subjects and judgments (Barclay and Weaver, 1963; Nunnally, 1967).

Guttman.   The cumulative scale analysis method suggested by Guttman (1956) approaches the measurement of attitudes differently. It is based on a deterministic model that assumes there is no variation in the response to an attitudinal statement or set of statements. Statements for this scale are constructed as either highly positive, positive, negative, or highly negative, but any one statement presumably reflects only one predetermined attitude position. In a series of statements, if a respondent answers one statement as positive, he can then be predicted to answer the others in a similar manner (Nunnally, 1967).

Initially, attitudinal statements varying on a conceptual dimension are formulated. A group of subjects are asked to respond to the statements, after which the statements are analyzed to determine if they form a scale and are arranged as theoretically constructed. In essence, the attitudinal statements are arranged in such an order that an individual responding positively to one statement also responds positively to all other items with a lower rank (Shaw and Wright, 1966).

According to Shaw and Wright (1967), each of these three major techniques for attitude measurement yields satisfactory scales; however, controversy exists as to whether they include equality of intervals or an arbitrary zero point. Thus, all of these techniques may produce ordinal level rather than interval level measurement scales.

Role attitudes, as a type of subjective phenomena, have been difficult to operationalize. Two factors have contributed to the problem of operationalization: the amount of measurement error involved in the scales for measuring role attitudes and their use in designs that do not allow control over a number of extraneous variables. For example, the measurement of patient satisfaction with nursing care may be made by a Likert-type scale within the context of a quasiexperimental or descriptive design. The Likert scale, at best, can be assumed to yield interval data; in the researcher's mind there may be a question, however, as to whether the data are only ordinal. In addition, validity and reliability estimates are necessary for the satisfaction scale in order to judge the degree of measurement error from those sources. The use of prior developed and tested role-attitude scales, such as for patient satisfaction, in descriptive or quasiexperimental designs introduces another source of error that, when compounded with the measurement error from the scales, makes it very difficult to operationalize or tap the "real world" attitude that is of theoretical interest.

Magnitude estimation is a measurement technique developed in the field of psychophysics (Stevens, 1960). The technique purports to yield a ratio level of measurement. In addition, it is used within the context of mathematical correlational or experimental designs that allow the researcher increased control over extraneous variables. Because of these two features for decreasing operational error, magnitude estimation is being tested for use in the social sciences for the measurement of subjective phenomena such as role attitudes.

PSYCHOPHYSICAL PARADIGM AND THE METHOD OF MAGNITUDE ESTIMATION

Psychophysical methods for scaling were developed to study the relation between physical properties of objects or stimuli and the sensory sensation they produce (Hays, 1967). *Physical stimuli* refers to presenting respondents with varying levels of events or objects—such as degrees of sound, tactile stimulation, light, etc.—and asking them to judge the sensory response that is evoked. One basic characteristic of the physical stimuli used for each of these examples is that they are scaled on a ratio scale, e.g., degree of loudness is delivered to the respondent in terms of decibels of sound. The magnitude of the sensory sensation that is evoked has been measured in a variety of ways, including assigning a number of various degrees of response, drawing lines proportional to the sensation evoked, and squeezing a hand dynamometer to describe responses. These magnitude-judging techniques are among the best-known and simplest techniques for constructing magnitude scales.

Developed in the field of psychophysics, the purpose of the magnitude-estimation technique is to form a ratio scale mapping the magnitude of a sensory sensation to the magnitude of a physical stimulus for each individual subject. In the social sciences and in nursing, magnitude estimation has been used to produce scales describing subjective or attitudinal responses to socially relevant stimuli that are assumed to produce ratio scales (Hamblin, 1974). The work with magnitude-estimation measurement technique has evolved concurrently with study of the function of the relationship between sensory or subjective responses and physical or social stimuli.

Psychophysical Paradigm: Form of the Stimulus-Response Relationship

Since the 1930s, psychophysicist S.S. Stevens and his colleagues have conducted a number of experiments to determine the form of the relationship between sensory responses and physical stimuli (Stevens, 1960; Stevens and Mack 1959). Their results consistently have indicated that a power function best describes the relationship:

$$\psi = \phi^n$$

where the magnitude of the sensory response (ψ) increases as a power function of the magnitude of the physical stimuli (ϕ) with c and n as parameters that can be empirically estimated. By 1960, Stevens had documented the existence of this function between at least 22 sensory responses and their physical stimuli (Stevens, 1960). These studies used magnitude-scaling techniques for producing ratio-level data. From this base of research, Stevens postulated the power law of psychophysics; i.e., the magnitude of sensory responses increases as a power function of the magnitude of the physical stimuli (Stevens, 1960). Stevens suggests the power function is a necessary consequence of the ratio invariance: "equal stimulus ratios produce equal perceptual or sensation ratios" (Stevens, 1966).

Psychophysical Paradigm
Adapted to Social Sciences

Apparently, one of the first generalizations of Stevens' psychophysical methods and theory to the relationship between social stimuli and subjective attitudinal responses was by Hamblin et al. (1963). These authors, who were investigating the influence of interference on aggressive behaviors, produced measureable amounts of interference and frustration in the subjects. The subjective aggression responses were scaled using magnitude-estimation techniques. The form of the relationship between interference and frustration and agression was best described the the power function. Using magnitude-estimation scaling techniques for the variables under study, Hamblin and Smith (1966), Hamblin (1971), Rainwater (1972), and Shinn (1969) have further substantiated the generalization of Stevens' psychophysical law to social stimuli and subjective responses. In addition, a series of studies indirectly substantiating the power-law phenomenon between social stimuli and attitudinal responses were summarized by Stevens (1966). These studies examined subjective preferences for wristwatches, aesthetic value of music, seriousness of criminal offenses, and levels of punishment.

From these earlier studies, Hamblin and Smith (1966) suggested a general form of the power relationship or power law:

$$R = cS^n$$

where the magnitude of any conditioned response (R) increases as a power function of the eliciting stimulus (S) with c and n as parameters that can be empirically estimated. In addition, Hamblin and Smith (1966) suggested the power-law phenomenon governing behavioral stimulus-response relationships could be logically extended to the multivariate form:

$$R = cS_1^{n_1} \times S_2^{n_2} \cdots S_k^{n_k}$$

where the magnitude of the response (R) will be a multivariate power function of the magnitudes of the eliciting stimuli $(S_1, S_2 \cdots S_k)$.

Their hypothesis concerning the multivariate power relationships was subsequently supported in several studies on values, status, and professors (Hamblin and Smith, 1966), components of general status (Hamblin, 1971; Rainwater, 1972), and components of national power (Shinn, 1969). Shinn (1969) contends the power-law phenomenon can be expected to describe relationships in at least two classes of response variables: (1) those reflecting cultural conditioning and (2) those reflecting technical expertise or educational conditioning. Like Stevens (1966), he labels these "consensus" variables, since the study of them reflects group values and norms, not just individual perceptions and standards. Studies investigating the components of general status are examples of the first category of consensus variables. The subjective responses to social stimuli—such as amount of income, types of occupations and levels of education—can be generated by a variety of subjects, since such responses are based on cultural conditioning (e.g., college students and navy seamen, Hamblin, 1971; and adults in metropolitan Boston, Rainwater, 1972). Shinn's (1969) *Components of National Power* serves to illustrate the second type of consensus relationship, since educational expertise was necessary for an individual to give opinions on the political stimuli.

The definition of attitude as an implicit cue-drive-producing response qualifies the concept as a subjective response to certain socially relevant stimuli. This also suggests the relationship of role attitudes to social stimuli can (1) be described with the psychophysical paradigm as adapted to the social sciences and thus (2) be measured through the use of magnitude-scaling devices; e.g., magnitude estimation. For example, studies determining nurses', doctors', or other health care workers' subjective responses to certain professionally (socially) relevant stimuli, such as their opinions of what defines quality health care, are tapping role attitudes and opinions reflecting professional socialization processes based on education and experience. Investigations focused on client attitudes and responses, such as their opinions of health care, are tapping cultural socialization processes and experiences of the patients. In both instances, the psychophysical paradigm allows the researcher to identify the general attitude pattern of the collective group that reflects values and norms of prior types of socialization.

Magnitude-Estimation Method

Magnitude estimation is one of the most useful of the magnitude-judgment methods for producing ratio scales because of its relative simplicity. Essentially, the method asks an individual or subject to estimate the apparent strength or intensity of his sensory responses relative to a set of stimuli (Stevens, 1960). Here the technique will be discussed from the perspective of subjective responses to social stimuli, particularly in terms of role attitude and expectation responses. Expectations of a role, or of role performance by others in contact with the role, are defined as respondents' opinions or attitudes toward role and role performance.

Hamblin (1971) suggests magnitude estimation should be used in conjunction with mathematical experimental or correlational designs. He states: "While it is generally recognized that ratio measurement is in many ways superior to the lower levels of measurement, its power is limited in anything less than the mathematical experiment" (Hamblin, 1971). The conditions of a mathematical experiment are summarized as follows: (1) manipulation of one or a multiple number of independent variables, (2) control by constancy (all subjects respond to all research treatments or independent variables), (3) simultaneous ratio measurements of all independent and dependent variables (magnitude estimation), (4) average out random measurement error, and (5) summarize the relationship(s) between variables with the best-fitting algebraic equation(s) (Hamblin, 1971). If condition (1) cannot be fulfilled, then the design is one of mathematical correlation.

Scaling through magnitude estimation requires the identification of (1) a set of social stimuli, (2) a population of appropriate respondents or subjects, (3) identifying operational definitions for the attitudinal variables under study, (4) training the respondents to give proportional judgments, and (5) having all subjects on all the attitudinal variables give numbers to describe their subjective reactions to the set of stimuli.

Set of Social Stimuli.   Two models have been used for providing the set of social stimuli; i.e., either a list of objects or events or a list of people to be judged on the attitudinal variables. Several basic principles must be observed in constructing the social stimuli set. As in general attitude measurement, the stimuli must be clearly and concisely stated in order to decrease the "noise" in the stimulus. Social stimuli tend to be quite noisy; i.e., they contain multiple cues including cues the researcher does not intend. The stimuli need to be precisely stated in order not to be confusing to the respondents. Another principle needs to be considered; i.e., the set of stimuli must vary on at least one major attitudinal dimension. If all the stimuli in the set evoke neutral or all evoke extreme responses, there will be no variation in attitudinal responses. The magnitude judgments assume the sets of stimuli vary and can be scaled on some empirical range. A series of pretests are usually necessary to clarify the social stimuli and insure their variation.

Appropriate Respondents.   Not everyone is an appropriate subject for magnitude-estimation techniques. The crucial criterion to be satisfied in selecting a group of respondents or subjects is that they possess the knowledge or experience needed to give the required judgments. As was noted earlier, magnitude scaling depends on some type of prior conditioning—either cultural, educational, or both. For example, if patients are to judge nurses on the quality of care they give, they must have experience in the patient role as well as have a knowledge of the nurses to be judged. If nurses are to judge a set of patient care tasks in terms of their professional complexity, then they must have experienced prior professional nursing socialization. Another problem to consider is: what size sample or population of respondents is desirable? Essentially, the focus is on identifying the central or general pattern of responses across a group. The researcher is confronted with the problem of how large a sample size is necessary to identify such a pattern. Hamblin and Smith (1966) suggest that samples should include 20 to 30 respondents.

Operational Definitions.   Broad definitions are constructed for each attitudinal variable to be measured. The definitions, while containing only *one* theoretical dimension to be measured or scaled, are developed broadly in order to stimulate subjective valuing or attitudinal processes from prior conditioning. For example, a definitional cue used by Hinshaw and Field (1974) when doing magnitude scaling reads:

> *Professional Creativity: You probably have noticed that some nurses on the unit are more successful in working out effective and creative solutions to nursing problems and others are less able to be creative in this way.*

Note the definitional cue is deliberately broad but contains only one conceptual dimension to be judged or scaled. As a result, individual variation in response is expected. One of the major problems with magnitude estimation as used in the social sciences is the difficulty of precisely defining attitudinal variables so as to insure that there is a single conceptual dimension to be scaled and simultaneously being able to leave the operational definitions fairly broad. Several pretests are usually necessary before the definitions are clearly defined so as to contain only one dimension.

Training Session.   Magnitude scaling requires that respondents or subjects be able to give proportional judgments on the set of social stimuli. In order to insure that subjects are prepared to give this type of judgment, a training session is conducted. Several methods have been used for training purposes (Hinshaw, 1975; Hinshaw and Field, 1975). Hinshaw (1975) used the following training session in a study to discriminate between a professional versus technologic basis for patient care decisions.

> *Let's work first on the method by which I'd like you to give your responses. For these responses, I'd like you to be thinking in proportional terms. Now, this may sound simple and rather silly, but to be sure we are together in our thinking, let's practice with a few numbers. O.K.?*

Given the number 10, I'd like you to give me a number:

Twice as large (20)
Half as large (5)
One-third as large (3.3)
Five times as large (50)

Now, note what you have done. You have given all these numbers in proportion or in relationship to the first number 10; i.e., the 20 is twice as large as the first number and five is one-half as large, etc.

Let's practice for a few more minutes, thinking in proportional terms. Take a look at this graph (Fig. 1). There are seven points on this graph. Point #1 is 10 units above the base line. If point #1 is 10 units above the base line, then how many units above is each of points 2 through 7?

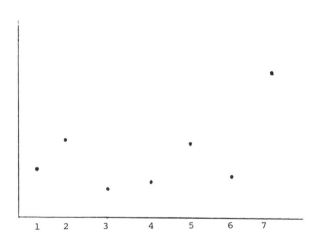

FIGURE 1. Seven-point graph used in training subjects to make proportional judgments. No scale on the y axis was presented to subjects. The investigator judged respondent's estimate against centimeter markings on the y axis. From Hinshaw, *Professional Decisions: A Technological Perspective.* Unpublished Doctoral Dissertation, University of Arizona, 1975.

The graph was presented to the subjects on a five-by-eight card. The correct responses were: #1 = 10; #2 = 16; #3 = 6; #4 = 7.5; #5 = 15; #6 = 9; #7 = 30.

As subjects gave estimates, they were plotted on log-log coordinates in relationship to the actual physical measurement from the baseline, which is consistent with work by Hamblin (1974). If the estimates given by the subject varied markedly from a straight line on the log-log coordinates, then an additional training session was conducted. Thus, the training session had the advantage of allowing the subject to visualize his progress through the use of a graph.

The additional training session was as follows:

I will present you with a series of lines. The first line will be considered average and is equal to 10 units. With each one of these lines, I'd like you to proportionally estimate it in terms of the average line; e.g., if you think it is twice as long, give it 20 units, or one-fourth as long, give it 2.5 units. You may compare the lines as closely as you like.

Series of lines: Twice as long
Half as long
One-fourth as long
Four times as long
(Observer checks accuracy.)

Any questions about giving your responses in these terms? We will use this principle for the rest of the responses.

The training session is crucial since the ability to produce magnitude scales depends on the use of the proportional judgment technique. If the researcher suspects later in the measurement protocol that proportional judgments are not being given, then the training session can be repeated.

Attitudinal Variable Scaling.   All respondents or subjects judge the set of social stimuli on all independent, dependent, and control variables (control by constancy principle). Magnitude scaling or proportional judgments are given on the set of social stimuli for each variable. The numbers assigned to each stimulus form the respondent's scale for the variable. The ratio or proportional concept requires the subject or respondent to select a standard or average stimulus for each variable. That standard stimulus is assigned an arbitrary number of units that is easily treated in calculating proportions or ratios, e.g., 10, 50, 100, etc. Then all the remaining stimuli are judged proportional to the standard; twice as much equals 20, 100, or 200, respectively, and one-half as much equals 5, 25, or 50. The attitudinal variables and the set or social stimuli are presented to each respondent or subject in a random order. This is done in order to counter any systematic initial excitement, fatigue, or ordering bias.

A set of instructions are given to the respondents to direct their magnitude-scaling efforts. For example, Hinshaw (1975) gave the following set of instructions to her subjects of registered nurses as they judged 16 patient care tasks on the basis of several professional and technologic variables:

I would like you to use the same technique of proportional judging that you practiced in the training session while estimating the placement of a set of patient care tasks on a series of characteristics. I will present you with a set of 16 cards, each one containing the description of a patient care task. You are to take a professional orientation to the tasks and consider both the techniques involved and the judgments required for their implementation and modification. Here is a list of the patient care tasks, take a minute to read through it before we start. (Pause.) With each characteristic, you will be asked to select one of these tasks as a standard or average. It will be assigned 10 units, just like in the training session. Then you will be asked to judge the other 15 tasks in proportion to the standard. For example, if you think a task has three times as much of the characteristic as the standard, then assign 30 units. If you think it has one-fifth as much of the characteristic, give it a 2. If the task has none, give it a 0.

Task Complexity: Some patient care tasks are more complex and require more professional knowledge, skill, and experience than others—others are relatively simple. Among these tasks, which would you consider average in complexity? If this task has 10 units of complexity, how much would this one have (1-15)?

The magnitude-estimation technique described encompasses the original dicta used by Stevens in psychophysics. Field and Hinshaw (1977) summarize these as adapted for the social sciences:

1. *Start the measurement series by giving or having the subject select a standard stimulus condition whose level of magnitude is in the middle of the stimulus range.*
2. *Present other variable stimuli that are both above and below the standard.*
3. *Call the standard by a number such as 10 that is easily multiplied and divided.*
4. *Assign a number to the standard only and leave the subject completely free to decide what he will call the rest of the stimuli.*
5. *Use only one standard in any experiment (an arbitrary number).*
6. *Randomize the order of presentation of the stimuli.*
7. *Keep the experimental session short as possible or give breaks periodically.*
8. *Let the subject present the stimuli to himself.*
9. *Use a group of subjects large enough to produce a stable median (N = 20-30 observers is recommended).*

These instructions and the magnitude-estimation technique can be used either with individuals in private interviews or in a group. In a group, the most difficult aspect of the protocol is the random ordering of both variables and sets of stimuli for all subjects.

Reliability and Validity

Magnitude estimation is treated in similar way to other measurement techniques in terms of validity and reliability. Validity is generally approached through face, content, predictive, and construct techniques. Face and content techniques have been used primarily to clarify and estimate the content of social stimuli sets when objects or events have made up the set. Ultimately, validity of the operational definitions are estimated through predictive and construct validity, since magnitude estimation is generally used in a mathematical design to test theoretical models with predicted relationships.

Reliability is generally approached through the use of test-retest techniques. Usually, the major disadvantage of the test-retest technique is memory bias; i.e., the respondent remembers what he answered in the initial test and he deliberately repeats that decision, thus giving a biased, inflated reliability score. However, when using magnitude-estimation techniques, this source of bias is minimized since the respondents are making approximately 100 judgments (judging 10 to 16 stimuli on 6 to 10 variables) in a random order in both the test and retest period. Under these conditions, the likelihood of recalling the judgment on any one stimulus with any one variable is minimized.

Hamblin's (1974) investigations do not report results of reliability and validity testing. However, the studies in nursing (Field, 1975; Hinshaw, 1974; Hinshaw and Field, 1975; Oakes, 1976) suggest fairly high reliability under test-retest conditions ($r \cong .90$). Both Oakes' (1976) and Hinshaw's (1975) research use predictive and construct validity and suggest that the broad operational definitions used for magnitude estimation tend to produce empirical results that substantiate the theoretical relationships predicted.

Analysis Protocol
for Magnitude-Estimation Data

The general protocol for analyzing data from magnitude-estimation scaling techniques consists of standardizing the data methodologically, averaging out random measurement error, logarithmically transforming the averaged data, and then using appropriate statistics—statistics requiring linear assumptions from the data. The data are standardized through the instructions given to the respondents. They are asked to select an average stimulus from the set of social stimuli that is assigned an arbitrary number (e.g., 10, 50, 100). This average becomes the standard against which all other stimuli are proportionally judged.

The data from individual respondents are usually averaged since the researcher is primarily interested in identifying the general attitudinal pattern based on the respondent's socialization and conditioning background. This requires averaging or obtaining a "central tendency" statistic; i.e., the geometric mean or the median. In attempting to identify a central pattern, nonsystematic individual variations and preferences can be considered to be random error that needs to be eliminated in order to see the general pattern.

Thus, all subjects' responses to each stimulus on each attitudinal variable are averaged to a set of geometric means or medians. The set of geometric means or medians becomes the basic data base with which further analysis is done.

One characteristic of data obtained by magnitude scaling and described by a power function is that it is linear in log-log space (Stevens, 1966). Thus, the basic set of data needs to be logarithmically transformed before linear statistical techniques can be utilized.

This section has reviewed the procedures involved in using magnitude-estimation scaling techniques. In summary, several procedural elements are required for the use of magnitude estimation; i.e., a set of social stimuli, a population of appropriate respondents as subjects, a set of broad operational definitions for the study variables, a structured training plan, and a procedure that allows all subjects to respond to all the variables in relation to the social stimuli. These elements are operationalized in correlational or experimental mathematical designs. The precision of scales produced by magnitude estimation is maximized (ratio-level scales) and variation from intrasubject variables is decreased since the subject is his own control. In addition, intersubject variation is decreased by averaging the data obtained from individual respondents. These design and scaling techniques for reducing measurement error have been used in several role attitude and expectation studies in nursing.

NURSING INVESTIGATIONS USING MAGNITUDE ESTIMATION

Two nursing studies that have used the magnitude-estimation techniques to measure role attitudes or expectations will be presented. The purpose of describing these two studies is to exemplify the use of magnitude-estimation techniques in role situations relevant to nursing and to operationalize the general ideas that were discussed previously.

The first study, "Professional Decisions: A Technological Perspective" (Hinshaw 1975) posed the question: "Do staff nurses make direct patient care decisions based on professional role attitudes and/or on organizational role attitudes?" The question: "How do patient, nurse, and doctor's role expectations of quality nursing care vary?" guided the second investigation to be reported on here (Hinshaw and Oakes, 1977). In both studies the variables measured are subjective phenomena. In the first study, two sets of role attitudes that guide decision making but originate in different socialization processes are the subjective phenomena under study. With the second investigation, occupants of complementary roles to nurses (patients and physicians) as well as role occupants themselves (registered nurses) give their opinion of what defines quality nursing care or quality role performance.

Professional Decisions: A Technologic Perspective (Hinshaw, 1975)

The purpose of this investigation was to study the dominant role attitudes that influence the decisions of health care professionals functioning in an organization. The theory of limited rationality (March and Simon, 1958; Simon, 1955) outlined two factors that limit decision situations under these conditions: (1) environmental controls inculcated through organization socialization experiences and expectations and (2) prior socialization experiences of the decision maker. This theory provided the basis for suggesting two role perspectives that might guide the decision processes of health care professionals who are employees of organizations. The organizational model or perspective reflects environmental expectations and socialization influencing employee decisions, whereas the professional model identifies the affect of prior educational socialization on practitioner decisions.

The decision under study was the intensity of the professional's *search for alternatives*. Search was defined as the degree to which alternatives for problem solving are generated and considered before a decision is made. From the viewpoint of health care professionals, the search process is valued as a way of implementing the "service" norm; i.e., providing services for clients on the basis of their individual needs.

The organizational model of employee decisions was constructed from two theories, March and Simon's (1958) decision-making and Perrow's (1967) technologic perspectives on organizations. Basically, the model asserted (1) that the major predictor of employee decisions is the routine or *frequent* nature of work tasks, (2) that the *complexity* or amount of professional knowledge and skill needed for the task indirectly influenced search alternatives, and (3) discretion or control over the tasks mediated the influence of both task frequency and complexity of search intensity.

The professional model was constructed from Wilensky's (1964) statement of professional characteristics. It suggested that (1) *complexity* and (2) *importance* of professional responsibilities or tasks are most predictive of search intensity and (3) *discretion* or control is an intervening variable between complexity or importance and the search. The organizational and professional models were similar on two of the role attitude variables (complexity and discretion) that are presumed to influence decisions, but on two variables (importance and frequency) they differed (Fig. 2).

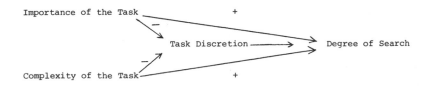

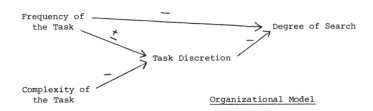

FIGURE 2. Professional and organizational models for decision making, with the signs (±) of the relationships between the variables indicated.

The theoretical relationships between search intensity and the organizational and professional variables fit Shinn's (1969) description of "consensus" variables. The judgments or responses were expected to reflect attitudes that are based on cultural, professional, and organizational socialization. Thus, the theoretical relationships between variables in both models were presumed to be described by a power function rather than a linear, exponential, or log function.

Since the variables of the decision model could be assumed to reflect role attitudes based on prior socialization, use of the principles and techniques of a mathematical correlation design and the measurement procedures of magnitude estimation were appropriate. For the set of social stimuli, subjects were asked to judge a series of 16 patient care tasks. The set of patient care tasks was selected as the stimuli conditions for several reasons: (1) the decision-making perspective (March and Simon, 1958) and the technologic perspective (Perrow 1967) for organizations suggest that the tasks an employee performs are major factors in determining the nature of search decisions and (2) the core of professional service is the tasks (patient care responsibilities) and decisions involved in the delivery of such service.

Recall that if a set of objects of events was to serve as the set of social stimuli, then two concerns must be satisfied, i.e., maximizing variability on a major dimension and decreasing the noise or multiple cues in the stimuli. In constructing the set of tasks, it was necessary to ensure variability on one major dimension; frequency of patient care tasks was the dimension selected. The set of tasks was obtained by requesting a group of staff nurses (n = 6) on a medical and surgical ward to list five tasks in each of three frequency categories (high, moderate, and infrequent). In order to decrease the noise in the set of tasks, they were clarified and redefined through two pretests and one pilot study.

The *population* consisted of 88 registered nurses employed on seven medical and surgical wards in a community medical center. All were professionally educated and could be expected to base nursing judgments on professional role attitudes reflecting that educational experience. However, the subjects were also organizational employees and had experienced organizational socialization as well.

Each of the subjects participated in a *structured training session* until the researcher was satisfied that the subject understood and could give proportional judgments (as described previously). The subjects responded to the *operational definitions constructed* for the professional and organizational variables. Specifically, each subject judged the set of patient care tasks on each variable (frequency, complexity, importance, discretion or control, and search intensity). A data collection sheet illustrating a set of data from one individual after the completion of this procedure is shown in Table 1. Thus, the *control by constancy principle* of the mathematical design was operationalized.

The reliability and validity of the scales produced by the magnitude-estimation techniques were assessed. Reliability in the form of stability was estimated through the test-retest technique. The reliability coefficients ranged from .75 to .93 (Frequency = .92, Complexity = .88, Importance = .75, Discretion = .87, and Search = .93). Since the theoretical models predicted the variable relationships, validity was estimated by the degree to which the empirical results supported the predicted relationships. Each of the variables was estimated to be valid except for the *task importance* concept.

The *data were standardized* by the instructions given to the subjects. They were asked to select an average task from the list of stimulus conditions, which was given the arbitrary number 10. The subjects were requested to judge the other tasks in proportion to the standard. Second, the *data were averaged* by obtaining the median judgment for each stimulus on each variable. Since this study focused on the systematic decision pattern representative of a professional group, averaging was quite appropriate. *Logarithmic transformations* of the data allowed the use of statistics requiring linear additive assumptions. Path analysis (Duncan, 1966; Heiss, 1975) was the statistical technique utilized.

FINDINGS

The results indicated that the professional model rather than the organizational model provided the most accurate description of the decision

TABLE 1

ONE SUBJECT'S MAGNITUDE ESTIMATION OF 16 PATIENT CARE TASKS (SOCIAL STIMULI) ON 5 TASK VARIABLES*

Task Condition	Task Feature				
	Fre-quency	Complex-ity	Impor-tance	Con-trol	Search
Teach simple Rx's	8	15	12	15	12
Cope with long-term immobility	8	15	18	8	20
Talk of patient fears/ anxieties	12	20	15	8	20
Insert Foley catheter	12	5	5	15	8
Check surgical/test site	20	15	12	20	5
Teach turn, cough, etc.	15	10[†]	15	20	12
Counsel hostile patients	2	30	30	5	30
Cope with pain measures	15	20	20	5	20
Explain tests/surgery to patient	10[†]	20	15	10[†]	20
Teaching complex Rx's	8	18	15	20	10[†]
Nursing rounds	20	8	15	20	12
Vital signs	20	2	8	20	2
Start IV	20	15	12	20	8
Explain tests/surgery to family	8	15	10[†]	8	15
Patient Rx tubes	20	5	12	20	5
Dying patient and family	5	20	20	5	20

Note: *Data from Field and Hinshaw (1977).*

The numbers represent magnitude-estimation judgments of the task on each variable.

[†]*Standard stimuli = 10 units.*

responses of practitioners functioning in organizations (R^2 of professional model = .76, while R^2 of organizational model = .61; difference significance at $p > .05$. In the professional model, the major variable influencing search was the complexity or amount of professional knowledge and skill required to perform the tasks. Further, discretion negatively influenced search intensity as well as provided an indirect path through which task complexity exerted a positive influence on search. Only limited support for the organizational model was evident in the results of the study. The data showed that repetitiveness exerted only a slight to moderate influence on search. Complexity had a moderate positive and frequency a slight negative effect on search through discretion or control.

This investigation illustrates the use of mathematical designs and magnitude-estimation techniques in the study of role attitudes as they guide decision processes in nursing. The conditions of the mathematical correlational design are operationalized; i.e., magnitude-estimation techniques are used to produce ratio scales of the variables; the control by constancy principle is satisfied, with all subjects responding to the professional and organizational variables in relation to a set of social stimuli (patient care tasks); and the data were averaged to decrease random measurement error and the best-fitting function for the data was tested. The elements required in the use of magnitude-estimation techniques were clearly delineated.

Expectations of Quality Nursing Care (Hinshaw and Oakes, 1977)

Hinshaw and Oakes' (1977) research used magnitude estimation to measure the attitudes of patients, nurses, and physicians about the expectations of quality nursing care. (Quality nursing care was defined as the degree of excellence that is rendered in the actual service or care given to patients.) The expectations of each group were assumed to reflect their prior socialization experiences. Patients are culturally conditioned to have certain expectations of health care and to hold certain stereotypes of such health care workers as nurses. Physicians and nurses are expected to base their judgments on their professional educational programs as well as on their experience as health care workers. This study operationalized the magnitude-estimation techniques differently and compromised one condition of the mathematical design—averaging of data was not done.

Three theoretical models were constructed to predict the characteristics that would define the quality of nursing care expectations for each of the three subpopulations. The theoretical predictors are primarily guided by the care-cure coordinate taxonomy of nursing role functions (ANA, 1965). Eight dimensions of nursing care were hypothesized to be valued differently by the three subpopulations; i.e., competency in technical skills, personalized care, information source, leadership abilities, cooperation with other personnel, professional creativity, professional knowledge, and professional demeanor.

Each group of occupants (physicians and patients) in complementary roles and actual role occupants (nurses) was predicted to value certain dimensions of patient care more than others. Patients were expected

to value competency in technical skills, personalized care, professional demeanor, and being an information source. This suggests clients adhere basically
to a care-and-cure concept of quality nursing care. Nurses' expectations of
quality nursing care were predicted to be multifunctional from all categories.
Physicians were expected to include primarily cure and coordinate functions:
competency in technical skills, leadership abilities, and professional knowledge.

A mathematical correlational design with magnitude-estimation
measurement techniques was used to estimate the expectations of quality
nursing care for clients, physicians, and nurses. The elements of the magnitude-
estimation techniques were operationalized as in the earlier investigation;
i.e., subjects experienced a formal training session, all subjects responded to
all the role variables defining quality nursing care, and broad definitional cues
were constructed for each variable. The *subjects* were selected for their
ability to judge the role performance of the role occupants. Two groups of
subjects (the nine patients and nine physicians) occupying complementary
roles to the nursing role and nine registered nurses actually occupying the
role were selected as respondents.

The *set of social stimuli* were constructed on a procedural model
suggested by an earlier study of Hamblin and Smith (1966). The social
stimuli consisted of the occupants of the role position *registered nurse*, who
also formed one group of respondents. The occupants were assumed to vary
in their ability to enact certain role functions, e.g., providing personal care,
being professionally creative, or providing a source of information for patients.
The different subject groups' opinion of the stimulus (registered nurse's role
performance) was predicted to vary according to their attitudes and expectations of the nursing role.

The measurement protocol had each subject presented pictures of
the nurses with whom he or she had had contact on a general medical unit.
Each subject selected one nurse (by photograph) as "average" according to
the variable. The subjects then ranked the other randomly presented nurses
in proportion to the average standard. Each independent, dependent, and
control variable was measured in the same manner to satisfy the *control by
constancy principle*. Table 2 shows data collected for one hypothetical
individual during this procedure.

Both reliability and validity tests were conducted with the
magnitude-estimation scales. A test-retest technique was employed to estimate the reliability of each individual subject's responses given twice. No
significant differences were noted between the two test periods. In assessing
patients', nurses', and physicians' perceptions of quality nursing care, predictive validity was estimated by the degree to which the theoretically predicted
expectations matched the empirical findings. Only the predictions for professional knowledge and professional creativity were inaccurate.

TABLE 2

ONE SUBJECT'S MAGNITUDE ESTIMATION OF 9 NURSES
(SOCIAL STIMULI) ON 9 ROLE-PERFORMANCE VARIABLES

Variables for Judgment

Nurse Stimuli	Competency with Technical Skills	Leadership Ability	Cooperation with Others	Personalized Care	Information Source	Professional Knowledge	Professional Creativity	Professional Demeanor	Personal Liking
A	15	12	5	20	5	10	20	15	5
B	10*	30	25	17.5	10*	10*	10	5	30
C	10	7.5	5	10*	7.5	10	10*	7.5	35
D	10	15	15	10	20	15	15	20	20
E	7.5	10*	10*	3	12	10	5	15	17.5
F	10	20	35	35	15	5	7.5	10*	10*
G	30	5	15	12	20	25	35	2.5	5
H	7.5	10	10	5	3	0	3	5	15
I	5	3	20	7.5	15	25	12.5	20	10

Note: *Data are from Field and Hinshaw (1977).*

Standard stimuli = 10 units.

301

The *data were standardized* as described earlier; however, averaged data could not be used in this investigation. The number of individuals was held to nine per subpopulation because that was the largest number of nurses that were available on one unit who could be employed for the judging process. However, there were 11 variables in the theoretical framework. If the data were averaged there would be fewer cases than variables. Multiple-regression solutions cannot be obtained under these conditions. Otherwise, the data were treated as described earlier; i.e., *logarithmic transformations* and *linear statistics* were applied.

The results of this study suggest that individuals occupying a specific role and individuals occupying complementary roles held a combination of differing, as well as similar, expectations of quality role performance. Patients, physicians, and nurses all considered competency in technical skills basic to quality nursing care. The expectations of those in roles complementary to nursing differed in several ways from the expectations held by the role occupants. Patients and physicians both expected personalized care as part of quality nursing care. Patients expected staff to be cooperative and willing to work with others; however, they *negatively* valued the professional knowledge base of the nurse as a needed part of delivering quality care. Physicians expected several coordination functions of nurses. Nurses expected themselves to be a source of information to patients and also valued professional demeanor as an attitude style to adopt in the delivery of care. Nurses' and physicians' expectations were in direct conflict with the information source role function. Nurses expected to provide information to their patients as part of quality care while physicians *did not* wish nurses to serve as sources of information to the patients. Thus, the role perspectives of three groups involved in the health care system were both convergent and divergent in terms of role expectations defining quality performance.

Comparison of the Studies

The two studies cited utilized magnitude-estimation scaling techniques within mathematical designs. The measurement protocols have been presented for both. The studies differed on two points; i.e., the decision-making investigation used a set of objects or events (patient care tasks) as social stimuli, while the quality-of-nursing-care study used nurses as the basic set. The decision study averaged the data, while the quality-of-nursing-care study worked with individual scores.

The use of nurses or other individuals as the social stimuli set was found to be easier to use, since it did not require pretesting a set of objects or events for clarity. However, this usage has an inherent problem. Individuals,

as stimuli, are often viewed as being "very good" or "not so good" *in general.*
For this reason, subjects judging them tend to judge them the same on all
variables. As a consequence, independent measurements may not be obtained
for each variable and statistical multicolinearity (Gordon, 1968) may result.
Thus, the use of nurses as stimuli is apt to give an inflated estimate of the
interaction between variables. When individuals (e.g., nurses) are used as
stimuli conditions, care must be taken to remind the respondents that individuals will differ on the variables under study; that is, they may be quite
creative but possibly not be as skillful as other colleagues.

One issue in the use of magnitude-estimation techniques not
considered in either of the reported studies is whether the technique produces
ratio-level scales as past research claims. According to Stevens (1966), "equal
(physical) stimulus ratios will produce equal (sensory) sensation ratios."
Thus, in psychophysics as ratio-scaled physical stimuli (i.e., decibels of sound)
were presented to subjects, they produced ratio scales of sensory sensation in
response. Research substantiating the production of ratio scales was first
initiated in the cross-modality studies of Stevens and Mack (1959). In the
social sciences, the validity of producing ratio scales has been questioned,
since the social stimuli are not always ratio scaled. When social stimuli are not
ratio scaled, then the basic principle cited by Stevens is violated. What happens
to the production of ratio-level scales under these conditions? Several of
Hamblin's investigations attempted to test for ratio-response scales when the
stimuli were not ratio level. Thus far, the results suggest that ratio scales of
subjective responses are formed under these conditions; however, the research
for these tests is minimal. Thus, whether ratio-level scales of attitudinal
responses are actually formed is still controversial.

SUMMARY

Nursing investigations often involve the measurement of subjective attitudes
related to health care roles. Frequently, subjective, attitudinal questions are
asked as, for example, What attitudes basically guide the delivery of health
care? Or, for a client, What constitutes quality health care? Understanding
and predicting answers to these questions is hindered by the inherent difficulty of operationalizing or measuring role attitudes in the empirical or
"real" world. The measurement of role attitudes is likely too biased, therefore, due to several basic sources of error; i.e., measurement error due to
level of scale measurement and design error from intersubject error.

Magnitude estimation, a measurement technique adapted to the social sciences from psychophysics, shows promise for coping with several of the traditional sources of error in attitude measurement. This technique can increase the precision or sensitivity of measurement by producing ratio-level scales. Further, the technique is used in the context of mathematical design, which decreases error due to intersubject variation.

This chapter has presented the general techniques used for magnitude estimation and those mathematical designs used in the study of subjective phenomena. Several nursing investigations of role attitudes have illustrated the use of these designs and techniques in health care research. The importance of role attitude research flows from the need to understand basic role expectations. Such understanding will increase the reality of what persons can expect of each other in the delivery of health care and demonstrate where sources of conflict may be generated due to divergent expectations of role performance. Both the ability to deliver and to accept health care are hampered by the generation of conflict.

Bibliography

Abdellah F: Nurse practitioners and nursing practice. Am J Public Health 66:245, 1976

Adams JS: Inequity in social exchange. Adv Exp Social Psychol 2:267, 1965

Adams JS, Jacobsen PR: Effects of wage inequities on work quality. J Abnormal Social Psychol 69:19, 1964

Ainsworth MD: The effects of maternal deprivation: review of findings and controversy in the context of research strategy. In Heise DR (ed): Personality and Socialization. Chicago, Rand McNally, 1972

Allport GW: Becoming. New Haven, Yale Univ Press, 1955

Amendments to Social Security Act (P.L. 92–603): Professional Standards Review Organization. Bethesda, Md, DHEW, 1973

American Medical Association: Directory of Approved Internships and Residencies 1973–74. Chicago, AMA, 1974

American Medical Association: Directory of Approved Residencies 1974–75. Chicago, AMA, 1975

American Nurses' Association: First position paper on education for nursing. Am J Nursing 65:106, 1965

American Psychological Association: Standards for Educational and Psychological Tests. Washington, DC, APA, 1974

Andersen R, Andersen O: A Decade of Health Services. Chicago, Univ of Chicago Press, 1967

Anderson SB, Ball E, Murphy R, et al.: Encyclopedia of Educational Evaluation. San Francisco, Jossey-Bass, 1975

Andrews P, Yankauer A: The pediatric nurse practitioner: growth of the concept. Am J Nursing 71:503–509

Argyris C: Management and Organizational Development: New York, McGraw-Hill, 1971

Arndt C, Laeger E: Role strain in a diversified role set: the director of nursing service. Part 1. Nursing Res 19:253, 1970

Arndt C, Laeger E: Role strain in a diversified role set: the director of nursing service. Part 2: Sources of stress. Nursing Res 19:495, 1970

Aronfreed J: The concept of internalization. In Goslin DA (ed): Handbook of Socialization Theory and Research. Chicago, Rand McNally, 1969

Ashley J: Hospitals, Paternalism, and the Role of the Nurse. New York, Teachers College Press, 1976

Backman C, Secord P: The self and role selection. In Gordon C, Gergen KJ (eds): The Self in Social Interaction. New York, Wiley, 1968

Bandura A: The role of modeling processes in personality development. In Hartup WW, Smothergill NL (eds): The Young Child: Reviews of Research. Washington, DC, Nat Assoc for the Education of Young Children, 1967

Bandura A: Social-learning theory of identificatory processes. In Goslin DA (ed): Handbook of Socialization Theory and Research. Chicago, Rand McNally, 1969

Bandura A, Walters R: Social Learning and Personality Development. New York, Holt, Rinehart and Winston, 1963

Bandura A, Walters RN: The development of self control. In Gordon C, Gergen KJ (eds): The Self in Social Interaction. New York, Wiley, 1968

Barclay JE, Weaver HB: Comparative reliabilities and ease of construction of Thurstone and Likert attitude scales. J Social Psychol 58:109, 1962

Barry JR, Wingrove CR (eds): Let's Learn about Aging: A Book of Readings. New York, Wiley, 1977

Barry WA: Marriage research and conflict: an integrative review. In Heise DR (ed): Personality and Socialization. Chicago, Rand McNally, 1972

Bar-Yosef R, Shild EO: Pressures and defenses in bureaucratic roles. Am J. Sociol 71:663, 1966

Becker HS, Geer B, Hughes EC, Strauss AL: Boys in White: Student Culture in Medical School. Chicago, Univ of Chicago Press, 1961

Becker MH (ed): The health belief model and personal health behavior. Health Educat Monog 2:2–30, 1974

Becker MH, Drachman RH, Kirscht JP: A new approach to explaining sick-role behavior in low-income populations. Am J Public Health 64:205, 1974

Becker MH, Drachman RH, Kirscht JP: Predicting mothers' compliance with pediatric medical regimens. J Pediatr 81:843, 1972

Becker MH, Green LW: A family approach to compliance with medical treatment: a selective review of the literature. Int J Health Educat 18:173, 1975

Becker MH, Haefner DP, Kasl SV, Kirscht JP, Maimon LA, Rosenstock IM: Selected psychosocial models of individual health-related behaviors. Med Care 15 (Suppl):27, 1977

Becker MH, Kaback MM, Rosenstock IM, Ruth MV: Some influences on public participation in a genetic screen program. J Comm Health 1:3, 1975

Becker MH, Maimon LA: Socio-behavioral determinants of compliance with health and medical care recommendations. Med Care 13:10, 1975

Becker TA: Perceived situational moderators of the relationship between subjective role ambiguity and role strain. J Appl Psychol 61:35, 1976

Becker WC: Consequences of different kinds of parental discipline. In Hoffman ML, Hoffman LW (eds): Review of Child Development Research. Vol. 1. New York, Russell Sage, 1964

Becker WC: Consequences of different kinds of parental discipline. In Heise DR: Personality and Socialization. Chicago, Rand McNally, 1972

Beckhouse LS: Behavioral Resolution of Role Incongruity: An Interactional Approach. Unpublished dissertation, Vanderbilt University, 1969

Beehr T: Role ambiguity as a role stress: some moderating and intervening variables. Unpublished dissertation, University of Michigan, 1974

Ben-David J: The professional role of the physician in bureaucratized medicine: a study in role conflict. Human Relations 11:255, 1963

Bendix R, Lipset SM: Class Status and Power, 2nd ed. New York, Free Press, 1966

Berger BM: Adolescence and beyond: an essay review of three books on the problems of growing up. Soc Prob 10:394, 1963

Berger P. Luckman T: The Social Construction of Reality. New York, Anchor, 1967

Berni R, Fordyce WE: Behavior Modification and the Nursing Process, 2nd ed. St. Louis, Mosby, 1977

Berrien, KF: General Social Systems. New Brunswick, NJ: Rutgers Univ Press, 1968

Berry J, Kushner R: A critical look at the Queen Bee Syndrome. J Nat Assoc Women Deans, Administrators, Counselors 38:173, 1975

von Bertalanffy L: The theory of open systems in physics and biology. Science 3:23, 1950

Bible BL, McComas JD: Role consensus and teacher effectiveness. Soc Forces 42:225, 1963

Biddle B, Thomas E (eds): Role Theory: Concepts and Research. New York, Wiley, 1966

Bidwell C: The young professional in the army: a study of occupational identity. Am Sociol Res 26:360, 1961

Biller HB: Father dominance and sex-role development in kindergarten-age boys In Heise DR: Personality and Socialization. Chicago, Rand McNally, 1972

Bixenstine VE, Douglas J: Effect of psychopathology on group consensus and cooperative choice in a six-person game. J Pers Soc Psychol 5:32, 1967

Blackwell E: Pioneer Work in Opening the Medical Profession to Women. London, Longmans, Green, 1895

Blake J, Davis K: Norms, values, and sanctions. In Faris, REL (ed): Handbook of Modern Sociology. Chicago, Rand McNally, 1964

Blankenship R: Colleagues in Organization: The Social Construction of Professional Work. New York, Wiley, 1977

Blau P: Bureaucracy in Modern Society. New York, Randon House, 1956

Blau P: Dynamics of Bureaucracy, rev ed. Chicago, Univ of Chicago Press, 1961

Blau PM: Exchange and Power in Social Life. New York, Wiley, 1964

Blau PM, Duncan OD: The American Occupational Structure. New York, Wiley, 1967

Blau P, Schoenherr RH: The Structure of Organizations. New York, Basic Books, 1971

Blau P. Scott WR: Formal Organizations. San Francisco, Chandler, 1962

Bloom SW: The process of becoming a physician. Ann Am Acad Pol Soc Sci 87:346, 1963

Bloom SW: The medical school as a social system: a case study of faculty-student relations. Milbank Mem Fund Q 49:1–196, 1971

Blumer H: Society as symbolic interaction. In Rose A (ed): Human

Behavior and Social Processes. Boston, Houghton Mifflin, 1962, pp 179–192

Bogue DV: Skid Row in American Cities. Chicago, Univ of Chicago Press, 1963, App B, pp 516–521

Bohrnstedt GW: Reliability and validity assessment in attitude measurement. In Summers GF (ed): Attitude Measurement. Chicago, Rand McNally, 1970

Bolton CD: Is sociology a behavioral science? In Manis J, Meltzer B (eds): Symbolic Interaction. Boston, Allyn & Bacon, 1967

Borgotta E: Role playing specification, personality and performance. Sociometry 24:218, 1961

Bragg BW, Allen VL: Ordinal position and conformity: a role theory analysis. Sociometry 33:371, 1970

Brault L: Primary Nursing: The Variable of Accountability. Unpublished Thesis, California State Univ, Long Beach, 1977

Brim OG Jr: The parent-child relation as a social system: parent and child roles. Child Dev 28:345, 1957

Brim OG Jr: Personality development as role learning. In Iscoe I, Stevenson H (eds): Personality Development in Children. Austin, Univ of Texas Press, 1960

Brim OG Jr: Socialization through the life cycle. In Brim OG Jr, Wheeler S (eds): Socialization After Childhood: Two Essays. New York, Wiley, 1966

Brim OG Jr: Adult socialization. In Sills DL (ed): International Encyclopedia of the Social Sciences, 1968, pp 555–562

Brim OG Jr: Adult socialization. In Clausen JA (ed): Socialization and Society. Boston, Little, Brown, 1968

Brim OG Jr: Family structure and sex role learning by children: a further analysis of Helen Koch's data. Sociometry 21:1, 1968

Brim OG Jr, Glass DC, Lanvin DE, Goodman N: Personality and Decisions Processes: Studies in the Social Psychology of Thinking. Stanford, Stanford Univ Press, 1962

Bronfenbrenner U: Socialization and social class through time and space. In Maccoby EE, Newcomb TM, Hartley EL (eds): Readings in Social Psychology. New York, Holt, Rinehart & Winston, 1958

Brown EL: Nursing for the Future. New York, Russell Sage Foundation, 1948

Brown B (ed): Primary nursing. Nurs Admin Q 1:2, 1977

Brunetto E, Birk P: The primary care nurse: the generalist in a structured health team. Am J. Public Health 62:785, 1972

Buckley W: Sociology and Modern Systems Theory. Englewood Cliffs, NJ, Prentice-Hall, 1967, p. 47

Bulger W: Some humanistic issues in health professions. Health Care Dimensions (Fall):29, 1974

Bullough B: Alienation and school segregation. Integrated Edu 10 (March–Apr):29, 1972

Bullough B: Influences on role expansion. Am J Nurs 1976, p. 1476

Bullough B: The law and the expanding nursing role. Am J Public Health 66:249, 1976

Bullough B, Bullough V: The causes and consequences of differentiation of the nursing role. In Stewart PL, Cantor MG (eds): Varieties of Work Experience: The Social Control of Occupational Groups and Roles. New York, Wiley, 1974

Bullough B, Bullough V: Sex discrimination in health care. Nurs Outlook 23:40, 1975

Burchard W: Role conflict of military chaplains. Am Sociol Rev 19:228, 1954

Bureau of Health Resources Development. Minorities and Women in Health Fields: Applicants, Students, and Workers. DHEW Publ No. (HRA) 75–22. Washington, DC, 1974

Cain LD Jr: Life course and social structure. In Faris REL (ed): Handbook of Modern Sociology. Chicago, Rand McNally, 1964

Caldwell BM: The effects of infant care. In Hoffman ML, Hoffman LW (eds): Review of Child Development Research. Vol. 1. New York, Russell Sage Foundation, 1964

Campbell E: Adolescent socialization. In Goslin DA (ed): Handbook of Socialization Theory and Research. Chicago, Rand McNally, 1969

Campbell JD: Peer relations in childhood. In Hoffman ML, Hoffman LW (eds): Review of Child Development Research. Vol. 1. New York, Russell Sage Foundation, 1964

Campbell JP, Dunnette M, Lawler E, Weick KE Jr: Managerial Behavior, Performance, and Effectiveness. New York, McGraw-Hill, 1970

Caplan RD, Jones KW: Effects of work load, role ambiguity, and type A personality on anxiety, depression and heart rate. J Appl Psychol 60:713, 1975

Caplan RD, Robinson EAR, French JRP, Caldwell JR, Shinn M: Adhering to Medical Regimens: Pilot Experiments in Patient Education and Social Support. Ann Arbor, Institute for Social Research, University of Michigan, 1976

Caplow T: The Sociology of Work. New York, McGraw-Hill, 1954

Caplow TA: Two against One: Coalition in Triads. Englewood Cliffs, NJ: Prentice-Hall, 1968

Carnegie Commission on Higher Education: College Graduates and Jobs. New York, McGraw-Hill, 1973

Carnegie ME: Are Negro schools of nursing needed today? Nurs Outlook 12:52, 1964

Carr-Saunders AM, Wilson PA: The Professions. Oxford: Clarendon Press, 1933

Cermak A: Community based learning in occupational therapy. Am J Occup Ther 30:157, 1976

Chesler P: Are we a threat to each other? Ms. 1 (8):88, 1972

Chomsky N: The Logical Structure of Linguistic Theory. Cambridge, Mass., MIT Press, 1961

Christensen HT (ed): Handbook of Marriage and the Family. Chicago, Rand McNally, 1964

Clausen JA: Family structure, socialization, and personality. In Hoffman LW, Hoffman ML (eds:) Review of Child Development Research. Vol. 2. New York, Russell Sage Foundation, 1966

Clausen JA (ed): Socialization and Society. Boston, Little, Brown, 1968, pp. 18–72

Clay RN: The Medieval Hospitals of England, London, Methuen, 1909

Cogan L:Negroes for Medicine: Report of a Macy Conference. Baltimore, Johns Hopkins Univ Press, 1968

Cogswell B: Rehabilitation of paraplegics: processes of socialization. Sociol Inquiry 37:3, 1967

Coleman JS Campbell EQ, Hobson C, et al: Equality of Educational Opportunity. Washington, DC: Office of Education, DHEW, 1966

Colton MR: Nursing's leadership vacuum. Supervisor Nurse 6:29, 1976

Cooley CH: Human Nature and the Social Order. New York, Schocken Books, 1964

Cooley CH (ed): Social Organization. New York, Schocken Books, 1962

Conway MH: Management effectiveness and the role making process. J Nurs Admin 4(Nov–Dec):25, 1974

Corwin R: The professional employee: a study of conflict in nursing roles. Am J Sociol 66:604, 1961

Coser R: Role distance, sociological ambivalence, and transitional status systems. Am J Sociol 72:173, 1966

Cottrell L: The adjustment of the individual to his age and sex roles. Am Sociol Rev 7:617, 1942

Cotttrell LS Jr: Interpersonal interaction and the development of the self. In Goslin DA (ed): Handbook of Socialization Theory and Research, Chicago, Rand McNally, 1969

Coutu W: Role-playing vs role-taking: an appeal for clarification. Am Sociol Rev 16:180, 1951

Croog S, Ver Steeg D: The hospital as a social system. In Freeman HE, Levine S, Reeder LG (eds): Handbook of Medical Sociology. Englewood Cliffs, NJ: Prentice-Hall, 1972, pp 274–314

Cronbach LJ, Meehl PE: Construct validity in psychological tests. Psychol Bull 52:281, 1955

Cullen JW, Fox BH, Isom RN (eds): Cancer: The Behavioral Dimensions. New York, Raven, 1976

Dabbs JM, Kirscht JP: Internal control and the taking of influenza shots. Psychol Rep 28:959, 1971

D'Andrade RG: Sex differences and cultural institutions. In Maccoby EE (ed): The Development of Sex Differences. Stanford, Stanford University Press, 1966

Daniels AK: How free should professions be? In Freidson E (ed): The Professions and Their Prospects. Beverly Hills, Calif, Sage, 1971

Davis F, Olesen V: Initiation into a women's profession: identity problems in the status transition coed to nursing students. Sociometry 26:89, 1963

Davis J: Conceptions of official leader roles in the air force. Social Forces 32:253, 1954

Davis K: Final note of a case of extreme isolation. In Heiss J (ed): Family Roles and Interaction: An Anthology, 2nd ed. Chicago, Rand McNally, 1976

Davis K, Moore WE: Some Principles of Stratification. Am Sociol Rev 10:242, 1945

Delafuente J: How to help customers choose the right OTC medication. AM Druggist 174:57, 1976

Department of Graduate Medical Evaluation: Graduate medical education. JAMA 236:2974, 2989

Deutsch M: Trust and suspicion. J Conflict Resolution 2:265, 1958

Deutsch M, Krauss RM: The effect of threat upon interpersonal bargaining. J Abnor Soc Psychol 61:181, 1960

Deutsch M, Krauss RM: Studies of interpersonal bargaining. J Conflict Resolution 6:52, 1962

Dixon J: Personal communication to Mary E. Conway in Salt Lake City, Utah, 1977

Dollard J, Doob L, Miller NE, Mowrer OH, Sears RR: Frustration and Aggression. New Haven, Yale Univ Press, 1939

Dorsey JL: Physician distribution in Boston and Brookline 1940 and 1961. Med Care 7:429, 1969

Douvan E, Gold M: Modal patterns in American adolescence. In Hoffman LW, Hoffman ML (eds): Review of Child Development Research. Vol. 2. New York, Russell Sage Foundation, 1966

Dragastin SF, Elder GH Jr (eds): Adolescence in the Life Cycle: Psychological Change and Social Context. New York, Wiley, 1975

Dreitzel HP (ed): Childhood and Socialization; Recent Sociology No. 5. New York, MacMillan, 1973, pp. 22–35

Dua PS: Comparison of effects of behaviorally oriented action and psychotherapy re-education on introversion-extraversion, emotionality and internal-external control. J Counseling Psychol 6:567, 1970

Dube WF: Women enrollment and its minority component in US medical schools: datagram. J Med Educ 51:691, 1976

Duff RS, Hollingshead AB: Sickness and Society. New York, Harper & Row, 1968

Duncan B, Smith AN, Silver HK: Comparison of the physical assessment of children by pediatric nurse practitioners and pediatricians. Am J Public Health 67:1170, 1971

Duncan OD: Path analysis: Sociological examples. Causal Models Soc Sci 72:115, 1966

Durkheim E: The Division of Labor in Society. New York, Free Press, 1964

Educational Preparation for Nursing, 1975: Nurs Outlook 24:568, 1976

Ehrlich HJ, Rinehart JW, Howell JC: The study of role conflict: explorations in methodology. Sociometry 25:85, 1962

Elder GH Jr: Adolescent Socialization and Personality Development. Chicago, Rand McNally, 1968

Elder GH Jr. Role relations, sociocultural environments, and autocratic family ideology. In Heise DR (ed): Personality and Socialization. Chicago, Rand McNally, 1972

Elkin F: Socialization and the presentation of self. In Heiss J (ed): Family Roles and Interaction: An Anthology, 2nd ed. Chicago, Rand McNally, 1976

Elkin F, Handel G: The Child and Society: The Process of Socialization, 2nd ed. New York, Random House, 1972

Elkin F, Westley WA: The myth of adolescent culture. Am Sociol Rev 20:680, 1955

Emerson RM: Operant psychology and exchange theory. In Burgess R, Bushnell D (eds): Behavioral Sociology. New York, Columbia Univ Press, 1969

Enelow AJ, Henderson JB (eds): Applying Behavioral Science to Cardiovascular Risk. American Heart Association, 1975

Engel GV: Professional autonomy and bureaucratic organization, Admin Sci Q 30:12, 1970

Etzioni A: Modern Organization. Englewood Cliffs, NJ: Prentice-Hall, 1964

Etzioni A: A Comparative Analysis of Complex Organization. New York, Free Press, 1975

Evan WM: Role strain and the norm of reciprocity in research organizations. Am J Sociol 68:346, 1962

Extending the Scope of Nursing Practice: A Report of the Secretary's Committee to Study Extended Roles for Nurses. DHEW Publ no. (HSM) 73–2037, November, 1971

Fabrega H: Toward a Model of Illness Behavior. Med. Care 13:470–484

Fahs IJ, Peterson OL: The decline of general practitioners. Pub Health Rep 83:26, 1968

Faley T Tedeschi JT: Status and reactions to threats. J Pers Soc Psychol 17:192, 1971

Fein R: The Doctor Shortage: An Economic Diagnosis, Studies in Social Economics. Washington, DC: The Brookings Institute, 1967

Ferguson LR: Dependency motivation in socialization. In Hoppe RA, Milton GA, Simmel EC (eds): Early Experiences and the Processes of Socialization. New York, Academic, 1970

Field MA, Hinshaw AS: Magnitude estimation: a method for measuring subjective phenomena. Communicating Nursing Research. Boulder, Colo: Western Interstate Commission for Higher Education, 1977

Finnerty FA, Shaw LW, Himmelsbatch CK: Hypertension in the inner city. Circulation 47:76, 1973

Fishbein M: Attitude and the prediction of behavior. In Fishbein M (ed): Readings in Attitude Theory and Measurement. New York, Wiley, 1967

Flanders JP: A review of research on imitative behavior. Psychol Bull 69:316, 1968

Ford L, Silver H, Day P: The pediatric nurse-practitioner program. JAMA 204:298, 1968

Forward Plan for Health, FY 1978–82: DHEW, Publ no. (OS) 76–50056, 1978

Fox RC: Experiment Perilous. Glencoe, Ill, Free Press, 1959

Frake CO: The ethnographic study of cognitive systems. In Gladwin T, Sturtevant WC (eds): Anthropology and Human Behavior. Washington DC: Anthropological Society of Washington, 1962.

Freeman J: Growing up girlish. Trans-action 8:36, 1970

Freidson E: Client control and medical practice. Am J Soc 65:374, 1960

Freidson E: Patient Views of Medical Practice. New York, Russell Sage Foundation, 1961

Freidson E: Dominant professions, bureaucracy and client services. In Rosengren, W, Lifton M (eds): Organizations and Clients. Columbus, Ohio, Merrill, 1970

Freidson E: Professional Dominance: The Social Structure of Medical Care. New York, Atherton, 1970

Freidson E (ed): The Professions and Their Prospects. Beverly Hills, Calif, Sage Publ 1971

Gamson WA: Experimental studies of coalition formation. Ad Ex Soc Psychol 1:82–110, 1964

Geertz C: Religion as a cultural system. Reprinted from Banton M (ed): Anthropological Approaches to the Study of Religion. London, Tavistock, 1965

Gentry WD (ed): Applied Behavior Modification. St. Louis, Mosby, 1975

Georgopoulos BS (ed): Organization Research on Health Institutions. Ann Arbor, Mich, Institute for Social Research, 1972

Georgopoulos BS, Christian L: The clinical nurse specialist: a role model. In Riehl PO, McVay JW (eds): The Clinical Nurse Specialist: Interpretations, New York, Appleton, 1973

Gerard HB, Rabbie JM: Fear and social comparison. J Abnorm Soc Psychol 63:586, 1961

Gergen KJ: The Concept of Self. New York, Holt, Rinehart and Winston, 1971

Getzels JW, Guba EG: Role, role conflict and effectiveness: an empirical study. Am Sociol Rev 19:164, 1954

Gewirtz JL: Mechanisms of social learning: some roles of stimulation and behavior in early human development. In Goslin DA (ed): Handbook of Socialization Theory and Research. Chicago, Rand McNally, 1969

Geyman JP: The Modern Family Doctor and Changing Medical Practice. New York, Appleton-Century-Crofts, 1971

Gibson JL, Ivancevich J, Donnelly JH Jr: Organizations. Dallas, Business, 1973

Glenn ND: Social stratification. In Broom L, Selznick P (eds): Sociology, 4th ed. New York, Harper & Row, 1968

Goffman E: The Presentation of Self in Everyday Life. Garden City, NY, Doubleday, 1959

Goldman P: A theory of conflict processes and organizational offices. J Conflict Resolution 10:328, 1966

Goode W: Community within a community: the professions. Am Sociol Rev 22:194, 1957

Goode W: Norm commitment and conformity to role status obligations. In Biddle B, Bruce J, Thomas E (eds): Role Theory: Concepts and Research. New York, Wiley, 1966

Goode W: A theory of role strain. Am Sociol Rev 25:483, 1960

Goode W: The protection of the inept. Am Sociol Rev 32:5, 1967

Goodman M: Expressed self-acceptance and interpersonal needs: a basis for mate selection. In Heiss J (ed): Family Roles and Interaction: An Anthology, 2nd ed. Chicago, Rand McNally, 1976

Goodman P, Friedman A: An examination of the effect of wage inequity in the hourly condition. Org Behav Human Perf 3:340, 1968

Gorden R: Issues in multiple regression. Am J Sociol 73:592, 1968

Gordis L: Methodologic issues in the measurement of compliance. In Sackett DL, Haynes RB (eds): Compliance with Therapeutic Regimens. Baltimore, Md.: John Hopkins Univ Press, 1976

Gordon C: Role and value development across the life-cycle. In Jackson JA (ed): Role. Cambridge, Eng, Cambridge University Press, 1972

Gortner SR: Research for a practice profession. Nurs Res 24:193, 1975

Goslin DA (ed): Handbook of Socialization Theory and Research. Chicago, Rand McNally, 1969

Goss M: Influences and authority among physicians. Am Sociol Rev 26:39, 1961

Gouldner A: Toward an analysis of latent social roles. Admin Sci Q 2:281, 1957

Gove WR: The relationship between sex roles, marital status, and mental illness. In Heiss J (ed): Family Roles and Interaction: An Anthology, 2nd ed. Chicago, Rand McNally, 1976

Gray RM, Kesler JP, Moddy PM: The effects of social class and friends' expectations on oral polio vaccination participation. Am J Public Health 56:2028, 1966

Green LW: Should health education abandon attitude change strategies? Perspectives from recent research. Health Educ Monogr 30:25, 1970

Greenberg J, Leventhal GS: Violating equity to prevent group failure. Proceedings of the 81st Annual Convention of the American Psychological Association. City Publisher, 1973, pp 215–16

Greenberg S (ed): The Quality of Mercy. New York, Atheneum, 1971

Greene C, Organ D: An evaluation of causal models linking the received role and job satisfaction. Administrative Sci Q 18:95, 1973

Greenwood E: Attributes of a Profession. Social Work. July, 1957

Grief S, MacDonald R: Role Relationships Between Nonphysicians and Treatment Team Leaders and Team Psychiatrists. Comm Ment Health J 9:378–387, 1973

Gross N, Ward M, McEachern A: Exploration in Role Analysis. New York, Wiley, 1958

Gross N, McEachern A, Mason WS: Role conflict and its resolution. In Biddle B, Thomas E (eds): Role Theory: Concepts and Research. New York, Wiley, 1966

Gullahorn J: Measuring role conflict. Am J Sociol 61:299, 1956

Gunter L, Crecraft HJ, Kennedy EJ: Mental health in a segregated setting. In Bullough B, Bullough V (eds): New Directions for Nurses. New York, Springer, 1974

Guttman L: Best possible systematic estimates at commonalities. Psychometrika 21:273, 1956

Haefner D, Kirscht JP: Motivational and behavioral effects of modifying health beliefs. Public Health Rep 85:478, 1970

Hall R: Social influence on the aircraft commander role. Am Sociol Rev 20:292, 1955

Hall R: Professionalization and bureaucratization. Am Sociol Rev 33:92, 1968

Halsey S: The Queen Bee Syndrome in Progressive Levels of Nursing Management. Unpublished Masters Thesis, Boston University, 1977

Hamblin RL: Ratio measurement for the social sciences. Soc Forces 50:191, 1971

Hamblin RL: Mathematical experimentation and sociological theory: a critical analysis. Sociometry 34:423, 1971

Hamblin RL: Social attitudes: magnitude measurement and theory. Blalock HM (ed): Measurement in the social sciences. Chicago, Aldine, 1974

Hamblin RL, Bridges; DA, Day RC, Yancy W: The interference-agression law? Sociometry 26:190, 1963

Hamblin RL, Clarimont DH, Chadwick BA: Utility and gambling decisions: experiments and equations. Soc Sci Res 4:1, 1975

Hamblin RL, Smith CR: Values, status and professors. Sociometry 29:183, 1966

Hammer WC, Tosi HW: Relationship of role conflict and role ambiguity to job involvement measures. J Appl Psychol 59:497, 1974

Hardy ME: Role overload and inequity: their consequences for social exchange. Dissertation, University of Washington, Seattle, 1971. Dissertation 33:16–0468020, 1971 (University Microfilm No. 72–20, 870)

Hardy ME: Role problems, role strain, job satisfaction and nursing care. Paper presented at the annual meeting of the American Sociological Association, New York, August 1976

Hartley RE: A developmental view of female sex-role identification. In Biddle BJ, Thomas EJ (eds): Role Theory: Concepts and Research. New York, Wiley, 1966

Hartup WW, Coates B: The role of imitation in childhood socialization. In Hoppe RA, Milton GA, Simmel EC (eds): Early Experiences and the Process of Socialization. New York, Academic, 1970

Haynes MA, Garvey MR: Physicians, hospitals and patients in the inner city. In Norman JC (ed): Medicine in the Ghetto. New York, Appleton, 1969

Haynes RB: A critical review of the "determinants" of patient compliance with therapeutic regimens. In Sackett DL, Haynes RB (eds): Compliance with Therapeutic Regimens. Baltimore, Md: Johns Hopkins Univ Press, 1976

Haynes RB, Sackett DL, Gibson ES, Taylor DW, Hackett BC, Roberts RS, Johnson AL: Improvement of medication compliance in uncontrolled hypertension. Lancet 1:1265, 1976

Hays WL: Measuring stimulus characteristics. In Hays WL (ed):

Quantification in Psychology. Belmont, Calif: Brooks/Cole, 1967

Heiman E, Dempsey M: Independent behavior of nurse practitioners: a survey of physician and nurse attitudes. Am J Public Health 66:587, 1976

Heise D: Causal Analysis. New York, Wiley, 1975

Heiss J: An introduction to the elements of role theory. In Heiss J (ed): Family Roles and Interaction: An Anthology, 2nd ed. Chicago, Rand McNally, 1976

Herzberg F: Work and the Nature of Man. Cleveland, World, 1966

Hetherington M, Deur J: The effects of father absence on child development. In Hartup WW (ed): The Young Child: Reviews and Research Vol. 2. Washington, DC, Nat Assoc for the Education of Young Children, 1972

Hewitt JP: Self and Society: A Symbolic Interactionist Social Psychology. Boston, Allyn & Bacon, 1976

Hill R, Aldous J: Socialization for marriage and parenthood. In Goslin DA (ed): Handbook of socialization Theory and Research. Chicago, Rand McNally 1969

Himmelfarb S, Eagly AH: Orientations to the study of attitudes and their change. In Himmelfarb S, Eagly AH (eds): Readings in Attitude Change. New York, Wiley, 1974

Hinshaw AS: Professional Decisions: A Technological Perspective. Unpublished dissertation, Univ of Arizona, 1975

Hinshaw AS, Field MA: An investigation of variables that underlie collegial evaluation. Nurs Res 23:292, 1974

Hinshaw AS, Oakes D: Theoretical model testing: patients' nurses' and physicians' expectations for quality nursing care. In Batey M (ed): Communicating Nursing Research. Vol. 10. Boulder, Colo: Western Interstate Commission for Higher Education, 1977, pp 163–91

Hochbaum GM: Public Participation in Medical Screening Programs: A Socio-psychological Study. Publ no. 572. Bethesda, Md: Public Health Service, 1958

Hodge RW, Seigel PM, Rossi PH: Occupational prestige in the United States, 1925–1963. Am J Social 70:286, 1964

Hoffman AM: The Daily Needs and Interests of Older People. Springfield, Ill: Thomas, 1970

Hoffman LW: Effects on children: summary and discussion. In Nye FI, Hoffman LW (eds): The Employed Mother in America. Chicago, Rand McNally, 1963

Hoffman LW: The decision to become a working wife. In Heiss J (ed):

Family Roles and Interaction: An Anthology, 2nd ed. Chicago, Rand McNally, 1976

Hoffman ML: Parent practices and moral development: generalizations from empirical research. Child Dev 34:295, 1963

Hogness JR: The Administration of Education for the Health Professions: A Time for Reappraisal. Third David D. Henry Lecture, University of Illinois Medical Center Campus, Chicago, Ill, April 8–9, 1976

Holder AR: Medical Malpractice Law. New York, Wiley, 1975

Holland M, Knobel R, Parrish I: The health field concept: its implications for educating health professionals. J Allied Health 5(Winter):47, 1976

Hollander EP, Hunt RGA (eds): Current Perspectives in Social Psychology. New York, Oxford Univ Press, 1972

Hollingshead AB: Elmtown's Youth. New York, Wiley, 1949

Homans GC: Social Behavior: Its Elementary Forms. New York: Harcourt, Brace and World, 1961

Homans, GC: Social Behavior: Its Elementary Forms, rev ed. New York, Harcourt, Brace, Jovanovich, 1974

House RJ, Rizzo JR: Role conflict and ambiguity as critical variables in a model of organizational behavior. Org Behav Human Perf 7:467, 1972

Howard A, Scott R: A proposed framework for analysis of stress in the human organism. Behav Sci 10:141, 1965

Hughes EC: Introduction. Hughes EC, Thorne B, DeBaggis AM, Williams D (eds): Education for the Professions of Medicine, Law, Theology, and Social Welfare. New York, McGraw-Hill, 1973

Hunt RG: Role and role conflict. In Hartley JH, Holloway GF (eds): Focus on Change and the School Administration. Buffalo, NY, State Univ of New York, School of Education, 1965

Huntington MJ: The development of a professional self-image. In Merton RK, Reader GG, Kendal PL (eds): The Student-Physician. Cambridge, Mass, Harvard Univ Press, 1957

Hyman HH: The psychology of status. Arch Psychol 38, no. 267:6, 1942

Inkeles A: Society, social structure, and child socialization. In Clausen JA (ed): Socialization and Society. Boston, Little, Brown, 1968

Inkeles A: Social structure and socialization. In Goslin DA (ed): Handbook of Socialization Theory and Research. Chicago, Rand McNally, 1969

Institute of Medicine: Social Security Studies Final Report Medicare-Medicaid Reimbursement Policies. Washington, DC, Nat Academy of Sciences, 1976

Jaccard J: A theoretical analysis of selected factors important to health education strategies. Health Educ Monogr 3:152, 1975

Jackson J: Structural characteristics of norms. In Biddle B, Thomas E (eds): Role Theory. New York, Wiley, 1966

Jackson JA: Professions and Professionalization. Cambridge, Eng, Cambridge University Press, 1970

Jacobson AH: Conflict of attitudes toward the roles of the husband and wife in marriage. In Biddle B, Thomas E (eds): Role Theory Concepts and Research. New York, Wiley, 1966

Jacobson E, Chambers W, Lieberman S: The use of the role concept in the study of complex organizations. J Soc Issues 7:18, 1951

JAMA 234:1344, 1975

James WH, Woodruff AB, Werner W: Effect of internal and external control upon changes in smoking behavior. J Consult Psychol 29:184, 1965

Janis I: Effect of fear arousal on attitude change: recent developments in theory and experimental research. Adv Exp Soc Psychol 3:166, 1967

Janowitz M: Sociological theory and social control. Am J Sociol 81:82, 1975

Jenkins JJ: The acquisition of language. In Goslin DA (ed): Handbook of Socialization Theory and Research. Chicago, Rand McNally, 1969

Johnson D: A philosophy of nursing. Nurs Outlook 8:198, 1959

Johnson TW, Stinson JE: Role ambiguity, role conflict, and satisfaction: moderating effects of individual differences. J Appl Psychol 60:329, 1975

Johnson WL: Educational preparation for nursing. Nurs Outlook 24:568, 1976

Jones EE: Ingratiation: A Social Psychological Analysis. New York, Wiley, 1964

Kagan J: Acquisition and significance of sex typing and sex role identity. In Hoffman ML, Hoffman LW (eds): Review of Child Development Research. Vol. 1. New York, Russell Sage Foundation, 1964

Kahn R: Some propositions toward researchable conceptualization of stress. In McGrath J (ed): Social and Psychological Factors in Stress. New York, Holt, Rinehart & Winston, 1970

Kahn R, Wolfe D: Role conflict in organizations. In Kahn R, Boulding E (eds): Power and Conflict in Organizations. New York, Basic, 1964

Kahn R, Wolfe DM, Quinn RP, Snoek JD, Rosenthal RA: Organizational Stress. New York, Wiley, 1964

Kalish BJ, Kalish PA: A discourse on the politics of nursing. J Nurs Admin 6:29, 1976

Kane RL, Kane RA: Physicians attitudes of omnipotence in a university hospital. J Med Educ 44:684, 1969

Kasl SV, Cobb S: Health behavior, illness behavior, and sick role behavior. Arch Environ Health 12:246, 1966

Kast F, Rosenzweig J: Organization and Management. New York, McGraw-Hill, 1970

Katz D: The functional approach to the study of attitudes. Public Opinion Q 24:163, 1960

Katz D, Kahn R: The Social Psychology of Organizations. New York, Wiley, 1966

Katz RC, Zlutnick S (eds): Behavior Therapy and Health Care: Principles and Applications. New York, Pergamon, 1975

Kegeles SS: Why people seek dental care: a text of a conceptual framework. J Health Human Behav 4:166, 1963

Kegeles SS: A field experimental attempt to change beliefs and behavior of women in an urban ghetto. J Health Soc Behav 10:115, 1969

Kelley HH: Two functions of reference groups. In Proshansky H, Seidenberg B (eds): Basic Studies in Social Psychology. New York, Holt, Rinehart & Winston, 1965

Kemper TD: Reference groups, socialization and achievement. Am Sociol Rev 33:31, 1968

Kerckhoff AC: Socialization and Social Class. Englewood Cliffs, NJ: Prentice-Hall, 1972

Kerlinger FN: Foundations of Behavioral Research, 2nd ed. New York, Holt, Rinehart & Winston, 1973

Kerr C: Forward. In Hughes ED, Thorne B, DeBaggis AM, Williams D (eds): Education for the Professions of Medicine, Law, Theology, and Social Welfare. New York, McGraw-Hill, 1973

Kiesler SB, Baral RL: The search for a romantic partner: the effects of self-esteem and physical attractiveness on romantic behavior. In Heiss J (ed): Family Roles and Interaction: An Anthology. 2nd ed. Chicago, Rand McNally, 1976

Killian L: The significance of multiple group membership in disaster.

In Proshansky H, Seidenberg I (eds): Basic Studies in Social Psychology. New York, Holt, Rinehart & Winston, 1966

Kinlein ML: Independent nurse practitioner. Nurs Outlook 20:22, 1972

Kinlein ML: The self-care concept. Am J Nurs 77:598, 1977

Kirscht JP: The health belief model and illness behavior. Health Educ Monogr 2:387, 1974

Kirscht JP, Haefner DP, Eveland JD: Public response to various written appeals to participate in health screening. Public Health Rep 90:139, 1975

Kirscht JP, Haefner DP, Kegeles SS, Rosenstock IM: A national study of health beliefs. J Health Human Behav 7:248, 1966

Knowles J (ed): The Teaching Hospital. Cambridge, Mass, Harvard University Press, 1966

Knutson AL: The Individual, Society, and Health Behavior. New York, Russell Sage Foundation, 1965

Koch H: Personal communication. In Kangilaski J: A profile of office practice. Bull Am Coll Phys, 1977, p 18

Kohlberg L: Development of moral character and moral ideology. In Hoffman ML, Hoffman LW (eds): Review of Child Development Research. Vol. 1. New York, Russell Sage Foundation, 1964

Kohlberg L: A cognitive-development analysis of children's sex role concepts and attitudes. In Maccoby EE (ed): The Development of Sex Differences. Stanford, Stanford University Press, 1966

Kohlberg L: Stage and sequence: the cognitive-developmental approach to socialization. In Goslin DA (ed): Handbook of Socialization Theory and Research. Chicago, Rand McNally, 1969

Kohlberg L, Kramer R: Continuities and discontinuities in childhood moral development. In Heise DR (ed): Personality and Socialization. Chicago, Rand McNally, 1972

Kohn ML: Social class and parental values. Am J Sociol 64:337, 1959

Kohn ML: Social class and parent-child relationships: an interpretation. Am J Sociol 68:471, 1963

Kohn ML: Class and Conformity. Homewood, Ill: Dorsey, 1969

Kohn M: Bureaucratic man: a portrait and an interpretation. Am Sociol Rev 36:461, 1971

Kohn ML, Schooler C: Class, occupation, and orientation. In Heise DR (ed): Personality and Socialization. Chicago, Rand McNally, 1972

Komarovsky M: Cultural contradictions and sex roles. Am J Sociol 52:184, 1946

Komarovsky M: Learning conjugal roles. In Heiss J (ed): Family Roles and Interaction: An Anthology. 2nd ed. Chicago, Rand McNally, 1976

Kornhauser W: Scientists in Industry: Conflict and Accommodation. Berkeley, Univ of California Press, 1962

Kramer M: Role models, role conceptions, and role deprivation. Nurs Res 17:115, 1968

Kramer M: Collegiate graduate nurses in medical center hospitals: mutual change or duel. Nurs Res 18:196, 1969

Kramer M: Role conceptions of baccalaureate nurses and success in hospital nursing. Nurs Res 19:428, 1970

Kramer M: Reality Shock: Why Nurses Leave Nursing. St Louis, Mosby, 1974

Krauss RM, Deutsch M: Communication in interpersonal bargaining. J Pers Soc Psychol 4:572, 1964

Kuhn A: The Logic of Social System. San Francisco, Jossey-Bass, 1974

Kuhn T: The Structure of Scientific Revolutions. 2nd ed. Chicago, Univ of Chicago Press, 1972

Ladner JA: Becoming a woman in the black lower class. In Heiss J (ed): Family Roles and Interaction: Anthology. 2nd ed. Chicago, Rand McNally, 1976

Lalonde M: A New Perspective on the Health of Canadians: A Working Document. Ottawa, Canada, 1974

Lambertson EC: Nursing Team Organization and Functioning: Results of a Study of the Division of Nursing Education. New York, Teachers College, Columbia Univ, 1953

Langlie JK: Social networks, health belief, and preventive health behavior. J Health Soc Behav 18:244, 1977

Lasagna L (ed): Patient Compliance. Mount Kisco, NY: Futura Press, 1976

Lauer RH, Boardman L: Role-taking: theory, typology, and propositions. Sociol Soc Res, 1971

Lawler EE: Pay and Organizational Effectiveness: A Psychological View. New York, McGraw-Hill, 1971

Lawler EE, Kopkin CA, Young TF, Fadem JA: Inequity reduction over time in an induced over payment situation. Organizational Behavior and Human Performance, 3:253–68, 1968

LeBow MD: Approaches to Modifying Patient Behavior. New York, Appleton, 1976

Leff HS: Interpersonal behavior in a non-zero-sum experimental game as a function of cognitive complexity, environmental complexity, and predispositional variables. Dissertation Abs 29:4103–A, 1969

Leininger M: Ecological Behavior Variability: Cognitive Images and Sociocultural Expressions in Two Gadsup Villages. Unpublished dissertation, Univ of Washington, Seattle, 1966

Leininger M: The significance of cultural concepts in nursing. Minnesota League Nurs Bull 16(2):3, 1968

Leininger M: Ethnoscience: A new and promising research approach for the health sciences. Image 3(1):2, 1969

Leininger M: This I believe . . . about interdisciplinary health education for the future. Nurs Outlook 19:787, 1971

Leininger M: Humanism, health, and cultural values. Health Care Dimensions, Health Care Issues (Fall):29, 1974

Leininger M: The leadership crisis in nursing: a critical problem and and challenge. J Nurs Admin 4(2):28, 1974

Leininger M: Survey of the function and organization of evolving health science centers in University contexts. Unpublished report, Univ of Utah, Salt Lake City, 1974, 1976

Leininger M: Psychopolitical and ethnocentric behaviors in emerging health science centers. Paper presented at the University of Utah Department of Anthropology, Salt Lake City, Utah, March 20, 1975

Leininger M: Two strange health tribes: the Gnisrun and Enicidem in the United States. Human Org 35:253, 1976

Lennard H, Bernstein A: Expectations and behavior in therapy. In Biddle B, Thomas E (eds): Role Theory: Concepts and Research. New York, Wiley, 1966

Lenski G: Power and Privilege: A Theory of Social Stratification. New York, McGraw-Hill, 1966

Leventhal H: Findings and theory in the study of fear communications. Adv Exp Soc Psychol 5:120, 1970

Leventhal H, Rosenstock IM, Hochbaum GM, Carriger BK: Epidemic impact on the general population in two cities. In: The Impact of Asian Influenza on Community Life: A Study in Five Cities. Public Health Service publication no. 766. Washington, DC, 1960

Leventhal H, Singer R, Jones S: Effects of fear and specificity of recommendations upon attitudes and behavior. J Pers Soc Psychol 2:20, 1965

Levin LS, Katz AH, Holst E: Self-care: Lay Incentives for Health. New York, Neale Watson Academic, 1976

Levin T: American Health: Professional Privilege vs. Public Need. New York, Praeger, 1974

Levine DM et al: The role of new health practitioners in a prepared group practice: provides differences in process and outcomes of medical care. Med Care 14:326, 1976

Levine RA: Culture, personality, and socialization: an evolutionary view. In Goslin DA (ed): Handbook of Socialization Theory and Research. Chicago, Rand McNally, 1969

Levine RA, Campbell DT: Ethnocentrism: Theories of Conflict, Ethnic Attitudes and Group Behavior. New York, Wiley, 1972

Levy MJ: The Structure of Society. Princeton, NJ, Princeton Univ Press, 1952

Lewin K: Field Theory in Social Science: Selected Theoretical Papers. New York, Harper & Row, 1951

Lewis RA: A developmental framework for the analysis of premarital dyadic formation. In Heiss J (ed): Family Roles and Interaction: An Anthology. 2nd ed. Chicago, Rand McNally, 1976

Light E, Keller S: Sociology. New York, Knopf, 1975

Likert RA: A technique for the measurement of attitudes. Arch Psychol, no. 140, 1932

Lindesmith AR, Strauss AL: Social Psychology. New York, Holt, Rinehart & Winston, 1968

Lindesmith AR, Strauss AL: Readings in Social Psychology. New York, Holt, Rinehart & Winston, 1969

Linn LS: Patient acceptance of the family nurse practitioner. Med Care 14:357, 1976

Linton R: The Study of Man. New York, Appleton, 1936

Linton R: The Cultural Background of Personality. New York, Appleton, 1945

Linton R: The status-role concept. In Hollander EP, Hunt GR (eds): Classic Contributions to Social Psychology. New York, Oxford University Press, 1972

Loether HJ: Problems of Aging: Sociological and Social Psychological Perspectives. Belmont, Calif: Dickenson, 1967

Lowery BJ, DuCette JP: Disease-related learning and disease control as a function of locus of control. Nurs Res 25:358, 1976

Lyons T: Role clarity, need for clarity, satisfaction, tension and withdrawal. Org Behav Human Perf 6:99, 1971

MacBride O: An overview of the health professions educational assistance act, 1963–1971. Health Manpower Policy Discussion Paper Series, no. D.I. Ann Arbor, Mich, Univ of Michigan Press, 1973

Maccoby EE: Role-taking in childhood and its consequences for social learning. Child Dev 30:239, 1959

Maccoby EE: The taking of adult roles in middle childhood. J Abnorm Soc Psychol 63:493, 1961

Maccoby EE: The Development of Sex Differences. Stanford, Stanford University Press, 1966

Maccoby EE: The development of moral values and behavior in childhood. In Clausen JA (ed): Socialization and Society. Boston, Little, Brown, 1968

Maccoby N, Farquhar JW: Communication for health: unselling heart disease. J Commun 25:114, 1975

MacDonald AP: Internal-external locus of control and the practice of birth control. Psychol Rep 27:206, 1970

MacDonald AP: Internal-external control change technics. Rehabil Lit 33:44, 1972

Manno B, Marston AP: Weight reduction as a function of negative reinforcement (sensitization) versus positive convert reinforcement. Behav Res Ther 10:201, 1972

March J, Simon HA: Organizations. New York, Wiley, 1958

Marram GD, Schlegel MW, Bevis EO: Primary Nursing: A Model for Individualized Care. St Louis, Mosby, 1974

Marston MV: Compliance with medical regimens: a review of literature. Nurs Res 19:312, 1970

Martin H, Katz F: The professional school as a moulder of motivation. J Health Soc Behav 2:106, 1961

Martin MW Jr: Some effects of communication on group behavior in Prisoner's dilemma. Dissertation Abs 27:231–B, 1966

Maslow A: Motivation and Personality. New York, Harper & Bros, 1954

Matza D: Position and behavior patterns of youth. In Faris REL (ed): Handbook of Modern Sociology. Chicago, Rand McNally, 1964

McCandless BR: Childhood socialization. In Goslin DA (ed): Handbook of Socialization Theory and Research. Chicago, Rand McNally, 1969

McDermott W: General medical care identification and analysis of alternative approaches. Johns Hopkins Med J 135:292, 1974. Reprinted in Prospects for Health Care, The First

Dartmouth-Hitchcock Conference on Health Care, Dartmouth College, Hanover, NH, 1974

McGrath J (ed.): Social and Psychological Factors in Stress. New York, McGraw-Hill, 1970

McGee R, and others. Sociology, an Introduction. Hinsdale, Ill: Dryden, 1977

McGlothlin WJ: The Professional Schools. New York, Center for Applied Research in Education, 1964

McGregor D: The Human Side of Enterprise. New York, McGraw-Hill, 1960

McKinlay JB: The business of good doctoring or doctoring as good business: reflections on Freidson's view of the medical game. Int J Health Serv (to be published)

Mead GH: The genesis of the self and social control. Int J Ethics 35:251, 1925

Mead GH: Mind, Self and Society. Chicago, Univ of Chicago, 1934

Mead GH: The genesis of self. In Gordon C, Gergen KJ (eds): The Self in Social Interaction. New York, Wiley, 1968

Mead GH: The development of the self through play and games. In Stone GP, Farberman HA (eds): Social Psychology Through Symbolic Interaction. Waltham, Mass, Xerox College, 1970

Mechanic D: Some problems in developing a social psychology of adaptation to stress. In McGrath J (ed): Social and Psychological Factors in Stress. New York, Holt, Rinehart & Winston, 1970

Mechanic D: Public Expectations and Health Care. New York, Wiley, 1972

Medical curriculum. JAMA 234:1344, 1975

Meeker RJ, Shure GH: Pacifist bargaining tactics: some "outsider" influences. J Conflict Resolution 13:487, 1969

Mehrens WA, Lehmann IJ: Measurement and Evaluation in Education and Psychology. New York, Holt, Rinehart & Winston, 1973

Merton RK: The Role-set: problems in sociological theory. Sociol 8:106–20, 1957

Merton RK: On Theoretical Sociology. New York, Free Press, 1967

Merton RK: Social Theory and Social Structure. New York, Free Press, 1968

Merton RK, Kitt AS: Contributions to the theory of reference group behavior. In Merton RK, Lazarsfeld PF (eds): Continuities in Social Research: Studies in the Scope and Method of "The American Soldier." Glencoe, Ill, Free Press, 1959

Merton RK, Reader J, Kendall P (eds): The Student Physician. Cambridge, Mass, Harvard Univ Press, 1957

Miles RH: An empirical test of causal inference between role perceptions of conflict and ambiguity and various personal outcomes. J Appl Psychol 60:334, 1975

Miller G: Patient Types and Role Strain in Three Organizational Settings. Unpublished dissertation, Univ of Washington, Seattle, 1964

Miller J: The nature of living systems. Behav Sci 16:278, 1971

Miller J: Living systems: the organization. Behav Sci 17:1, 1972

Miller LK, Hamblin RL: Interdependence, differential rewarding and productivity. Am Sociol Rev 28:768, 1963

Mills CW: The Power Elite. New York, Oxford Univ Press, 1956

Mishler E: Personality Characteristics and the Resolution of Role Conflicts. Public Opinion Quarterly 17:115–135, 1953

Mitchell W: A social-learning view of sex differences in behavior. In Maccoby EE (ed): The Development of Sex Differences. Stanford, Stanford University Press, 1966

Mitchell, W: Occupational role strain: the American elective official. Admin Sci Q 3:210, 1958

Moore WE: Occupational socialization. In Goslin DA (ed): Handbook of Socialization Theory and Research. Chicago, Rand McNally, 1969

Moore WE: The Profession: Roles and Rules. New York, Russell Sage Foundation, 1970

Morais HM: History of the Negro in Medicine. New York, Publishers, 1968

Moreno J: Psychodramatic treatment of psychosis. Sociometry 3:115.

Mumford E: Interns, from Students to Physicians. Cambridge, Mass, Harvard Univ Press, 1970

Mussen PH: Early sex-role development. In Goslin DA (ed): Handbook of Socialization Theory and Research. New York, Rand McNally, 1969

Myrdal G: An American Dilemma: The Negro Problem and American Democracy. New York, Harper & Bros, 1944

National Center for Health Statistics, DHEW: Health Resources Statistics: Health Manpower and Health Facilities, 1972–1973. Bethesda, Md, US GPO, 1973

National Health Planning Resources and Development Act of 1974 (PL93–641), US DHEW. Bethesda, Md, US GPO, 1974

Neiman LJ, Hughes JW: The Problem of the concept of role—a resurvey of the literature. Soc Forces 30:141, 1951

Newcomb TM: Attitude development as a function of reference groups: the Bennington study. In Proshansky H, Seidenberg, B (eds): Basic Studies in Social Psychology. New York, Holt, Rinehart & Winston, 1965

Noble J (ed): Primary Care and the Practice of Medicine. Boston, Little, Brown, 1976

Norman JC: Medicine in the Ghetto. New York, Appleton, 1969

Norris CM: Direct access to the patient. Am J Nurs 1970, p 1006

Nunnally JC: Psychometric Theory. New York, McGraw-Hill, 1967

Nye FE, Hoffman LW: The Employed Mother in America. Chicago, Rand McNally, 1963

Oakes DL: Patients', Nurses' and Physicians' Perceptions of Quality Nursing Care. Unpublished Master's Thesis, Univ of Arizona, 1976

Olesen V, Whittaker E: The Silent Dialogue. San Francisco, Jossey-Bass, 1968

Olmsted AG, Paget MA: Some theoretical issues in professional socialization. J Med Educ 44:663, 1969

Orem DE: Nursing: Concepts of Practice. New York, McGraw-Hill, 1971

Oseasohn R: Primary care by a nurse practitioner in a rural clinic. Am J Nurs 75:267, 1975

Overall B, Aronson H: Expectations of psychotherapy in patients of lower socio-economic class. In Biddle B, Thomas E (eds): Role Theory: Concepts and Research. New York, Wiley, 1966

Palmer FH: Inferences to the socialization of the child from animal studies: a view from the bridge. In Goslin DA (ed): Handbook of Socialization Theory and Research. Chicago, Rand McNally, 1969

Palola E: Organization Types and Role Strains: A Laboratory Study of Complex Organization. Unpublished dissertation, Univ of Washington, Seattle, 1962

Park RE: Symbiosis and socialization: a frame of reference for the study of society. Am J Soc 45:1–25

Parke RD: The role of punishment in the socialization process. In Hoppe RA, Milton GA, Simmel EC (eds): Early Experiences and the Processes of Socialization. New York, Academic, 1970

Parke RD: Some effects of punishment on children's behavior. In Hartup WW (ed): The Young Child: Reviews of Research.

Vol. 2. Washington, DC: Nat Assoc for the Education of Young Children, 1972

Parker A: The dimensions of primary care: blue prints for change. In Andreopoulos S (ed): Care: Where Medicine Fails. New York, Wiley, 1974

Parsons T: Age and sex in the social structure of the United States. Am Sociol Rev 7:604, 1942

Parsons T: The Social System. New York, Free Press, 1951

Parsons T: Youth in the context of American society. Daedalus 91:97, 1962

Parsons T, Fox R: Therapy and the modern urban family. J Soc Issues 8:31, 1952

Paul BD: Anthropological perspectives on medicine and public health. Ann Am Acad Polit Soc Sci 346:34, 1963

Pavalko RM: Sociology of Occupations and Professions. Itasca, Ill, Peacock, 1971

Pellegrino ED: Acute and chronic illness. Rep R Soc Med and Josiah Macy Jr Fdn, New York, 1973

Pellegrino ED: The academic role of the vice-president for health sciences: can a walrus become a unicorn? J Med Educ 50:224, 1975

Perrow C: A framework for the comparative analysis of organization. Am Sociol Rev 32:194, 1967

Perrow C: Organizational Analysis. Belmont, Calif, Wadsworth, 1970

Perry S, Wynne LL: Role conflict, Role redefinition, and social change in a clinical research organization. Social Forces. 38:62–65, 1959

Phelan JG, Richardson E: Cognitive complexity, strategy of the other player, and two person game behavior. J Psychol 71:205, 1969

Piaget J: The Moral Judgment of the Child. Glencoe, Ill, Free Press, 1948

Piaget J: On the Development of Memory and Identity. Worcester, Mass, Clark Univ Press, 1968

Pratt L: Family Structure and Effective Health Behavior: The Energized Family. Boston, Houghton Mifflin, 1976

Preventive Medicine USA. Task force reports sponsored by the John E. Foggarty International Center for Advanced Study in the Health Sciences, National Institutes of Health and the American College of Preventive Medicine. New York, Neale Watson Academic, 1976

Pruitt DG, Johnson DF: Mediation as an aid to face saving in negotiation. J Pers Soc Psychol 14:239, 1970

Putnam L, Heinen JS: Women in management: the fallacy of the trait approach. MSU Business Topics 14(3):47, 1976

Quint JC: Institutionalized practices of information. Psychiatry 28 (May): 119, 1965

Rafky DM: Phenomenology and socialization: some comments on the assumptions underlying socialization theory. In Drieitzel HP (ed): Childhood and Socialization. Recent Sociology no. 5. New York, Macmillan, 1973

Rainwater L: The Social Meaning of Poverty, unpublished manuscript. Cambridge, Mass, Harvard Univ, 1972

Reeder LG, Berkanovic E: Sociological concomitants of health orientations: a partial replication of Suchman. J Health Soc Behav 14:134 1973

Reiter F: The nurse clinician. Am J Nurs 66:274, 1966

Rheingold HL: The social and socializing infant. In Goslin DA (ed): Handbook of Socialization Theory and Research. Chicago, Rand McNally, 1969

Rich W: Special role and role expectations of black administrators of neighborhood health programs. Comm Mental Health J 11:394–401, 1975

Richards ND: Methods and effectiveness of health education: the past, present and future of social scientific involvement. Soc Sci Med 9:141, 1975

Riehl PO, McVay JW: The Clinical Nurse Specialist: Interpretations. New York, Appleton, 1973

Riesman F: Strategies against Poverty. New York, Random House, 1969

Riley M, Foner A: Aging and Society: An Inventory of Research Findings. Vol. 1. New York, Russell Sage Foundation, 1968

Riley MW, Foner A, Hess B, Toby M: Socialization for the middle and later years. In Goslin DA (ed): Handbook of Socialization Theory and Research. Chicago, Rand McNally, 1969

Roberts MM: American Nursing: History and Interpretation. New York, Macmillan, 1961

Rogers DE: Medical academe and the problems of pirmary care. Proceedings of the Institute on Primary Care. Washington, DC, Assoc of American Medical Colleges, 1974

Rogers M: Reveille in Nursing. Philadelphia, Davis, 1964

Rogers ME: An Introduction to the Theoretical Basis for Nursing. Philadelphia, Davis, 1970

Rose A: Human Behavior and Social Processes. Boston, Houghton Mifflin, 1962

Rosen G: The hospital: historical sociology of a community institution. In Freidson E (ed): The Hospital in Modern Society. London, Free Press of Glencoe, Collier-Macmillan, 1963

Rosenberg CM, Raynss, AE: Keeping Patients in Psychiatric Treatment. Cambridge, Mass, Ballinger, 1976

Rosenstock IM: Historical origins of the health belief model. Health Educ Monogr 2:328, 1974

Rosenstock CM, Raynes AE: Keeping Patients in Psychiatric Treatment. Cambridge, Mass, Ballinger, 1976

Rosenstock IM: Why people use health services. Milbank Mem Fund Q 44:94, 1966

Rosenstock IM: Prevention of illness and maintenance of health. In Kosa J, Zola IK (eds): Poverty and Health: A Sociological Analysis, rev ed. Cambridge, Mass, Harvard Univ Press, 1975

Rosow I: Forms and functions of adult socialization. Soc Forces 44:35, 1965

Rosow I: Socialization to Old Age. Berkeley, Univ of California Press, 1974

Rossi AS: Transition to parenthood. In Heiss J (ed): Family Roles and Interaction: An Anthology. 2nd ed. Chicago, Rand McNally, 1976

Rotter JB: Generalized expectancies for internal versus external control of reinforcement. Psychol Monogr 80:1–28, 1966

Roy D: Quota restriction and goldbricking in a machine shop. Am J Sociol 57:427, 1952

Roy C Sr: The Roy adaptation model. In Riehl JP, Roy C Sr (eds): Conceptual Models for Nursing Practice. New York, Appleton, 1974

Rubin JR, Brown BR: The Social Psychology of Bargaining and Negotiation. New York, Academic, 1975

Rushing W: Differences in profit and non-profit organizations: a study of effectiveness and efficiency in general short-stay hospitals. Admin Sci Q 19:474, 1974

Sackett DL: The magnitude of compliance. Paper presented at Symposium on Compliance, Hamilton, Ontario, Canada, May 25, 1977

Sackett DL, Haynes RB (eds): Compliance with Therapeutic Regimens. Baltimore, Md, Johns Hopkins Univ Press, 1976

Sackett DL, Haynes RB, Gibson ES, et al: Randomized clinical trials of strategies for improving medication compliance in primary hypertension. Lancet 1:7918, 1975

Sales S: Organizational role as a risk factor in coronary disease. Admin Sci Q 14:325, 1969

Salisbury R: The pharmacist's duty to warn the patient of side effects. J Am Pharm Assoc 17:97, 1977

Sampson EE: The study of ordinal position: antecedents and outcomes. In Heise DR (ed): Personality and Socialization. Chicago, Rand McNally, 1972

Sanchez R, Bynum G: Health care in rural New Mexico. J Med Educ 48(Dec):124, 1973

Sarbin TR, Allen V: Role theory. In Lindzey G, Aronson E (eds): The Handbook of Social Psychology, New York, 1968

Satow RL: Value-rational authority and professional organizations: Weber's missing type. Admin Sci Q 20:526, 1975

Saunders L: Cultural Differences and Medical Care. New York, Russell Sage Foundation, 1954

Schacter S, Singer JE: Cognitive, social and physiological determinants of emotional state. Psychol Rev 69:379, 1962

Schlenker BR, Bonoma TV, Tedeschi JT Pivnick WP: Compliance to threats as a function of the wording of threat and the exploitiveness of the threatener. Sociometry 33:394, 1970

Schwartz SH, Amos RE: Positive and negative referent others as sources of influence: a case of helping. Sociometry 40:12, 1977

Scott RW: Professionals in bureaucracies—areas of conflict. In Vollmer H, Mills D (eds): Professionalization. Englewood Cliffs, NJ, Prentice-Hall, 1966

Scott R: Professional employees in a bureaucratic structure: social work. In Etzioni A (ed): The Semi-Professions and Their Organizations. New York, Free Press, 1969

Scott, WR: Social Processes and Social Structures: An Introduction to Sociology. New York, Holt, Rinehart & Winston, 1970

Seashore S, Yuchtman E: A system resource approach to organizational effectiveness. Am Sociol Rev 32:89, 1972

Secord PF, Backman CW: Social Psychology. New York, McGraw-Hill, 1964

Seeman M: Role conflict and ambivalence in leadership. Am Sociol Rev 18:373, 1953

Sewell WH: Social class and childhood personality. Sociometry 24:340, 1961

Sewell WH: Some recent developments in socialization theory and research. In Stone GP, Farberman HA (eds): Social Psychology Through Symbolic Interaction. Waltham, Mass, Xerox College, 1970

Shaw ME, Costanzo PR: Theories of Social Psychology. New York, McGraw-Hill, 1970

Shaw M, Wright JM: Scales for the Measurement of Attitudes. New York, McGraw-Hill 1967

Sherif M: An Outline of Social Psychology. New York, Harper & Row, 1948

Shibutani T: Reference groups as perspectives. Am J Sociol 60:562, 1955

Shibutani T: Reference group and social control. In Rose AM (ed): Human Behavior and Social Processes. Boston, Houghton Mifflin, 1962

Shibutani T: Self-control and concerted action. In Gordon C, Gergen KJ (eds): The Self in Social Interaction. New York, Wiley, 1968

Shinn AM Jr: An application of psychophysical scaling techniques to the measurement of national power. J Politics 31:932, 1969

Siegel AE: The working mother: a review of research. Child Dev 34:513, 1963

Siegel AE, Sieget S: Reference groups, membership groups, and attitude change. J Abnorm Soc Psychol 55:360, 1957

Simmel G: The Society of Georg Simmel, Wolf K (ed). New York, Free Press, 1950

Simmons R: The role conflict of the first-line supervisor, an experimental sutdy. Am J Sociol 73:482, 1968

Simon H: Administrative Behavior. New York, Macmillan, 1959

Simon HA: A behavioral model of rational choice. Q J Economics 69:99, 1955

Skinner BF: Science and Human Behavior. New York, Macmillan, 1953

Smelser W: Dominance as a factor in achievement and perception in cooperative problem solving interactions. J Abnorm Soc Psychol 62:535, 1961

Smith EE: The effects of clear and unclear role expectations on group productivity and defensiveness. J Abnorm Soc Psychol 55:213, 1957

Smith HL: Two lines of authority: the hospital's dilemma. Jaco EG (ed): Patients Physicians and Illness. New York, Free Press, 1958

Smith MB: Competence and socialization. In Clausen J (ed): Socialization and Society, Boston, Little, Brown, 1968

Snoek JD: Role strain in diversified role sets. Am J Sociol 71:363, 1966

Sofer C: Organizations in Theory and in Practice. New York, Basic, 1972

Spencer TD: Sex-role learning in early childhood. In Hartup WW, Smothergill NL (eds): The Young Child: Reviews of Research. Washington, DC, Nat Assoc for the Education of Young Children, 1967

Spengler C: Other women. In Grissum M, Spengler C (eds): Womanpower and Health Care. Boston, Little, Brown, 1976

Staines G, Tavris A, Jayaratne TE: The Queen Bee Syndrome. Psychol Today 7(8):55, 1974

Stanton M: Political action and nursing. Nurs Clin North Am 9:579, 1974

Stein LI: The doctor-nurse game. Arch Gen Psychiatry 16:699, 1967

Steiner ID: Group Process and Productivity. New York, Academic, 1972

Stevens CM: Strategy and Collective Bargaining Negotiation. New York, McGraw-Hill, 1963

Stevens JC, Mack J: Scales of apparent force. J Exp Psychol 58:405, 1959

Stevens SS (ed): Handbook of Experimental Psychology. New York, Wiley, 1952, pp 1–49

Stevens SS: On the averaging of data. Science 121:113, 1955

Stevens SS: On the psychophysical law. Psychol Rev 64:153, 1957

Stevens SS: The psychophysics of sensory function. Am Scientist 48:226, 1960

Stevens SS: A metric for the social sciences. Science 151:677, 1966

Stoeckle J: Developments and implications of technology in medicine. Paper presented at Boston University, April 1976

Stolz LM: Effects of maternal employment on children: evidence from research. Child Dev 31:749, 1960

Stouffer S, Toby J: Role conflict and personality. Am J Sociol 16:395, 1951

Stouffer SA, Suchman EA, DeVinney LC, Star S, Williams RN: The American Soldier; Studies in Social Psychology in World War II. Vols. I, II. Princeton, NJ, Princeton Univ Press, 1949

Streissguth AP, Bee HL: Mother-child interactions and cognitive development. In Hartup WW (ed): The Young Child: Reviews of Research. Vol. 2. Washington, DC, Nat Assoc for the Education of Young Children, 1972

Suchman EA: Social patterns of illness and medical care. J Health Behav 6:2, 1965

Suchman EA: Preventive health behavior: a model for research on community health campaigns. J Health Soc Behav 8:197, 1967

Sullivan HS: An Interpersonal Theory of Psychiatry. New York, Norton, 1953

Synopsis of Education for the Health Professions, Committee of Presidents of the Health Professions Educational Associations of the Association for Academic Health Centers, 1975

Taynor J, Deaux K: When women are more deserving than men: equity, attribution and perceived sex differences. J Pers Soc Psychol 28:360, 1973

Tedeschi JT, Bonoma TV, Brown RC Jr: A paradigm for the study of coercive power. J Conflict Resolution 15:197, 1971

Tedeschi JT, Schlenker BR, Bonoma TV: Cognitive dissonance: private ratiocination or public spectacle? Am Psychol 26:685, 1971

Tedeschi JT, Schlenker BR, Bonoma TV: Conflict, Power and Games: The experimental Study of Interpersonal Relations. Chicago, Aldine, 1973

Teevan JJ: Reference groups and premarital sexual behavior. In Heiss J (ed): Family Roles and Interaction: An Anthology. 2nd ed. Chicago, Rand McNally, 1976

Terhune KW: Motives, situation, and interpersonal conflict within prisoner's dilemma. J Pers Soc Psychol Monogr (Suppl) 8, 1968

Terreberry S: The evolution of organizational environments. In Baker F (ed): Organizational Systems. Homewood, Ill, Dorsey, 1973

Theodore CN, Haug JN: Selected characteristics of the physician population, 1963 and 1967. Chicago, AMA, 1968, p. 74

Thibault J, Kelley H: The Social Psychology of Groups. New York, Wiley, 1959

Thomas E, Biddle B: Basic concepts for classifying the phenomena of role. In Biddle B, Thomas E (eds): Role Theory Concepts and Research. New York, Wiley, 1966

Thomas WI, Znaniecki F: The Polish Peasant in Europe and America. Boston, Badger, 1918

Thompson J: Organizations in Action. New York, McGraw-Hill, 1967

Thurstone L, Chave E: The Measurement of Attitude. Chicago, Univ of Chicago Press, 1929

Tice LF: The next 100 years: where will pharmacy be at the tricentennial? J Am Pharm Assoc 17:22, 1977

Tillotson JL (ed): Proceedings of the Nutrition-Behavioral Research Conference, publ no. (NIH) 76–978. Bethesda, Md, US DHEW, 1976

Tosi HW: Organizational stress as a moderator of the relationship between influence and role response. Acad Mgt J 14:7, 1971

Turner RH: Role-taking, role standpoint, and reference group behavior. Am J Sociol 61:316, 1956

Turner RH: Role-taking: process versus conformity. In Rose AM (ed): Human Behavior and Social Process. An Interactionist Approach. Boston, Houghton Mifflin, 1962

Turner RH: Role: sociological aspects. In Sills DL (ed): International Encyclopedia of the Social Sciences. Vol. 13. New York: Macmillan, 1968a, p 552

Turner RH: The self-conception in social interaction. In Gordon C, Gergen KJ (eds): The Self in Social Interaction. New York, Wiley, 1968b

US Cadet Nurse Corps and Other Federal Nurse Training Programs 1943–1948. Washington, DC, US GPO, 1950

US Census Bureau: Census of the Population, 1970 Subject Reports, Occupational Characteristics, Final Report PC (2) 74. Washington, DC, US GPO, 1973, pp 1,3,10

US Census Bureau; Current Population Reports, 24 Million Americans —Poverty in United States—1969. Series P. 60, no. 76. Washington, DC, US GPO, 1970

US Department of Health, Education, and Welfare. The Supply of Health Manpower. Publication no. (HRA) 75–38. Bethesda, Md, U.S. DHEW, 1974

Vollmer HM, Mills DL (eds): Professionalization. Englewood Cliffs, NJ, Prentice-Hall, 1966

Vroom VH: Work and Motivation. New York, Wiley, 1964

Wallace A: Administrative forms of Social Organization. Addison Wesley Modular Publ 9. Reading, Mass, Cummings, 1971

Wallston BS, Wallston KA, Kaplan GD, Maides SA: Development and validation of the health locus of control (HLC) scale. J Consult Clin Psychol 44:580, 1976

Walster E, Berscheid E, Walster W: New directions in equity research. Adv Exp Soc Psychol 9:1, 1976

Wardwell W: Reduction of strain in a marginal social role. Am J Sociol 61:16, 1955

Warner W, Havighurst RJ, Loeb MB: Who Shall Be Educated? New York, Harper & Row, 1944

Warner WL, Lunt PS: The Social Life of a Modern Community. New Haven, Conn, Yale Univ Press, 1941

Warner WL, Meeter M, Eels K: Social Class in America. Chicago, Science Research Associates, 1949

Weber M: Essays on Sociology. Gerth HH, Mills CW (eds, trans). New York, Oxford Univ Press, 1946

Weber M: The Theory of Social and Economic Organization. Henderson AN, Parsons T (trans). New York, Free Press, 1947

Weber M: Types of social organization. In Parsons T, Shills E, Naegele K, Pitts J (eds): Theories of Society. Vol I. New York, Free Press of Glencoe, 1961

Webster M, Sobieszck, B: Sources of Self-Evaluation. New York, Wiley, 1974

Weiner B, Kukla A: An attributional analysis of achievement motivation. J Pers Soc Psychol 15:1, 1970

Weinstein EA, Deutschberger P: Tasks, bargains and identities in social interaction. Soc Forces 42:451, 1964

Weinstein EA: The development of interpersonal competence. In Goslin DA (ed): Handbook of Socialization Theory and Research. Chicago, Rand McNally, 1969

Weiss SS (ed): Proceedings of the National Heart and Lung Institute Working Conference on Health Behavior, publication no. (NIH) 76-868. Bethesda, Md, US DHEW, 1975

Weitz J: Job expectancy and survival. J Abnorm Soc Psychol 40:245, 1956

Westley WA, Elkin F: The protective environment and adolescent socialization. Soc Forces 35:243, 1957

Wheeler S: The structure of formally organized socialization settings. In Brim OG Jr, Wheeler S (eds): Socialization after Childhood: Two Essays, New York, Wiley, 1966

White KL: Article. In Greenberg S (ed): The Quality of Mercy. New York, Atheneum, 1971

White P: Motivation reconsidered: the concept of competence. Psychol Rev 66:297, 1959

Wilensky HL: The professionalization of everyone? Am J Sociol 69:488, 1964

Williams TR: Introduction to Socialization: Human Culture Transmitted. St Louis, Mosby, 1972

Wilensky H: Intellectuals in Labor Unions. Glencoe, Ill, Free Press, 1956

Windwer C: Relationship among prospective parents' locus of control, social desirability, and choice of psychoprophylaxis. Nurs Res 26:96, 1977

Wolfe D, Snoek JD: A study of adjustment under role conflict. J Soc Issues 18:102–127, 1962

Wolfe D, Snoek JD: A study of tensions and adjustment under role conflict. J Soc Issues 18(3):102–121

Wray D: Marginal men of industry: the foremen. Am J Sociol 54:298, 1949

Wright GE: More family physicians or more primary care? An analysis of the Family Practice Act (S. 3418). Health Manpower Policy Discussion Paper Series, no. D-1. Ann Arbor, Mich, Univ of Michigan, 1973

Yarrow LJ: Separation from parents during early childhood. In Hoffman ML, Hoffman LW (eds): Review of Child Development Research. Vol. 1. New York, Russell Sage Foundation, 1964

Zigler E, Child IL: Socialization. In Lindzey G, Aronson E (eds): The Handbook of Social Psychology, 2nd ed. Vol. 3. Reading, Mass, Addison-Wesley, 1969

Zigler E, Child IL (eds): Socialization and Personality Development. Reading, Mass, Addison-Wesley, 1973

Index

Nursing (*cont.*)
  in education, 262-263
  team, 162, 163
Nursing care expectations of quality of,
    199-303
Nursing role
  differentiation of, 149-150, 162-163,
    171-172, 173-174, 215
  rationalizing, 173
Nursing schools, 167, 262-263. *See also*
    Socialization, professional

Oakes, D. L., 293, 294, 299
Observational learning, 50
Occupational prestige, 159
Occupational therapist, 26
Olesen, V., 79, 82, 88, 99, 144, 147,
    149, 151, 152, 153
Olmstead, A. G., 155
Operant conditioning, 49, 50
Order, management of, 122
  types of control, 122-129
Ordinal scale, 281, 283
Orem, D. E., 263
Organ, D., 106
Organizations, 111-136
  closed, 114
  division of labor in, 120-122
  management of order in, 122
    motivation, 125-129
    types of control in, 122-124
  norms of, 107-108, 134-135
  open, 114
  rate of change in, 80
  resources needed by, 117, 120
  role conflict in, 246
  as systems, 111-115
    problems of, 115-120, 135
Oseasohn, R., 253
Osteopaths, 164
Outcome, 77, 78, 106, 126-128
Output, 105, 116
  definition of, 77, 112
Overall, B., 85, 98

Paget, M. A., 155
Palola, E., 85, 93
Park, R. E., 31
Parke, R. D., 50
Parker, A., 187
Parsons, T., 6, 19, 20, 124, 175, 214,
    215
Partial withdrawal, and role strain, 98,
    107

Patients' rights, 208
Patient role, 175-176. *See also* Sick role,
    Illness behavior
Paul, B. D., 253
Pavalko, R. M., 134
Pediatrics, 178
Pediatricians, 189, 194, 196
  primary care and, 164, 180, 182, 183
Peer group, 150, 244
Peer review, 133
Pellegrino, E. D., 178, 251
Perrow, C., 117, 295
Perry S., 99
Personality, 21
Personality theories, 57-61
Peterson, O. L., 180
Pharmacist, 26
Pharmacy, multidisciplinary efforts and,
    252, 263
Phelan, J. G., 102
Physicians
  foreign-trained, 189
  image of, 175-176
  number of, 163
  nurses and, 171
  power of, 257, 266
  role differentiation of, 163, 174-175
  role negotiation and, 97
  socialization of, 177-209. *See also*
    Socialization, professional
Physicians' assistants, 163, 174, 257
Piaget, J., 22, 52
Pivnick, W. P., 102
Play, 45-46
Political role behaviors, 260-266. *See
    also* Power
Position(s), 9, 35-36. *See also* Status
  definition of, 75
  reference group and, 138
  selecting, 95-96
Positive reference group, 139
Postulates, 11
Power, 158, 203. *See also* Political
    role behaviors
  national, 285-286
  of nurses, 231, 263
  of physicians, 257, 266
  of psychiatric nurses, 263
  of psychiatric social workers, 263
  role bargaining and, 102-103
  socialization and, 67
  and stratification, 159, 160
Power law of psychophysics, 284, 285
Pratt, L., 226
Precision, 280-281
Predictive validity, 279-280